ATRIAL FIBRILLATION - MECHANISMS AND TREATMENT

Edited by **Tong Liu**

Atrial Fibrillation - Mechanisms and Treatment
http://dx.doi.org/10.5772/46219
Edited by Tong Liu

Contributors
José Joaquín Rieta, Raúl Alcaraz, Atilla Bitigen, Vecih Oduncu, Tong Liu, Panagiotis Korantzopoulos, Guangping Li, Anna Chernova, Svetlana Nicoulina, Vladimir Abramovich Shulman, Dudkina Ksenya, Oksana Gavrilyuk, Hongtao Wang, Lucía Cid Conde, José López Castro, Stefano Perlini, Fabio Belluzzi, Francesco Salinaro, Francesco Musca, Hanan Ahmed Galal Azzam, Paul Wolkowicz, Patrick Umeda, OLeg Sharifov, Ferdinand Urthaler

Published by InTech
Janeza Trdine 9, 51000 Rijeka, Croatia

Publishing Process Manager Dejan Grgur
Technical Editor InTech DTP team
Cover InTech Design team

Additional hard copies can be obtained from orders@intechopen.com

Atrial Fibrillation - Mechanisms and Treatment, Edited by Tong Liu
p. cm.
ISBN 978-953-51-1023-1

For EU product safety concerns:
IN TECH d.o.o., Prolaz Marije Krucifikse Kozulić 3, 51000 Rijeka, Croatia,
info@intechopen.com or visit our website at intechopen.com.

Meet the editor

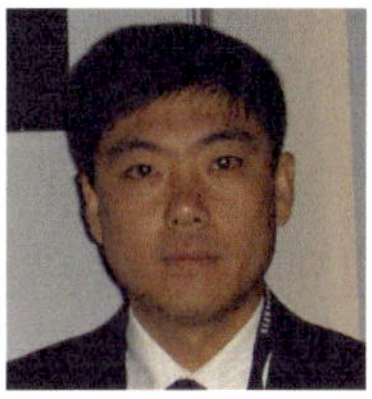

Dr. Tong Liu graduated from Tianjin Medical University in 2000, and got his PhD in 2006. He received training in the research of electrophysiology at the Heart Institute, Cedars-Sinai Medical Center, Los Angeles, from 2009 to 2010. He has particular interests in cardiac electrophysiology, and has focused on the research of atrial fibrillation over the past decade. Dr. Liu is the Youth Committee Member of Chinese Society of Pacing and Electrophysiology (CSPE). He is on the editorial boards of World Journal of Cardiology, Cardiovascular Diagnosis and Therapy, Chinese Journal of Cardiovascular Medicine and Chinese Journal of Evidence-Based Cardiovascular Medicine, as well as a peer reviewer for more than 15 scientific journals. He has published over 30 articles in peer reviewed medical journals.

Contents

Preface

Atrial fibrillation is a rapidly evolving epidemic associated with increased cardiovascular morbidity and mortality, and its prevalence has increased during the past few decades. In the past few years, the recent understanding of the diverse mechanisms of this arrhythmia has led to the improvement of our therapeutic strategies. However, many clinicians have still felt the frustration in management of this commonly encountered arrhythmia.

This book contains a spectrum of different topics from bench to bedside in atrial fibrillation. We try to introduce the most recent advancement of mechanisms and treatment of AF including genetics, calcium signaling, thrombogenesis, signal analysis, upstream therapies focus on renin-angiotensin-aldosterone system inhibitors, antioxidants and n-3 polyunsaturated fatty acids, and anticoagulation issues. I strongly believe that scientists, cardiologists and electrophysiologists will find this book very informative and useful. The references cited in each chapter will definitely act as additional source of information for readers.

I am grateful to the all the authors who contributed to this book with their valuable experience. I also appreciate the great help from InTech editorial office, Ms. Mirna Cvijic and Mr. Dejan Grgur, who guided me through the publication process step by step. I would also like to thank for the important contributions from the co-editors of this book – Prof. Guangping Li, my mentor, and Dr. Panagiotis Korantzopoulos, my best friend who guided me to explore the wonderful world of arrhythmia. Finally, special thanks to my family – wife, Lijian, and son, Yujie, who provided continuous inspiration and support to my work.

Tong Liu, MD, PhD
Department of Cardiology, Tianjin Institute of Cardiology
Second Hospital of Tianjin Medical University, Tianjin
People's Republic of China

Section 1

Pharmacological Management

Chapter 1

Atrial Fibrillation and the Renin-Angiotensin-Aldosterone System

Stefano Perlini, Fabio Belluzzi,
Francesco Salinaro and Francesco Musca

Additional information is available at the end of the chapter

http://dx.doi.org/10.5772/53917

1. Introduction

Atrial fibrillation (AF) is the most common cardiac arrhythmia, affecting approximately 1% of the general population and up to 8% of subjects over the age of 80 years.[1] AF is a major contributor to cardiovascular mortality and morbidity, being associated with decreased quality of life, increased incidence of congestive heart failure,[2] embolic phenomena, including stroke,[2,3] and a 30 % higher risk of death.[3,4] AF-associated morbidity includes a four- to five-fold increased risk for stroke, [2,5] a two-fold increased risk for dementia,[6,7] and a tripling of risk for heart failure.[5] According to the Framingham Study, the percentage of strokes attributable to AF increases steeply from 1.5% at 50–59 years of age to 23.5% at 80–89 years of age, [2] and the presence of AF accounts for a 50–90% increased risk for overall mortality.[3] From the viewpoint of the AF-related socio-economic burden, it has been estimated that it is consuming between 0.9% and 2.4% of total National Health Service expenditure in the UK,[8] while in the USA, total costs are 8.6–22.6% higher for AF patients in all age- and sex- population strata.[9] Therefore significant clinical, human, social and economical benefits are therefore expected from any improvement in AF prevention and treatment.

It has to be noted that although multiple treatment options are currently available, no single modality is effective for all patients.[10] AF can occasionally affect a structurally normal heart of otherwise healthy individuals (so-called "lone AF")[11], but most typically it occurs in subjects with previous cardiovascular damage due to hypertension, coronary artery disease and diabetes. Moreover, it can be associated with clinical conditions such as hyperthyroidism, acute infections, recent cardiothoracic or abdominal surgery, and systemic inflammatory diseases. Whatever the cause, AF is characterized by very rapid, chaotic electrical activity of the atria, resulting in accelerated and irregular ventricular activity, loss of atrial mechanical function and increased risk of atrial clot formation.

Many studies have shown that the recurrence of AF may be partially related to a phenomenon known as "atrial remodeling", in which the electrical, mechanical, and structural properties of the atrial tissue and cardiac cells are progressively altered, creating a more favorable substrate for AF development and maintenance.[12,13] Atrial remodeling is both a cause and a consequence of the arrhythmia, and in recent years it has become more and more evident that treatment should also be based on an "upstream" therapy[14,10] aimed at modifying the arrhythmia substrate and at reducing the extent of atrial remodelling.

2. Atrial remodeling: electrical and structural factors

According to Coumel's triangle of arrhythmogenesis, three cornerstones are required in the onset of clinical arrhythmia[15] – the arrhythmogenic substrate, the trigger factor and the modulation factors such as autonomic nervous system or inflammation. Once established, AF itself alters electrical and subsequently structural properties of the atrial tissue and these changes cause or "beget" further AF self-perpetuation.[12] The mechanisms responsible for the onset and persistence of the arrhythmia involve electrical as well as structural determinants, that are very complex and yet poorly understood. From the electrical standpoint, there is still debate on the three models that were proposed in 1924[16] by Garrey for describing the mechanisms of spatiotemporal organization of electrical activity in the atria during AF. According to the *focal mechanism theory,* AF is provoked and perhaps also driven further by the rapid firing of a single or multiple ectopic foci, whereas the *single circuit re-entry theory* assumes the presence of a single dominant re-entry circuit, and the *multiple wavelet theory* postulates the existence of multiple reentry circuits with randomly propagating wave-fronts that must find receptive tissue in order to persist.[17] It has to be recognized that all three models are non-exclusive and each may be applicable to certain subgroups of AF patients, or that they may even coexist in the same subject during different stages of AF development. Moreover, AF persistence is associated with modifications in the atrial myocyte electrical properties (the so-called *electrical remodeling*), that may stabilize the arrhythmia by decreasing the circuit size. The electrophysiological properties of the atrial myocardium may be further modified by changes in autonomic nervous system activity as well as by the interference of drugs and hormones, that may therefore participate in arrhythmogenesis.

Beyond these electrical determinants, AF onset and persistence may be affected by the structural factors, such as the dimensions and geometry of the atrial chambers, the atrial tissue structure and the amount and the composition of the extracellular matrix surrounding the atrial myocytes (i.e. *structural remodeling).* Together, these alterations create an arrhythmogenic substrate essential for the persistence of AF. Atrial structure is modified by volume

http://dx.doi.org/10.5772/53917

and pressure overload, due to either mitral valve disease or left ventricular diastolic dysfunction in the setting of arterial hypertension, coronary artery disease or aortic valve disease. Also diabetes is associated with changes in atrial structure and function. It is not therefore surprising that all these clinical conditions are associated with an increased AF incidence and prevalence. Beyond being a possible substrate for AF onset, atrial structure is profoundly altered by the effects of rapid atrial rate. Prolonged rapid atrial pacing induces changes in atrial myocytes such as an increase in cell-size, myocyte lysis, perinuclear accumulation of glycogen, alterations in connexin expression, fragmentation of sarcoplasmic reticulum and changes in mitochondrial shape.[18] Moreover, structural remodeling is characterized by changes in extracellular matrix composition, with both diffuse interstitial and patchy fibrosis.[19] All these alterations results in electrical tissue non-homogeneity, slowed conduction and electrical uncoupling, that facilitate AF continuation. In contrast to electrical remodeling, structural changes are far less reversible and they tend to persist even after sinus rhythm restoration. Among the several mechanisms and signaling pathways involved in structural remodeling and atrial fibrosis, a key role is played by the renin-angiotensin system, and by the transforming growth-factor β_1 (TGF-β_1) pathway, associated with tissue inflammation[19] and reactive oxygen species production.[20,21]

Profibrotic signals act on the balance between matrix metalloproteinases (MMPs) – the main enzymes responsible for extracellular matrix degradation – and their local tissue inhibitors (TIMPs), that can be differentially altered in compensated as opposed to decompensated pressure-overload hypertrophy.[22-25] Furthermore, profibrotic signals stimulate the proliferation of fibroblasts and extracellular deposition of fibronectin, collagens I and III, proteglycans and other matrix components. In a canine model of congestive heart failure, Li *et al.* showed that the development of atrial fibrosis is angiotensin-II dependent,[26] via mechanisms that are partly mediated by the local production of cytokine TGF-β_1.[27] In transgenic mice, overexpression of the latter cytokine has been shown to lead to selective atrial fibrosis, increased conduction heterogeneity and enhanced AF susceptibility, despite normal atrial action potential duration and normal ventricular structure and function.[28]

3. The renin-angiotensin-aldosterone system (RAAS) as a "novel" risk factor for AF

Among many others, two factors contribute to the search of different therapeutic approaches to AF specifically targeting substrate development and maintenance:[29] the recognition of novel risk factors for the development of this arrhythmia and the well-known limitations of the current antiarrhythmic drug therapy to maintain sinus rhythm, still having inadequate efficacy and potentially serious adverse effects.[30] In this setting, the inhibition of the renin-angiotensin-aldosterone system (RAAS) has been considered useful in both primary and secondary prevention of AF, particularly in patients presenting left ventricular hypertrophy (LVH) or heart failure. The RAAS is a major endocrine/paracrine system involved in the regulation of the cardiovascular system.[31] Its key mediator is angiotensin II, an octapeptide that is cleaved from the liver-derived 485-aminoacid precursor angiotensinogen through a process involving the enzymatic activities of renin and angiotensin converting enzyme (ACE). Two main angiotensin II receptors exist, i.e angiotensin II type 1 (AT_1) and type 2 (AT_2). AT_1-receptor mediated pathways lead to vasoconstriction, water retention, increased renal tubular sodium reabsorption, stimulation of cell growth and connective tissue deposition, and impaired endothelial function. AT_2-receptor has opposing effects, inasmuch as it mediates vasodilation, decreases renal tubular sodium reabsorption, inhibits cell growth and connective tissue deposition, and improves endothelial function. These two angiotensin receptors have different expression patterns, AT_1 being constitutively expressed in a wide range of tissues of the cardiovascular, renal, endocrine, and nervous system, and AT_2 expression being activated during stress conditions.[32] It is becoming increasingly evident that all these mechanisms are involved in atrial remodeling and hence in AF development and maintenance. Moreover, among the other biologically active RAAS components that are involved in these processes, angiotensin-(1-7) [Ang-(1-7)] seems to be particularly important. In an experimental canine model of chronic atrial pacing, Ang-(1-7) has been shown to reduce AF vulnerability and atrial fibrosis,[33] influencing atrial tachycardia-induced atrial ionic remodeling. [34]

Among the compounds that may interfere RAAS four classes of drugs are particularly relevant in cardiovascular therapy: angiotensin receptor blockers (ARBs), ACE inhibitors (ACEIs), aldosterone antagonists and direct renin inhibitors. ARBs directly block AT_1 receptor activation, ACEIs inhibit ACE-mediated production of angiotensin II, and the recently developed direct renin inhibitor aliskiren blocks RAAS further upstream.[32,35,36] Over the last decade, these drugs have been tested in the setting of AF treatment and prevention.

4. The role of RAAS in the pathogenesis of AF

4.1. Atrial stretch and AF

Atrial arrhythmias frequently occur under conditions associated with atrial dilatation and increased atrial pressure, causing atrial tissue stretch and modifying atrial refractoriness, and it has been shown in several animal as well as clinical models.[37-40] These factors increase susceptibility to AF, that is associated with shortening of the atrial effective refractory period (AERP), possibly by opening of stretch-activated ion channels. In the setting of arterial hypertension and congestive heart failure (CHF), angiotensin II has been associated with increased left atrial and left ventricular end-diastolic pressure,[41] and both ACEIs and ARBs have been shown to reduce left atrial pressure.[42-45] Therefore, one potential mechanism by which ACEIs and ARBs may reduce atrial susceptibility to AF is by reducing atrial stretch. Many other mechanisms appear to be involved in the antiarrhythmic properties of RAAS inhibition, and in an animal model of ventricular tachycardia-induced CHF it has been shown that ACE inhibition is more successful than hydralazine/isosorbide mononitrate association in reducing burst pacing-induced AF promotion, despite a similar reduction in left atrial pressure.[26] As described below, angiotensin II-mediated mechanisms contribute to both *structural* and *electrical remodeling* of the atrial tissue.

4.2. The role of RAAS in structural remodeling

Atrial fibrosis causes conduction heterogeneity, hence playing a key role in the development of a vulnerable *structural* substrate for AF, and the proinflammatory and profibrotic effects of angiotensin II have been extensively described.[46-48] Excessive fibrillar collagen deposition, resulting from deregulated extracellular matrix metabolism, leads to atrial fibrosis, and it has been shown that angiotensin II has a direct effect in stimulating cardiac fibroblast proliferation and collagen synthesis, via AT_1 receptor – mediated mechanisms involving a mitogen-activated protein kinases (MAPKs) phosphorylation pathway. [49-51] The latter cascade is inhibited by AT_2 receptor activation, that has an antiproliferative effects.[52] Moreover, cardiac fibroblast function is modulated by angiotensin II through mechanisms involving TGF- • $_1$, osteopontin (OPN), and endothelin-1 (ET-1). [49,53-55] Interestingly, Nakajima and coworkers showed that selective atrial fibrosis, conduction heterogeneity, and AF propensity are enhanced in a $TGF\beta_1$ cardiac overexpression transgenic mice model,[56] as also confirmed by others.[27,28]

Beyond having both direct and indirect effects on collagen synthesis, angiotensin II interferes with collagen degradation by modulating interstitial matrix metalloproteinase (MMP) activity and tissue inhibitor of metalloproteinase (TIMP) concentrations,[52] and an atrial tissue imbalance between MMPs and TIMPs has been reported in both clinical and animal studies on AF. [52,57] Goette and coworkers showed increased atrial expression of ACE and increased activation of the angiotensin II-related intracellular signal transduction pathway in human atrial tissue derived from AF patients,[58] and atrial overexpression of angiotensin II has also been shown in a canine model of ventricular tachycardia-induced CHF[26,59] In transgenic mice experiments with cardiac-restricted ACE overexpression, Xiao et al. have demonstrated that elevated atrial tissue angiotensin II concentrations stimulates atrial fibrosis and hence an AF-promoting substrate.[60] In contrast, RAAS inhibition reduces tissue angiotensin II concentration, and attenuates atrial structural remodeling and fibrosis, thereby contrasting AF maintenance.[26,59,61-64]

4.3. The role of RAAS in electrical remodeling

Electrical remodeling has been hypothesized as a main mechanism by which, once established, "AF begets further AF" self-perpetuation.[12] In the clinical practice, this phenomenon is evident when considering that over time it becomes more and more difficult to keep in sinus rhythm a patient with AF. The concept of electrical remodeling has been originally proposed by Wijffels et al.[12] to explain the experimental observation that when AF is maintained artificially, the duration of burst pacing-induced paroxysms progressively increases until AF becomes sustained. This indicates that AF itself alters the atrial tissue electrical properties, thereby developing a functional substrate that promotes AF perpetuation and may involve alterations in ionic currents and in excitability cellular properties.[65] In their study, Wijffels et al. demonstrated that the increased propensity to AF is associated with shortening of the atrial effective refractory period (AERP) in accordance with the multiple wavelet theory,[12] a mechanism that was subsequently attributed to a reduction of action potential duration (APD) secondary to the progressive downregulation of the transient outward current (Ito) and of the L-typeCa^{2+} current (ICa,L).[66] As to the modulation of the ICa,L current, the role of angiotensin II is controversial, with studies reporting increase, decrease, or even no effect.[29,67] In contrast, angiotensin II has been demonstrated to downregulate Ito current,[68,67] inasmuch as AT_1 receptor stimulation leads to internalization of the Kv4.3 (i.e., the pore-forming α-subunit underlying Ito), regulating its cell-surface expression.[68] As shown by Liu and coworkers, chronic Ang-(1-7) infusion prevented the decrease of Ito, ICa,L, and of Kv4.3 mRNA expression induced by chronic atrial pacing, [34] thereby contributing to reduce AF vulnerability.[33] Subsequently, Nakashima et al. showed that ACEI or ARB treatment results in complete inhibition of the shortening of AERP, that is normally induced by rapid atrial pacing.[69] A further mechanism by which the RAAS may exert a proarrhythmic effect is the modulation of gap junctions, that are low-resistance pathways for the propagation of impulses between cardiomyocytes formed by connexins (Cx).[70] Cx40 gene polymorphisms have been associated with the development of non familial AF,[71] and angiotensin II has been implicated in Cx43 downward remodeling. [72-74] Moreover, angiotensin II directly induces delayed after-depolarizations and accelerates the automatic rhythm of isolated pulmonary vein cardiomyocytes.[75] These cells are considered an important source of ectopic beats and of atrial fibrillation bursts, representing the target of AF treatment with radio-frequency ablation.[76] Therefore these experimental results demonstrate that angiotensin II may play a role in the pathophysiology of atrial fibrillation also by modulating the pulmonary vein electrical activity via an electrophysiological effect that was shown to be AT_1 receptor – mediated, being inhibited by losartan, [75] and that is attenuated by heat-stress responses.[77] Recently, also the direct renin inhibitor aliskiren was shown to reduce the arrhythmogenic activity of pulmonary vein cardiomyocytes.[36] It has also been demonstrated that aldosterone promotes atrial fibrillation, causing a substrate for atrial arrhythmias characterized by atrial fibrosis, myocyte hypertrophy, and conduction disturbances,[78] and the specific antagonist spironolactone has been shown to prevent aldosterone-induced increased duration of atrial fibrillation in a rat model.[79]

4.4. RAAS gene polymorphisms and AF

The ACE DD (deletion/deletion) genotype of the ACE gene has been shown to be a predisposing factor for persistent AF,[80] and it was recently reported that the same genotype is associated with lowest rates of symptomatic response in patients with lone AF.[81] Moreover, polymorphisms of the angiotensinogen gene have also been associated with nonfamilial AF,[82] and it has been shown that significant interactions exist between angiotensinogen gene haplotypes and ACE I/D (insertion/deletion) polymorphism resulting in increased susceptibility to AF.[83,84] Also aldosterone synthase (CYP11B2) T-344C polymorphism, which is associated with increased aldosterone activity, was shown to be an independent predictor of AF in patients with HF.[85] According to Sun and coworkers, this aldosterone synthase gene polymorphism might also be associated with atrial remodelling in hypertensive patients.[86]

5. Atrial fibrillation and the renin-angiotensin-aldosterone system (RAAS): Clinical observations

A possible relationship between the RAAS and the risk of developing AF was brought about by several clinical data, derived from patient series in different settings, that are here summarized.

5.1. Heart failure

In heart failure, several observations indicate a possible effect of RAAS inhibition in reducing the incidence of new onset AF. In a retrospective analysis of the SOLVD trial, Vermes et al. showed that enalapril reduces the risk of AF development in patients with various degrees of heart failure.[87] Similarly, Maggioni et al. demonstrated that use of the ARB valsartan is associated with a reduction in the risk of AF in the Val-HeFT trial population.[88] Since the vast majority of these patients (92.5%) were already receiving an ACEI, a combination effect was hypothesized, and the benefit of combined treatment with both an ARB and an ACEI was also supported by the results of the CHARM trial with candesartan.[89] The latter study was composed by three component trials based on left ventricular ejection fraction (LVEF) and ACEI treatment. CHARM-Alternative trial enrolled patients with LVEF ≤40% not treated with ACEIs because of prior intolerance, CHARM-Added recruited patients with LVEF ≤40% already treated with an ACEI, and CHARM-Preserved included patients with LVEF >40%, independent of ACEI treatment. The incidence of new-onset AF was reduced in candesartan-treated patients, especially (but not exclusively) in the CHARM-Alternative trial.[89] These data indicate additional benefits in AF prevention, on the top of the already known effects of ACEI/ARB treatment in patients with heart failure.

5.2. Post-MI

After an acute myocardial infarction, treatment with the ACEI trandolapril reduced the incidence AF in patients with impaired left ventricular function, irrespective of the effects on ejection fraction per se.[90] Similar results were reported by Pizzetti et al. with lisinopril in their analysis of the GISSI-3 trial.[91]

5.3. Hypertension

The issue of the possible role of ACEI/ARB drug treatment in the primary prevention of AF in hypertensive patients derives from several conflicting observations. According to the CAPPP and the STOP-H2 trials, ACEIs were comparable to other antihypertensive regiments in preventing AF.[92,93] In contrast, a retrospective, longitudinal, cohort study by L'Allier et al. reported a benefit of ACEIs over calcium channel blockers in terms of new onset AF and AF-related hospitalizations.[94] Similar results were derived from the LIFE trial, showing that when compared with the β-blocker atenolol, patients receiving the ARB losartan had significantly lower incidence of new-onset AF and associated stroke.[95] A recent nested case-control observational study showed that compared with treatment with calcium channel blockers, long-term antihypertensive treatment with ACEIs, ARBs, or β-blockers may decrease the risk of new-onset AF.[96]

5.4. Increased cardiovascular risk

In patients with increased cardiovascular risk, the rate of new onset AF was not reduced by ramipril in a subanalysis of the HOPE clinical trial by Salehian and coworkers,[97] although in a population with a rather low incidence of AF (2.1%). Also in the ACTIVE I trial, there was no benefit of irbesartan treatment in preventing hospitalization for atrial fibrillation or atrial fibrillation recorded by 12-lead electrocardiography, nor was there a benefit in a subgroup of patients who underwent transtelephonic monitoring.[98] In contrast, according to Schmieder et al. the VALUE trial showed that valsartan-based antihypertensive treatment reduced the development of new-onset AF compared to amlodipine,[99] in subjects at higher risk of this arrhythmia due to an almost 25% prevalence of electrocardiographically-defined left ventricular hypertrophy. These conflicting data may indicate that a possible benefit of ACEI or ARB treatment can at best be observed in patients with the highest probability of increased RAAS activation.

5.5. Postoperative AF

A reduced incidence of new-onset AF was observed in patients undergoing coronary artery bypass graft surgery who were treated with ACEIs,[100] in a large multicenter prospective trial recruiting 4,657 subjects. These results were confirmed with the use of ACEIs alone or associated with candesartan,[101] whereas the reduced risk of developing postoperative AF did not reach the statistical significance in the *post hoc* evaluation of patients enrolled in the AFIST II and III trials.[102]

5.6. Secondary prevention after cardioversion and after catheter ablation

In the setting of secondary prevention, patients undergoing AF cardioversion represent a group in which the potential role of RAAS inhibition has been first investigated by van den Berg et al.[103], iwho studied 30 CHF patients treated with lisinopril or placebo before and after the procedure. Although the reduced incidence of recurrent AF in ACE-I treated patients did not reach the statistical significance, this study was followed by many others. Dagres et al. [104] demonstrated that treatment with the ARB irbesartan is associated with attenuated left atrial stunning after cardioversion. Subsequent studies showed that the association of an ACEI or an ARB with amiodarone prevents AF recurrences after cardioversion when compared with amiodarone alone.[105-107] Interestingly, irbesartan showed a dose-dependent preventive effect.[106] In contrast, Tveit and coworkers did not find any benefit by treating with the ARB candesartan for 3-6 weeks before and 6 months after electrical cardioversion.[108] We contributed to this debate by showing that also in the setting of lone AF,[11] long-term treatment with the ACE-I ramipril is effective in preventing relapses of AF after successful cardioversion.[109] Moreover, at the end of a 3-year follow-up, ramipril treatment also prevented left atrium enlargement,[109] which has been demonstrated to occur in the natural history of lone AF.[110]

In patients undergoing catheter ablation for drug refractory AF, ACEIs or ARBs did not show the same promising results,[111-115] raising the question whether these interventions are indeed able to revert atrial remodeling in this clinical setting.[116]

5.7. Paroxysmal AF prevention

Both ACEIs and ARBs have shown some promise in the setting of the prevention of paroxysmal AF recurrences. In two long-term clinical trials on amiodarone-treated patients, losartan or perindopril were more effective than amlodipine in the maintenance of sinus rhythm. [117,118] The same held true for telmisartan, that Fogari et al. showed as more effective than ramipril in reducing AF recurrence and severity as well as in improving P-wave dispersion, suggesting a possible specific effect of telmisartan on atrial electric remodeling.[119] In a retrospective analysis of patients with predominantly paroxysmal AF, Komatsu and coworkers showed that the enalapril added to amiodarone reduced the rate of AF recurrence and prevented the development of atrial structural remodeling.[120] In a post hoc subgroup analysis of the AFFIRM trial, Murray et al. showed that ACEIs and ARBs reduced the risk of AF recurrence in patients with a history of CHF or impaired left ventricular function. [121] The GISSI-AF trial did not show any significant effect of valsartan treatment on the rate of AF recurrences in a cohort of 1,442 patients with a history of recent AF.[122] Although it has to be noted that valsartan-treated patients had a significantly higher prevalence of coronary artery disease and peripheral artery disease, and that more than half of the patients were already taking concomitant ACEI treatment, the GISSI-AF shed some doubt on the whole issue of the preventive role of RAAS inhibition in AF prevention.[122] In the same line, the very recent ANTIPAF trial concluded that 12-month treatment with the ARB olmesartan did not reduce the number of AF episodes in patients with documented paroxysmal AF without structural heart disease.[123] Similar results were shown by the J-RHYTHM II study comparing the ARB candesartan with the calcium antagonist amlodipine in the treatment of paroxysmal AF associated with hypertension.[124] Both studies used daily transtelephonic monitoring to examine asymptomatic and symptomatic paroxysmal AF episodes. [123,124]

5.8. Emerging role for aldosterone antagonists

In the recent years, it has been suggested that upstream therapy using aldosterone antagonists, such as spironolactone or eplerenone, may reduce the deleterious effect of excessive aldosterone secretion on atrial tissue, thereby contributing to modify the risk of developing and of maintaining AF.[125] Dabrowski et al. showed that combined spironolactone plus beta-blocker treatment might be a simple and valuable option in preventing AF episodes in patients with normal left ventricular function and history of refractory paroxysmal AF.[126] In patients with AF, spironolactone treatment was associated with a reduction in the AF burden, as reflected by a combination of hospitalizations for AF and electrical cardioversion.[127] In a recent trial in patients with systolic heart failure and mild symptoms (EMPHASIS-HF), the aldosterone antagonist eplerenone reduced the incidence of new-onset AF or atrial flutter.[128]

5.9. Meta-analyses

The promise of a protective role of RAAS inhibition is largely based on the analysis of retrospective data, although on several thousands of patients. Another limitation is the fact that in most cases, the detection of AF recurrences is based on annual electrocardiograms, periodical 24-hour Holter analysis, or patient self-reported symptoms symptoms. In recent years, with the analysis of data from patients with an implanted pacemaker, it is becoming increasingly clear that continuous monitoring is much more reliable in identifying the presence of asymptomatic recurrences, with a mean sensitivity in detecting an AF episode lasting >5 minutes that was 44.4%, 50.4%, and 65.1% for 24-hour Holter, 1-week Holter, and 1-month Holter monitoring, respectively.[129] To partially overcome some of these limitations, several meta-analyses of the available trials have been conducted.[130-141] In synthesis, despite the promising preliminary experimental and clinical data, the efficacy of RAAS inhibition in the prevention of atrial fibrillation recurrences is still under debate, leading Disertori et al. in a very recent review article to the definition of "an unfulfilled hope".[136] In meta-analysis including 92,817 randomized patients, Khatib and coworkers concluded that although RAAS inhibition appears to reduce the risk of developing new onset atrial fibrillation in different patient groups, further research with stronger quality trials is required to draw definitive conclusions.[141]

Indeed, ACE-I or ARBs cannot be considered as an alternative to the established antiarrhythmic agents and transcatheter ablation. However, since they are recommended for most concomitant cardiovascular diseases that are associated with an increased risk of AF (i.e., hypertension, heart failure, ischemic heart disease) and since there are several lines of evidence that increased angiotensin II tissue levels are involved in both structural and electrical remodeling of the atrial tissue, it appears reasonable to use these drugs. In general, no substantial difference was found in the comparison between ACE-I and ARB treatment, a finding that was confirmed also by the results of the the ONTARGET and TRANSCEND trials.[142]

5.10. Atrial remodeling as a therapeutic target: modulation of the renin-angiotensin-aldosterone system

Since angiotensin II plays a central role in the development of atrial fibrosis, inhibition of atrial angiotensin converting enzyme (ACE) and AT_1 angiotensin receptors might be beneficial in AF. In experimental models, AF susceptibility and atrial fibrosis were decreased by candesartan or enalapril, but not by hydralazine or isosorbide mononitrate despite similar hemodynamic effects,[26,63] thus suggesting a key role of targeting renin-angiotensin system, rather than of improving the hemodynamics. This concept was further underscored after demonstrating a preventive role of ramipril treatment in patients with lone AF.[109] Also spironolactone was able to prevent AF episodes in patients with normal left ventricular function and a history of refractory paroxysmal AF.[126] With the notable exception of the GISSI-AF,[122] ANTIPAF,[123] and J-RHYTHM II[124] trials, the majority of the available studies showed that modulation of the renin-angiotensin-aldosterone system is able to reduce the incidence of AF, as well as its recurrence after electrical cardioversion.[134] These data are summarized in several meta-analyses,[131,132,140,143] also including the GISSI-AF data.[135] In a broader view, although ACE inhibitors and angiotensin-II receptor blockers (ARBs) are not to be considered antiarrhythmic drugs, several studies have shown that they are associated with a lower incidence of ventricular arrhythmias in patients with ischemic heart disease and left ventricular (LV) dysfunction,[90,144,145] possibly because of the adverse effects of angiotensin II on the cardiac remodeling process. Indeed, it must be recognized that in the presence of a cardiac disease causing atrial overload and/or dysfunction, the effectiveness of ACE inhibitors and/or ARBs might be attributable either to a direct antiarrhythmic effect or to an effect on atrial structure and/or function likely able to favorably modify the arrhythmic substrate, such as the increase in left atrial (LA) dimensions that is frequently observed in patients with arterial hypertension and/or LV dysfunction.

In the setting of AF, it has to be remembered that angiotensin II not only has several effects on the *structure* of the atrial myocardium, but also on its *electrical* properties, as it has been elegantly shown in isolated pulmonary vein cardiomyocytes,[75] and in instrumented animal studies.[69] Therefore, the protective effect of ACE inhibition or angiotensin II antagonists on the electrical and structural remodeling of the atria is very likely, due to a combination of their actions on atrial distension/stretch, sympathetic tone, local renin-angiotensin system, electrolyte concentrations, and cardiac loading conditions.

6. Conclusions

The onset of atrial fibrillation results from a complex interaction between triggers, arrhythmogenic substrate, and modulator factors. Once established, AF itself alters the electrical and structural properties of the atrial myocardium, thereby perpetuating the arrhythmia. Among many other factors, angiotensin II and aldosterone play an important role not only in determining atrial fibrosis, but also in modulating the electrical properties of the atrial myocardium. These aspects may be relevant in explaining the many clinical observations indicating the role of drugs modulating the renin-angiotensin-aldosterone system in preventing atrial fibrillation in different settings.

Author details

Stefano Perlini[1], Fabio Belluzzi[2], Francesco Salinaro[1] and Francesco Musca[1,3]

*Address all correspondence to: stefano.perlini@unipv.it

1 Clinica Medica II, Department of Internal Medicine, Fondazione IRCCS San Matteo, University of Pavia, Italy

2 Department of Cardiology Fondazione IRCCS Ospedale Maggiore, Milan, Italy

3 Department of Cardiology, IRCCS Fondazione Ca'Granda Ospedale Maggiore Policlinico, Milan, Italy

References

[1] Fuster V, Ryden LE, Cannom DS, Crijns HJ, Curtis AB, Ellenbogen KA, Halperin JL, Le Heuzey JY, Kay GN, Lowe JE, Olsson SB, Prystowsky EN, Tamargo JL, Wann S (2006) ACC/AHA/ESC 2006 guidelines for the management of patients with atrial fibrillation-executive summary: a report of the American College of Cardiology/American Heart Association Task Force on practice guidelines and the European Society of Cardiology Committee for Practice Guidelines (Writing Committee to Revise the 2001 Guidelines for the Management of Patients with Atrial Fibrillation). Eur Heart J 27 (16):1979-2030

[2] Wolf PA, Abbott RD, Kannel WB (1991) Atrial fibrillation as an independent risk factor for stroke: the Framingham Study. Stroke 22 (8):983-988

[3] Benjamin EJ, Wolf PA, D'Agostino RB, Silbershatz H, Kannel WB, Levy D (1998) Impact of atrial fibrillation on the risk of death: the Framingham Heart Study. Circulation 98 (10):946-952

[4] Stewart S, Hart CL, Hole DJ, McMurray JJ (2002) A population-based study of the long-term risks associated with atrial fibrillation: 20-year follow-up of the Renfrew/Paisley study. Am J Med 113 (5):359-364

[5] Krahn AD, Manfreda J, Tate RB, Mathewson FA, Cuddy TE (1995) The natural history of atrial fibrillation: incidence, risk factors, and prognosis in the Manitoba Follow-Up Study. Am J Med 98 (5):476-484. doi:10.1016/S0002-9343(99)80348-9

[6] Ott A, Breteler MM, de Bruyne MC, van Harskamp F, Grobbee DE, Hofman A (1997) Atrial fibrillation and dementia in a population-based study. The Rotterdam Study. Stroke 28 (2):316-321

[7] Miyasaka Y, Barnes ME, Petersen RC, Cha SS, Bailey KR, Gersh BJ, Casaclang-Verzosa G, Abhayaratna WP, Seward JB, Iwasaka T, Tsang TS (2007) Risk of dementia in stroke-free patients diagnosed with atrial fibrillation: data from a community-based cohort. Eur Heart J 28 (16):1962-1967. doi:10.1093/eurheartj/ehm012

[8] Wachtell K, Devereux RB, Lyle AP (2007) The effect of angiotensin receptor blockers for preventing atrial fibrillation. Curr Hypertens Rep 9 (4):278-283

[9] Wolf PA, Mitchell JB, Baker CS, Kannel WB, D'Agostino RB (1998) Impact of atrial fibrillation on mortality, stroke, and medical costs. Arch Intern Med 158 (3):229-234

[10] Camm AJ, Kirchhof P, Lip GY, Schotten U, Savelieva I, Ernst S, Van Gelder IC, Al-Attar N, Hindricks G, Prendergast B, Heidbuchel H, Alfieri O, Angelini A, Atar D, Colonna P, De Caterina R, De Sutter J, Goette A, Gorenek B, Heldal M, Hohloser SH, Kolh P, Le Heuzey JY, Ponikowski P, Rutten FH (2010) Guidelines for the management of atrial fibrillation: the Task Force for the Management of Atrial Fibrillation of the European Society of Cardiology (ESC). Eur Heart J 31 (19):2369-2429. doi:10.1093/eurheartj/ehq278

[11] Evans W, Swann P (1954) Lone auricular fibrillation. Br Heart J 16 (2):189-194

[12] Wijffels MC, Kirchhof CJ, Dorland R, Allessie MA (1995) Atrial fibrillation begets atrial fibrillation. A study in awake chronically instrumented goats. Circulation 92 (7): 1954-1968

[13] Allessie M, Ausma J, Schotten U (2002) Electrical, contractile and structural remodeling during atrial fibrillation. Cardiovasc Res 54 (2):230-246

[14] Smit MD, Van Gelder IC (2009) Upstream therapy of atrial fibrillation. Expert Rev Cardiovasc Ther 7 (7):763-778

[15] Farre J, Wellens HJ (2004) Philippe Coumel: a founding father of modern arrhythmology. Europace 6 (5):464-465

[16] Garrey WE (1924) Auricular Fibrillation. Physiological Reviews 4 (2):215-250

[17] Moe GK, Rheinboldt WC, Abildskov JA (1964) A Computer Model of Atrial Fibrillation. Am Heart J 67:200-220

[18] Ausma J, Wijffels M, Thone F, Wouters L, Allessie M, Borgers M (1997) Structural changes of atrial myocardium due to sustained atrial fibrillation in the goat. Circulation 96 (9):3157-3163

[19] Frustaci A, Chimenti C, Bellocci F, Morgante E, Russo MA, Maseri A (1997) Histological substrate of atrial biopsies in patients with lone atrial fibrillation. Circulation 96 (4):1180-1184

[20] Bruins P, te Velthuis H, Yazdanbakhsh AP, Jansen PG, van Hardevelt FW, de Beaumont EM, Wildevuur CR, Eijsman L, Trouwborst A, Hack CE (1997) Activation of the complement system during and after cardiopulmonary bypass surgery: postsurgery activation involves C-reactive protein and is associated with postoperative arrhythmia. Circulation 96 (10):3542-3548

[21] Kim YH, Lim DS, Lee JH, Shim WJ, Ro YM, Park GH, Becker KG, Cho-Chung YS, Kim MK (2003) Gene expression profiling of oxidative stress on atrial fibrillation in humans. Exp Mol Med 35 (5):336-349

[22] Tozzi R, Palladini G, Fallarini S, Nano R, Gatti C, Presotto C, Schiavone A, Micheletti R, Ferrari P, Fogari R, Perlini S (2007) Matrix metalloprotease activity is enhanced in the compensated but not in the decompensated phase of pressure overload hypertrophy. Am J Hypertens 20 (6):663-669. doi:10.1016/j.amjhyper.2007.01.016

[23] Falcao-Pires I, Palladini G, Goncalves N, van der Velden J, Moreira-Goncalves D, Miranda-Silva D, Salinaro F, Paulus WJ, Niessen HW, Perlini S, Leite-Moreira AF (2011) Distinct mechanisms for diastolic dysfunction in diabetes mellitus and chronic pressure-overload. Basic Res Cardiol 106 (5):801-814. doi:10.1007/s00395-011-0184-x

[24] Castoldi G, di Gioia CR, Bombardi C, Perego C, Perego L, Mancini M, Leopizzi M, Corradi B, Perlini S, Zerbini G, Stella A (2010) Prevention of myocardial fibrosis by N-acetyl-seryl-aspartyl-lysyl-proline in diabetic rats. Clin Sci (Lond) 118 (3):211-220

[25] Perlini S, Palladini G, Ferrero I, Tozzi R, Fallarini S, Facoetti A, Nano R, Clari F, Busca G, Fogari R, Ferrari AU (2005) Sympathectomy or doxazosin, but not propranolol, blunt myocardial interstitial fibrosis in pressure-overload hypertrophy. Hypertension 46 (5):1213-1218

[26] Li D, Shinagawa K, Pang L, Leung TK, Cardin S, Wang Z, Nattel S (2001) Effects of angiotensin-converting enzyme inhibition on the development of the atrial fibrillation substrate in dogs with ventricular tachypacing-induced congestive heart failure. Circulation 104 (21):2608-2614

[27] Kupfahl C, Pink D, Friedrich K, Zurbrugg HR, Neuss M, Warnecke C, Fielitz J, Graf K, Fleck E, Regitz-Zagrosek V (2000) Angiotensin II directly increases transforming growth factor beta1 and osteopontin and indirectly affects collagen mRNA expression in the human heart. Cardiovasc Res 46 (3):463-475

[28] Verheule S, Sato T, Everett Tt, Engle SK, Otten D, Rubart-von der Lohe M, Nakajima HO, Nakajima H, Field LJ, Olgin JE (2004) Increased vulnerability to atrial fibrillation in transgenic mice with selective atrial fibrosis caused by overexpression of TGF-beta1. Circ Res 94 (11):1458-1465

[29] Ehrlich JR, Hohnloser SH, Nattel S (2006) Role of angiotensin system and effects of its inhibition in atrial fibrillation: clinical and experimental evidence. Eur Heart J 27 (5): 512-518

[30] Lafuente-Lafuente C, Mouly S, Longas-Tejero MA, Mahe I, Bergmann JF (2006) Antiarrhythmic drugs for maintaining sinus rhythm after cardioversion of atrial fibrillation: a systematic review of randomized controlled trials. Arch Intern Med 166 (7): 719-728. doi:10.1001/archinte.166.7.719

[31] Iravanian S, Dudley SC, Jr. (2008) The renin-angiotensin-aldosterone system (RAAS) and cardiac arrhythmias. Heart Rhythm 5 (6 Suppl):S12-17

[32] Ram CV (2008) Angiotensin receptor blockers: current status and future prospects. Am J Med 121 (8):656-663

[33] Liu E, Yang S, Xu Z, Li J, Yang W, Li G (2010) Angiotensin-(1-7) prevents atrial fibrosis and atrial fibrillation in long-term atrial tachycardia dogs. Regul Pept 162 (1-3): 73-78. doi:10.1016/j.regpep.2009.12.020

[34] Liu E, Xu Z, Li J, Yang S, Yang W, Li G (2011) Enalapril, irbesartan, and angiotensin-(1-7) prevent atrial tachycardia-induced ionic remodeling. Int J Cardiol 146 (3): 364-370. doi:10.1016/j.ijcard.2009.07.015

[35] Perlini S, Salinaro F, Fonte ML (2008) Direct renin inhibition: another weapon to modulate the renin-angiotensin system in postinfarction remodeling? Hypertension 52 (6):1019-1021. doi:10.1161/HYPERTENSIONAHA.108.121590

[36] Tsai CF, Chen YC, Lin YK, Chen SA, Chen YJ (2011) Electromechanical effects of the direct renin inhibitor (aliskiren) on the pulmonary vein and atrium. Basic Res Cardiol 106 (6):979-993. doi:10.1007/s00395-011-0206-8

[37] Calkins H, el-Atassi R, Kalbfleisch S, Langberg J, Morady F (1992) Effects of an acute increase in atrial pressure on atrial refractoriness in humans. Pacing Clin Electrophysiol 15 (11 Pt 1):1674-1680

[38] Solti F, Vecsey T, Kekesi V, Juhasz-Nagy A (1989) The effect of atrial dilatation on the genesis of atrial arrhythmias. Cardiovasc Res 23 (10):882-886

[39] Murgatroyd FD, Camm AJ (1993) Atrial arrhythmias. Lancet 341 (8856):1317-1322

[40] Ravelli F, Allessie M (1997) Effects of atrial dilatation on refractory period and vulnerability to atrial fibrillation in the isolated Langendorff-perfused rabbit heart. Circulation 96 (5):1686-1695

[41] Matsuda Y, Toma Y, Matsuzaki M, Moritani K, Satoh A, Shiomi K, Ohtani N, Kohno M, Fujii T, Katayama K, et al. (1990) Change of left atrial systolic pressure waveform in relation to left ventricular end-diastolic pressure. Circulation 82 (5):1659-1667

[42] Chatterjee K, Parmley WW, Cohn JN, Levine TB, Awan NA, Mason DT, Faxon DP, Creager M, Gavras HP, Fouad FM, et al. (1985) A cooperative multicenter study of captopril in congestive heart failure: hemodynamic effects and long-term response. Am Heart J 110 (2):439-447

[43] Fitzpatrick MA, Rademaker MT, Charles CJ, Yandle TG, Espiner EA, Ikram H (1992) Angiotensin II receptor antagonism in ovine heart failure: acute hemodynamic, hormonal, and renal effects. Am J Physiol 263 (1 Pt 2):H250-256

[44] Rademaker MT, Charles CJ, Espiner EA, Frampton CM, Nicholls MG, Richards AM (2004) Combined inhibition of angiotensin II and endothelin suppresses the brain natriuretic peptide response to developing heart failure. Clin Sci (Lond) 106 (6):569-576. doi:10.1042/CS20030366

[45] de Graeff PA, Kingma JH, Dunselman PH, Wesseling H, Lie KI (1987) Acute hemodynamic and hormonal effects of ramipril in chronic congestive heart failure and comparison with captopril. Am J Cardiol 59 (10):164D-170D

[46] Burstein B, Nattel S (2008) Atrial structural remodeling as an antiarrhythmic target. J Cardiovasc Pharmacol 52 (1):4-10

[47] Burstein B, Nattel S (2008) Atrial fibrosis: mechanisms and clinical relevance in atrial fibrillation. J Am Coll Cardiol 51 (8):802-809

[48] Corradi D, Callegari S, Maestri R, Benussi S, Alfieri O (2008) Structural remodeling in atrial fibrillation. Nat Clin Pract Cardiovasc Med 5 (12):782-796. doi:10.1038/ncpcardio1370

[49] Sadoshima J, Izumo S (1993) Molecular characterization of angiotensin II--induced hypertrophy of cardiac myocytes and hyperplasia of cardiac fibroblasts. Critical role of the AT1 receptor subtype. Circ Res 73 (3):413-423

[50] Crabos M, Roth M, Hahn AW, Erne P (1994) Characterization of angiotensin II receptors in cultured adult rat cardiac fibroblasts. Coupling to signaling systems and gene expression. J Clin Invest 93 (6):2372-2378. doi:10.1172/JCI117243

[51] Zhou G, Kandala JC, Tyagi SC, Katwa LC, Weber KT (1996) Effects of angiotensin II and aldosterone on collagen gene expression and protein turnover in cardiac fibroblasts. Mol Cell Biochem 154 (2):171-178

[52] Lin CS, Pan CH (2008) Regulatory mechanisms of atrial fibrotic remodeling in atrial fibrillation. Cell Mol Life Sci 65 (10):1489-1508

[53] Dostal DE (2001) Regulation of cardiac collagen: angiotensin and cross-talk with local growth factors. Hypertension 37 (3):841-844

[54] Lee AA, Dillmann WH, McCulloch AD, Villarreal FJ (1995) Angiotensin II stimulates the autocrine production of transforming growth factor-beta 1 in adult rat cardiac fibroblasts. J Mol Cell Cardiol 27 (10):2347-2357

[55] Lijnen PJ, Petrov VV, Fagard RH (2000) Induction of cardiac fibrosis by transforming growth factor-beta(1). Mol Genet Metab 71 (1-2):418-435. doi:10.1006/mgme.2000.3032

[56] Nakajima H, Nakajima HO, Salcher O, Dittie AS, Dembowsky K, Jing S, Field LJ (2000) Atrial but not ventricular fibrosis in mice expressing a mutant transforming growth factor-beta(1) transgene in the heart. Circ Res 86 (5):571-579

[57] Kallergis EM, Manios EG, Kanoupakis EM, Mavrakis HE, Arfanakis DA, Maliaraki NE, Lathourakis CE, Chlouverakis GI, Vardas PE (2008) Extracellular matrix alterations in patients with paroxysmal and persistent atrial fibrillation: biochemical assessment of collagen type-I turnover. J Am Coll Cardiol 52 (3):211-215. doi:10.1016/j.jacc.2008.03.045

[58] Goette A, Staack T, Rocken C, Arndt M, Geller JC, Huth C, Ansorge S, Klein HU, Lendeckel U (2000) Increased expression of extracellular signal-regulated kinase and angiotensin-converting enzyme in human atria during atrial fibrillation. J Am Coll Cardiol 35 (6):1669-1677

[59] Cardin S, Li D, Thorin-Trescases N, Leung TK, Thorin E, Nattel S (2003) Evolution of the atrial fibrillation substrate in experimental congestive heart failure: angiotensin-dependent and -independent pathways. Cardiovasc Res 60 (2):315-325

[60] Xiao HD, Fuchs S, Campbell DJ, Lewis W, Dudley SC, Jr., Kasi VS, Hoit BD, Keshelava G, Zhao H, Capecchi MR, Bernstein KE (2004) Mice with cardiac-restricted angiotensin-converting enzyme (ACE) have atrial enlargement, cardiac arrhythmia, and sudden death. Am J Pathol 165 (3):1019-1032. doi:10.1016/S0002-9440(10)63363-9

[61] Sakabe M, Fujiki A, Nishida K, Sugao M, Nagasawa H, Tsuneda T, Mizumaki K, Inoue H (2004) Enalapril prevents perpetuation of atrial fibrillation by suppressing atrial fibrosis and over-expression of connexin43 in a canine model of atrial pacing-induced left ventricular dysfunction. J Cardiovasc Pharmacol 43 (6):851-859

[62] Li Y, Li W, Yang B, Han W, Dong D, Xue J, Li B, Yang S, Sheng L (2007) Effects of Cilazapril on atrial electrical, structural and functional remodeling in atrial fibrillation dogs. J Electrocardiol 40 (1):100 e101-106. doi:10.1016/j.jelectrocard.2006.04.001

[63] Okazaki H, Minamino T, Tsukamoto O, Kim J, Okada K, Myoishi M, Wakeno M, Takashima S, Mochizuki N, Kitakaze M (2006) Angiotensin II type 1 receptor blocker prevents atrial structural remodeling in rats with hypertension induced by chronic nitric oxide inhibition. Hypertens Res 29 (4):277-284

[64] Kumagai K, Nakashima H, Urata H, Gondo N, Arakawa K, Saku K (2003) Effects of angiotensin II type 1 receptor antagonist on electrical and structural remodeling in atrial fibrillation. J Am Coll Cardiol 41 (12):2197-2204

[65] Nattel S, Maguy A, Le Bouter S, Yeh YH (2007) Arrhythmogenic ion-channel remodeling in the heart: heart failure, myocardial infarction, and atrial fibrillation. Physiol Rev 87 (2):425-456. doi:10.1152/physrev.00014.2006

[66] Yue L, Feng J, Gaspo R, Li GR, Wang Z, Nattel S (1997) Ionic remodeling underlying action potential changes in a canine model of atrial fibrillation. Circ Res 81 (4): 512-525

[67] Laszlo R, Eick C, Rueb N, Weretka S, Weig HJ, Schreieck J, Bosch RF (2008) Inhibition of the renin-angiotensin system: effects on tachycardia-induced early electrical remodelling in rabbit atrium. J Renin Angiotensin Aldosterone System 9 (3):125-132. doi:10.1177/1470320308095262

[68] Doronin SV, Potapova IA, Lu Z, Cohen IS (2004) Angiotensin receptor type 1 forms a complex with the transient outward potassium channel Kv4.3 and regulates its gating properties and intracellular localization. J Biol Chem 279 (46):48231-48237. doi: 10.1074/jbc.M405789200

[69] Nakashima H, Kumagai K, Urata H, Gondo N, Ideishi M, Arakawa K (2000) Angiotensin II antagonist prevents electrical remodeling in atrial fibrillation. Circulation 101 (22):2612-2617

[70] Valderrabano M (2007) Influence of anisotropic conduction properties in the propagation of the cardiac action potential. Prog Biophys Mol Biol 94 (1-2):144-168. doi: 10.1016/j.pbiomolbio.2007.03.014

[71] Tsai CT, Lai LP, Hwang JJ, Lin JL, Chiang FT (2008) Molecular genetics of atrial fibrillation. J Am Coll Cardiol 52 (4):241-250

[72] Emdad L, Uzzaman M, Takagishi Y, Honjo H, Uchida T, Severs NJ, Kodama I, Murata Y (2001) Gap junction remodeling in hypertrophied left ventricles of aortic-banded rats: prevention by angiotensin II type 1 receptor blockade. J Mol Cell Cardiol 33 (2): 219-231. doi:10.1006/jmcc.2000.1293

[73] Fischer R, Dechend R, Gapelyuk A, Shagdarsuren E, Gruner K, Gruner A, Gratze P, Qadri F, Wellner M, Fiebeler A, Dietz R, Luft FC, Muller DN, Schirdewan A (2007) Angiotensin II-induced sudden arrhythmic death and electrical remodeling. American J Physiol Heart Circ Physiol 293 (2):H1242-1253. doi:10.1152/ajpheart.01400.2006

[74] Mayama T, Matsumura K, Lin H, Ogawa K, Imanaga I (2007) Remodelling of cardiac gap junction connexin 43 and arrhythmogenesis. Exp Clin Cardiol 12 (2):67-76

[75] Chen YJ, Chen YC, Tai CT, Yeh HI, Lin CI, Chen SA (2006) Angiotensin II and angiotensin II receptor blocker modulate the arrhythmogenic activity of pulmonary veins. Br J Pharmacol 147 (1):12-22. doi:10.1038/sj.bjp.0706445

[76] Haissaguerre M, Jais P, Shah DC, Takahashi A, Hocini M, Quiniou G, Garrigue S, Le Mouroux A, Le Metayer P, Clementy J (1998) Spontaneous initiation of atrial fibrillation by ectopic beats originating in the pulmonary veins. N Engl J Med 339 (10): 659-666

[77] Cheng CC, Huang CF, Chen YC, Lin YK, Kao YH, Chen YJ, Chen SA (2011) Heat-stress responses modulate beta-adrenergic agonist and angiotensin II effects on the arrhythmogenesis of pulmonary vein cardiomyocytes. J Cardiovasc Electrophysiol 22 (2):183-190. doi:10.1111/j.1540-8167.2010.01849.x

[78] Reil JC, Hohl M, Selejan S, Lipp P, Drautz F, Kazakow A, Munz BM, Muller P, Steendijk P, Reil GH, Allessie MA, Bohm M, Neuberger HR (2012) Aldosterone promotes atrial fibrillation. Eur Heart J 33 (16):2098-2108. doi:10.1093/eurheartj/ehr266

[79] Lammers C, Dartsch T, Brandt MC, Rottlander D, Halbach M, Peinkofer G, Ockenpoehler S, Weiergraeber M, Schneider T, Reuter H, Muller-Ehmsen J, Hescheler J, Hoppe UC, Zobel C (2012) Spironolactone prevents aldosterone induced increased duration of atrial fibrillation in rat. Cell Physiol Biochem 29 (5-6):833-840. doi: 10.1159/000178483

[80] Gensini F, Padeletti L, Fatini C, Sticchi E, Gensini GF, Michelucci A (2003) Angiotensin-converting enzyme and endothelial nitric oxide synthase polymorphisms in patients with atrial fibrillation. Pacing Clin Electrophysiol 26 (1 Pt 2):295-298

[81] Darbar D, Motsinger AA, Ritchie MD, Gainer JV, Roden DM (2007) Polymorphism modulates symptomatic response to antiarrhythmic drug therapy in patients with lone atrial fibrillation. Heart Rhythm 4 (6):743-749

[82] Tsai CT, Lai LP, Lin JL, Chiang FT, Hwang JJ, Ritchie MD, Moore JH, Hsu KL, Tseng CD, Liau CS, Tseng YZ (2004) Renin-angiotensin system gene polymorphisms and atrial fibrillation. Circulation 109 (13):1640-1646

[83] Ravn LS, Benn M, Nordestgaard BG, Sethi AA, Agerholm-Larsen B, Jensen GB, Tybjaerg-Hansen A (2008) Angiotensinogen and ACE gene polymorphisms and risk of atrial fibrillation in the general population. Pharmacogenet Genomics 18 (6):525-533. doi:10.1097/FPC.0b013e3282fce3bd

[84] Tsai CT, Hwang JJ, Chiang FT, Wang YC, Tseng CD, Tseng YZ, Lin JL (2008) Renin-angiotensin system gene polymorphisms and atrial fibrillation: a regression approach for the detection of gene-gene interactions in a large hospitalized population. Cardiology 111 (1):1-7. doi:10.1159/000113419

[85] Amir O, Amir RE, Paz H, Mor R, Sagiv M, Lewis BS (2008) Aldosterone synthase gene polymorphism as a determinant of atrial fibrillation in patients with heart failure. Am J Cardiol 102 (3):326-329. doi:10.1016/j.amjcard.2008.03.063

[86] Sun X, Yang J, Hou X, Li J, Shi Y, Jing Y (2011) Relationship between -344T/C polymorphism in the aldosterone synthase gene and atrial fibrillation in patients with essential hypertension. J Renin Angiotensin Aldosterone System 12 (4):557-563. doi: 10.1177/1470320311417654

[87] Vermes E, Tardif JC, Bourassa MG, Racine N, Levesque S, White M, Guerra PG, Ducharme A (2003) Enalapril decreases the incidence of atrial fibrillation in patients with left ventricular dysfunction: insight from the Studies Of Left Ventricular Dysfunction (SOLVD) trials. Circulation 107 (23):2926-2931

[88] Maggioni AP, Latini R, Carson PE, Singh SN, Barlera S, Glazer R, Masson S, Cere E, Tognoni G, Cohn JN (2005) Valsartan reduces the incidence of atrial fibrillation in pa-

tients with heart failure: results from the Valsartan Heart Failure Trial (Val-HeFT). Am Heart J 149 (3):548-557. doi:10.1016/j.ahj.2004.09.033

[89] Ducharme A, Swedberg K, Pfeffer MA, Cohen-Solal A, Granger CB, Maggioni AP, Michelson EL, McMurray JJ, Olsson L, Rouleau JL, Young JB, Olofsson B, Puu M, Yusuf S (2006) Prevention of atrial fibrillation in patients with symptomatic chronic heart failure by candesartan in the Candesartan in Heart failure: Assessment of Reduction in Mortality and morbidity (CHARM) program. Am Heart J 152 (1):86-92

[90] Pedersen OD, Bagger H, Kober L, Torp-Pedersen C (1999) Trandolapril reduces the incidence of atrial fibrillation after acute myocardial infarction in patients with left ventricular dysfunction. Circulation 100 (4):376-380

[91] Pizzetti F, Turazza FM, Franzosi MG, Barlera S, Ledda A, Maggioni AP, Santoro L, Tognoni G (2001) Incidence and prognostic significance of atrial fibrillation in acute myocardial infarction: the GISSI-3 data. Heart 86 (5):527-532

[92] Hansson L, Lindholm LH, Ekbom T, Dahlof B, Lanke J, Schersten B, Wester PO, Hedner T, de Faire U (1999) Randomised trial of old and new antihypertensive drugs in elderly patients: cardiovascular mortality and morbidity the Swedish Trial in Old Patients with Hypertension-2 study. Lancet 354 (9192):1751-1756

[93] Hansson L, Lindholm LH, Niskanen L, Lanke J, Hedner T, Niklason A, Luomanmaki K, Dahlof B, de Faire U, Morlin C, Karlberg BE, Wester PO, Bjorck JE (1999) Effect of angiotensin-converting-enzyme inhibition compared with conventional therapy on cardiovascular morbidity and mortality in hypertension: the Captopril Prevention Project (CAPPP) randomised trial. Lancet 353 (9153):611-616

[94] L'Allier PL, Ducharme A, Keller PF, Yu H, Guertin MC, Tardif JC (2004) Angiotensin-converting enzyme inhibition in hypertensive patients is associated with a reduction in the occurrence of atrial fibrillation. J Am Coll Cardiol 44 (1):159-164

[95] Wachtell K, Hornestam B, Lehto M, Slotwiner DJ, Gerdts E, Olsen MH, Aurup P, Dahlof B, Ibsen H, Julius S, Kjeldsen SE, Lindholm LH, Nieminen MS, Rokkedal J, Devereux RB (2005) Cardiovascular morbidity and mortality in hypertensive patients with a history of atrial fibrillation: The Losartan Intervention For End Point Reduction in Hypertension (LIFE) study. J Am Coll Cardiol 45 (5):705-711

[96] Schaer BA, Schneider C, Jick SS, Conen D, Osswald S, Meier CR (2010) Risk for incident atrial fibrillation in patients who receive antihypertensive drugs: a nested case-control study. Ann Intern Med 152 (2):78-84. doi: 10.1059/0003-4819-152-2-201001190-00005

[97] Salehian O, Healey J, Stambler B, Alnemer K, Almerri K, Grover J, Bata I, Mann J, Matthew J, Pogue J, Yusuf S, Dagenais G, Lonn E (2007) Impact of ramipril on the incidence of atrial fibrillation: results of the Heart Outcomes Prevention Evaluation study. Am Heart J 154 (3):448-453. doi:10.1016/j.ahj.2007.04.062

[98] Investigators AI, Yusuf S, Healey JS, Pogue J, Chrolavicius S, Flather M, Hart RG, Hohnloser SH, Joyner CD, Pfeffer MA, Connolly SJ (2011) Irbesartan in patients with atrial fibrillation. N Engl J Med 364 (10):928-938. doi:10.1056/NEJMoa1008816

[99] Schmieder RE, Kjeldsen SE, Julius S, McInnes GT, Zanchetti A, Hua TA (2008) Reduced incidence of new-onset atrial fibrillation with angiotensin II receptor blockade: the VALUE trial. J Hypertens 26 (3):403-411

[100] Mathew JP, Fontes ML, Tudor IC, Ramsay J, Duke P, Mazer CD, Barash PG, Hsu PH, Mangano DT (2004) A multicenter risk index for atrial fibrillation after cardiac surgery. Jama 291 (14):1720-1729

[101] Ozaydin M, Dede O, Varol E, Kapan S, Turker Y, Peker O, Duver H, Ibrisim E (2008) Effect of renin-angiotensin aldosteron system blockers on postoperative atrial fibrillation. Int J Cardiol 127 (3):362-367

[102] White CM, Kluger J, Lertsburapa K, Faheem O, Coleman CI (2007) Effect of preoperative angiotensin converting enzyme inhibitor or angiotensin receptor blocker use on the frequency of atrial fibrillation after cardiac surgery: a cohort study from the atrial fibrillation suppression trials II and III. Eur J Cardiothorac Surg 31 (5):817-820. doi:10.1016/j.ejcts.2007.02.010

[103] Van Den Berg MP, Crijns HJ, Van Veldhuisen DJ, Griep N, De Kam PJ, Lie KI (1995) Effects of lisinopril in patients with heart failure and chronic atrial fibrillation. J Card Fail 1 (5):355-363

[104] Dagres N, Karatasakis G, Panou F, Athanassopoulos G, Maounis T, Tsougos E, Kourea K, Malakos I, Kremastinos DT, Cokkinos DV (2006) Pre-treatment with Irbesartan attenuates left atrial stunning after electrical cardioversion of atrial fibrillation. Eur Heart J 27 (17):2062-2068

[105] Madrid AH, Bueno MG, Rebollo JM, Marin I, Pena G, Bernal E, Rodriguez A, Cano L, Cano JM, Cabeza P, Moro C (2002) Use of irbesartan to maintain sinus rhythm in patients with long-lasting persistent atrial fibrillation: a prospective and randomized study. Circulation 106 (3):331-336

[106] Madrid AH, Marin IM, Cervantes CE, Morell EB, Estevez JE, Moreno G, Parajon JR, Peng J, Limon L, Nannini S, Moro C (2004) Prevention of recurrences in patients with lone atrial fibrillation. The dose-dependent effect of angiotensin II receptor blockers. J Renin Angiotensin Aldosterone System 5 (3):114-120

[107] Ueng KC, Tsai TP, Yu WC, Tsai CF, Lin MC, Chan KC, Chen CY, Wu DJ, Lin CS, Chen SA (2003) Use of enalapril to facilitate sinus rhythm maintenance after external cardioversion of long-standing persistent atrial fibrillation. Results of a prospective and controlled study. Eur Heart J 24 (23):2090-2098

[108] Tveit A, Grundvold I, Olufsen M, Seljeflot I, Abdelnoor M, Arnesen H, Smith P (2007) Candesartan in the prevention of relapsing atrial fibrillation. Int J Cardiol 120 (1):85-91. doi:10.1016/j.ijcard.2006.08.086

[109] Belluzzi F, Sernesi L, Preti P, Salinaro F, Fonte ML, Perlini S (2009) Prevention of recurrent lone atrial fibrillation by the angiotensin-II converting enzyme inhibitor ramipril in normotensive patients. J Am Coll Cardiol 53 (1):24-29

[110] Katritsis DG, Toumpoulis IK, Giazitzoglou E, Korovesis S, Karabinos I, Paxinos G, Zambartas C, Anagnostopoulos CE (2005) Latent arterial hypertension in apparently lone atrial fibrillation. J Interv Card Electrophysiol 13 (3):203-207

[111] Richter B, Derntl M, Marx M, Lercher P, Gossinger HD (2007) Therapy with angiotensin-converting enzyme inhibitors, angiotensin II receptor blockers, and statins: no effect on ablation outcome after ablation of atrial fibrillation. Am Heart J 153 (1): 113-119. doi:10.1016/j.ahj.2006.09.006

[112] Al Chekakie MO, Akar JG, Wang F, Al Muradi H, Wu J, Santucci P, Varma N, Wilber DJ (2007) The effects of statins and renin-angiotensin system blockers on atrial fibrillation recurrence following antral pulmonary vein isolation. J Cardiovasc Electrophysiol 18 (9):942-946. doi:10.1111/j.1540-8167.2007.00887.x

[113] Park JH, Oh YS, Kim JH, Chung WB, Oh SS, Lee DH, Choi YS, Shin WS, Park CS, Youn HJ, Chung WS, Lee MY, Seung KB, Rho TH, Hong SJ (2009) Effect of Angiotensin converting enzyme inhibitors and Angiotensin receptor blockers on patients following ablation of atrial fibrillation. Korean Circ J 39 (5):185-189. doi:10.4070/kcj.2009.39.5.185

[114] Zheng B, Kang J, Tian Y, Tang R, Long D, Yu R, He H, Zhang M, Shi L, Tao H, Liu X, Dong J, Ma C (2009) Angiotensin-converting enzyme inhibitors and angiotensin II receptor blockers have no beneficial effect on ablation outcome in chronic persistent atrial fibrillation. Acta Cardiol 64 (3):335-340

[115] Patel D, Mohanty P, Di Biase L, Wang Y, Shaheen MH, Sanchez JE, Horton RP, Gallinghouse GJ, Zagrodzky JD, Bailey SM, Burkhardt JD, Lewis WR, Diaz A, Beheiry S, Hongo R, Al-Ahmad A, Wang P, Schweikert R, Natale A (2010) The impact of statins and renin-angiotensin-aldosterone system blockers on pulmonary vein antrum isolation outcomes in post-menopausal females. Europace 12 (3):322-330. doi:10.1093/europace/eup387

[116] Folkeringa RJ, Crijns HJ (2010) Do non-antiarrhythmic drugs have enough pleiotropic power to reduce atrial fibrillation? Europace 12 (3):299-300. doi:10.1093/europace/euq009

[117] Yin Y, Dalal D, Liu Z, Wu J, Liu D, Lan X, Dai Y, Su L, Ling Z, She Q, Luo K, Woo K, Dong J (2006) Prospective randomized study comparing amiodarone vs. amiodarone plus losartan vs. amiodarone plus perindopril for the prevention of atrial fibrillation recurrence in patients with lone paroxysmal atrial fibrillation. Eur Heart J 27 (15): 1841-1846. doi:10.1093/eurheartj/ehl135

[118] Fogari R, Mugellini A, Destro M, Corradi L, Zoppi A, Fogari E, Rinaldi A (2006) Losartan and prevention of atrial fibrillation recurrence in hypertensive patients. J Cardiovasc Pharmacol 47 (1):46-50

[119] Fogari R, Mugellini A, Zoppi A, Preti P, Destro M, Lazzari P, Derosa G (2012) Effect of telmisartan and ramipril on atrial fibrillation recurrence and severity in hypertensive patients with metabolic syndrome and recurrent symptomatic paroxysmal and persistent atrial fibrillation. J Cardiovasc Pharmacol Ther 17 (1):34-43. doi: 10.1177/1074248410395018

[120] Komatsu T, Ozawa M, Tachibana H, Sato Y, Orii M, Kunugida F, Nakamura M (2008) Combination therapy with amiodarone and enalapril in patients with paroxysmal atrial fibrillation prevents the development of structural atrial remodeling. Int Heart J 49 (4):435-447

[121] Murray KT, Rottman JN, Arbogast PG, Shemanski L, Primm RK, Campbell WB, Solomon AJ, Olgin JE, Wilson MJ, Dimarco JP, Beckman KJ, Dennish G, Naccarelli GV, Ray WA (2004) Inhibition of angiotensin II signaling and recurrence of atrial fibrillation in AFFIRM. Heart Rhythm 1 (6):669-675. doi:10.1016/j.hrthm.2004.08.008

[122] Disertori M, Latini R, Barlera S, Franzosi MG, Staszewsky L, Maggioni AP, Lucci D, Di Pasquale G, Tognoni G (2009) Valsartan for prevention of recurrent atrial fibrillation. N Engl J Med 360 (16):1606-1617

[123] Goette A, Schon N, Kirchhof P, Breithardt G, Fetsch T, Hausler KG, Klein HU, Steinbeck G, Wegscheider K, Meinertz T (2012) Angiotensin II-antagonist in paroxysmal atrial fibrillation (ANTIPAF) trial. Circ Arrhythm Electrophysiol 5 (1):43-51. doi: 10.1161/CIRCEP.111.965178

[124] Yamashita T, Inoue H, Okumura K, Kodama I, Aizawa Y, Atarashi H, Ohe T, Ohtsu H, Kato T, Kamakura S, Kumagai K, Kurachi Y, Koretsune Y, Saikawa T, Sakurai M, Sato T, Sugi K, Nakaya H, Hirai M, Hirayama A, Fukatani M, Mitamura H, Yamazaki T, Watanabe E, Ogawa S, Investigators JRI (2011) Randomized trial of angiotensin II-receptor blocker vs. dihydropiridine calcium channel blocker in the treatment of paroxysmal atrial fibrillation with hypertension (J-RHYTHM II study). Europace 13 (4):473-479. doi:10.1093/europace/euq439

[125] Dabrowski R, Szwed H (2012) Antiarrhythmic potential of aldosterone antagonists in atrial fibrillation. Cardiol J 19 (3):223-229

[126] Dabrowski R, Borowiec A, Smolis-Bak E, Kowalik I, Sosnowski C, Kraska A, Kazimierska B, Wozniak J, Zareba W, Szwed H (2010) Effect of combined spironolactone-beta-blocker +/- enalapril treatment on occurrence of symptomatic atrial fibrillation episodes in patients with a history of paroxysmal atrial fibrillation (SPIR-AF study). Am J Cardiol 106 (11):1609-1614

[127] Williams RS, deLemos JA, Dimas V, Reisch J, Hill JA, Naseem RH (2011) Effect of spironolactone on patients with atrial fibrillation and structural heart disease. Clin Cardiol 34 (7):415-419. doi:10.1002/clc.20914

[128] Swedberg K, Zannad F, McMurray JJ, Krum H, van Veldhuisen DJ, Shi H, Vincent J, Pitt B, Investigators E-HS (2012) Eplerenone and atrial fibrillation in mild systolic

heart failure: results from the EMPHASIS-HF (Eplerenone in Mild Patients Hospitalization And SurvIval Study in Heart Failure) study. J Am Coll Cardiol 59 (18): 1598-1603. doi:10.1016/j.jacc.2011.11.063

[129] Botto GL, Padeletti L, Santini M, Capucci A, Gulizia M, Zolezzi F, Favale S, Molon G, Ricci R, Biffi M, Russo G, Vimercati M, Corbucci G, Boriani G (2009) Presence and duration of atrial fibrillation detected by continuous monitoring: crucial implications for the risk of thromboembolic events. J Cardiovasc Electrophysiol 20 (3):241-248

[130] Madrid AH, Peng J, Zamora J, Marin I, Bernal E, Escobar C, Munos-Tinoco C, Rebollo JM, Moro C (2004) The role of angiotensin receptor blockers and/or angiotensin converting enzyme inhibitors in the prevention of atrial fibrillation in patients with cardiovascular diseases: meta-analysis of randomized controlled clinical trials. Pacing Clin Electrophysiol 27 (10):1405-1410. doi:10.1111/j.1540-8159.2004.00645.x

[131] Healey JS, Baranchuk A, Crystal E, Morillo CA, Garfinkle M, Yusuf S, Connolly SJ (2005) Prevention of atrial fibrillation with angiotensin-converting enzyme inhibitors and angiotensin receptor blockers: a meta-analysis. J Am Coll Cardiol 45 (11): 1832-1839

[132] Anand K, Mooss AN, Hee TT, Mohiuddin SM (2006) Meta-analysis: inhibition of renin-angiotensin system prevents new-onset atrial fibrillation. Am Heart J 152 (2): 217-222

[133] Jibrini MB, Molnar J, Arora RR (2008) Prevention of atrial fibrillation by way of abrogation of the renin-angiotensin system: a systematic review and meta-analysis. Am J Ther 15 (1):36-43. doi:10.1097/MJT.0b013e31804beb59

[134] Kalus JS, Coleman CI, White CM (2006) The impact of suppressing the renin-angiotensin system on atrial fibrillation. J Clin Pharmacol 46 (1):21-28

[135] Schneider MP, Hua TA, Bohm M, Wachtell K, Kjeldsen SE, Schmieder RE (2010) Prevention of atrial fibrillation by Renin-Angiotensin system inhibition a meta-analysis. J Am Coll Cardiol 55 (21):2299-2307

[136] Disertori M, Barlera S, Staszewsky L, Latini R, Quintarelli S, Franzosi MG (2012) Systematic review and meta-analysis: renin-Angiotensin system inhibitors in the prevention of atrial fibrillation recurrences: an unfulfilled hope. Cardiovasc Drugs Ther 26 (1):47-54. doi:10.1007/s10557-011-6346-0

[137] Liu T, Korantzopoulos P, Xu G, Shehata M, Li D, Wang X, Li G (2011) Association between angiotensin-converting enzyme insertion/deletion gene polymorphism and atrial fibrillation: a meta-analysis. Europace 13 (3):346-354. doi:10.1093/europace/euq407

[138] Huang G, Xu JB, Liu JX, He Y, Nie XL, Li Q, Hu YM, Zhao SQ, Wang M, Zhang WY, Liu XR, Wu T, Arkin A, Zhang TJ (2011) Angiotensin-converting enzyme inhibitors and angiotensin receptor blockers decrease the incidence of atrial fibrillation: a meta-analysis. Eur J Clin Invest 41 (7):719-733. doi:10.1111/j.1365-2362.2010.02460.x

[139] Bhuriya R, Singh M, Sethi A, Molnar J, Bahekar A, Singh PP, Khosla S, Arora R (2011) Prevention of recurrent atrial fibrillation with angiotensin-converting enzyme inhibitors or angiotensin receptor blockers: a systematic review and meta-analysis of randomized trials. J Cardiovasc Pharmacol Ther 16 (2):178-184. doi: 10.1177/1074248410389045

[140] Zhang Y, Zhang P, Mu Y, Gao M, Wang JR, Wang Y, Su LQ, Hou YL (2010) The role of renin-angiotensin system blockade therapy in the prevention of atrial fibrillation: a meta-analysis of randomized controlled trials. Clin Pharmacol Ther 88 (4):521-531

[141] Khatib R, Joseph P, Briel M, Yusuf S, Healey J (2012) Blockade of the renin-angiotensin-aldosterone system (RAAS) for primary prevention of non-valvular atrial fibrillation: A systematic review and meta analysis of randomized controlled trials. Int J Cardiol. doi:10.1016/j.ijcard.2012.02.009

[142] Kintscher U (2009) ONTARGET, TRANSCEND, and PRoFESS: new-onset diabetes, atrial fibrillation, and left ventricular hypertrophy. J Hypertens Suppl 27 (2):S36-39. doi:10.1097/01.hjh.0000354519.67451.96

[143] Coleman CI, Makanji S, Kluger J, White CM (2007) Effect of angiotensin-converting enzyme inhibitors or angiotensin receptor blockers on the frequency of post-cardiothoracic surgery atrial fibrillation. Ann Pharmacother 41 (3):433-437

[144] Campbell RW (1996) ACE inhibitors and arrhythmias. Heart 76 (3 Suppl 3):79-82

[145] Fletcher RD, Cintron GB, Johnson G, Orndorff J, Carson P, Cohn JN (1993) Enalapril decreases prevalence of ventricular tachycardia in patients with chronic congestive heart failure. The V-HeFT II VA Cooperative Studies Group. Circulation 87 (6 Suppl):VI49-55

Chapter 2

Antioxidant Therapies in the Prevention and Treatment of Atrial Fibrillation

Tong Liu, Panagiotis Korantzopoulos and
Guangping Li

Additional information is available at the end of the chapter

http://dx.doi.org/10.5772/53408

1. Introduction

Atrial fibrillation (AF) is the most common sustained arrhythmia encountered in clinical practice, representing a major public health problem. Accumulating evidence suggests oxidative stress may play an important role in the pathogenesis and perpetuation of AF [1-5]. There are several redox signaling pathways that are possibly related to increased oxidative stress in the setting of AF, including mitochondrial DNA damage, increased activity of enzymes such as NADPH oxidase and xanthine oxidase, nitric oxide synthase uncoupling, activation of pro-arrhythmic transcription factors such as peroxi-some proliferator-activated receptor, c-fos and NF-κB. In the past few years experimental data and clinical evidence have tested the concept of antioxidant interventions to prevent AF. Besides statins, ACEIs and/or ARBs, several other interventions with antioxidant properties, such as Vitamin C and E, thiazolidinediones, N-acetylcysteine, probucol, nitric oxide donors or precursors, NADPH oxidase inhibitors, Xanthine oxidase inhibitors have emerged as novel strategies in the prevention and treatment of AF [6-10]. In this chapter, we aim to summarize recent evidence regarding antioxidant therapies in the prevention and treatment of atrial fibrillation

2. Vitamin C and E

Recently, antioxidant vitamins C and E have been tested in the prevention of AF, especially postoperative AF (POAF) [11-14]. These dietary vitamin supplementations have been proven to protect against the development and progression of AF in experimental models [15, 16]. Vitamin C is a potent water-soluble antioxidant that protects against oxidative stress derived by reactive oxygen and nitrogen species. In a canine model of AF, Carnes et al. [15] were the first to demonstrate that ascorbate attenuates the pacing-induced atrial remodeling and atrial peroxynitrite production. However, Shiroshita-Takeshita [16] and colleagues did not confirm the protective effects of Vitamin C and E against AF in their study. Additionaly, tachypacing-induced atrial effective refractory period shortening and AF promotion were not influenced by antioxidant vitamins, whereas simvastatin attenuated atrial remodeling and prevented AF. Recently, Lin et al. [17] investigated whether Vitamin C has direct electrophysiological effects on isolated rabbit pulmonary vein (PV) preparations. They demonstrated that ascorbic acid decreases PV spontaneous activity and attenuates the arrhythmogenic effects of hydrogen peroxide (H_2O_2). Given that PVs represent major sources of ectopic beats that trigger paroxysmal AF, the potential preventive effects of vitamin C on AF recurrence after PV isolation should be tested in future clinical trials.

The clinical evidence regarding Vitamin C and E on AF prophylaxis is mainly limited in the setting of POAF prevention. In a retrospective observational study, Carnes et al. [15] evaluated the effects of supplemental ascorbate on POAF prevention. A series of 43 consecutive patients scheduled for coronary artery bypass graft (CABG) surgery were given 2 g ascorbic acid the night before surgery, followed by 500mg doses twice daily for the 5 days following CABG. Patients receiving ascorbate had a 16.3% incidence of POAF, in contrast to 34.9% in the control group (P=0.048). However, multivariate analysis after adjusting for other confounding factors demonstrated that β-blockers use exhibits the most protective effect (84% risk reduction, *P*=0.007) and ascorbate alone was not an independent protector for POAF. In particular, the two groups were not ideally matched regarding all risk factors for AF, and the incidence of diabetes, hypertension, and previous history of AF was higher in the control group compared to the treatment group. Finally, this study may not have enough power to evaluate POAF incidence.

Eslami et al [18] examined the effects of ascorbic acid as an adjunct to β-blockers in a prospective, randomized trial. One hundred patients undergoing CABG surgery were randomized to the ascorbic acid or to the control group. All patients had been treated with β-blockers for at least for one week. Patients in the ascorbic acid group received 2 g of ascorbic acid on the night before the surgery and 1 g twice daily for 5 days following surgery. Patients in the control group did not receive ascorbic acid. Patients in both groups continued to receive β-blockers postoperatively. The incidence of POAF was 4% in the Vitamin C group and 26% in the control group (P=0.002). The authors concluded that ascorbic acid can be prescribed as an adjunctive therapy to β-blockers for the prophylaxis of POAF. Finally, Papoulidis et al. [19] evaluated the preventive effects of Vitamin C on POAF incidence in 170 patients undergoing isolated on-pump CABG. Importantly, all the patients were under β-blockers therapy preoperatively. The incidence of POAF was 44.7% in the Vitamin C group and 61.2% in the control group (*P*=0.041). Notably, patients with Vitmain C had a shorter hospital stay as well as conversion time from AF into sinus rhythm.

Very recently, in another randomized clinical trial (RCT) [20] which enrolled 152 patients scheduled for cardiac surgery, the combination of vitamin C (1 g/d) plus vitamin E (400 IU/d) reduced the risk of POAF in patients aged over 60 years indicating that the efficacy of the antioxidant interventions may be improved with aging. In a recent meta-analysis including five randomized controlled trials with 567 patients, Harling et al. [13] showed that the prophylactic use of vitamins C and E significantly reduced the incidence of POAF (OR: 0.43, 95% CI: 0.21 to 0.89) as well as the all-cause arrhythmia (OR: 0.54, 95% CI: 0.29 to 0.99) following cardiac surgery. However, the overall quality of enrolled studies was relatively poor. Undoubtedly, further well-designed studies with enough sample size are warranted in order to to clarify this issue.

The clinical evidence relating to the potential role of antioxidant vitamins for secondary prevention of AF is sparse. Korantzopoulos et al. [21] prospectively studied 44 patients following successful electrical cardioversion of persistent AF. The patients randomized into Vitamin C group and control group. Within one week, AF recurred in 4.5% of patients in the vitamin C group and in 36.3% of patients in the control group (P=0.024). Moreover, inflammatory biomarkers decreased after cardioversion in patients receiving vitamin C. Another recently published study evaluated whether serum Vitamin E level was related to AF recurrence in patients undergoing electrical cardioversion (EC) [22]. One hundred fourty four consecutive patients who underwent successful EC were prospectively enrolled and followed for 3 months. It was indicated that low serum Vitamin E level is an independent predictor for the AF recurrence. Further studies are needed in order to examine the efficacy of antioxidant vitamin E in AF prevention.

3. Thiazolidinediones

Thiazolidinediones (TZDs) represent a class of insulin-sensiting agents with peroxisome proliferator-activated receptor-γ (PPAR-γ) activation effects, used to improve insulin resistance in patients with type 2 diabetes [23, 24]. Troglitazone, the first drug developed and used clinically, has been withdrawn from the market due to its liver toxicity. Pioglitazone and rosiglitazone are the only compounds that are available for clinical use now. Apart from their insulin-sensitizing effects, TZDs have several pleiotropic properties including anti-inflammatory and antioxidant [25, 26]. It has been demonstrated that PPAR-γ ligands inhibit the expression of inducible nitric oxide synthase (iNOS) and peroxynitrite production in mesangial cells and in cerebellar granule cells [27]. Also, TZDs enhance endothelial nitric oxide (NO) bioavailability, reducing nicotinamide adenine dinucleotide phosphate (NADPH) oxidase-dependent superoxide production, while they induce antioxidant enzymes such as Cu/Zn superoxide dismutase (Cu/Zn SOD) [28].

Recent experimental evidence indicates that TZDs, especially pioglitazone, prevent atrial electrical and structural remodeling through their anti-inflammatory and antioxidant properties. In a rabbit model of congestive heart failure, pioglitazone attenuated atrial structural remodeling and inhibited AF promotion, at the same degree as candesartan. Furthermore, the PPAR-γ activator suppressed transforming growth factor-β (TGF-β), tumor necrosis factor-α (TNF-α) and extracellular signal-regulated kinase (ERK) expression in atrial tissue. Therefore, the authors proposed that pioglitazone may inhibit AF by modulating inflammatory, oxidative stress, and hypertrophic signaling pathways involved in atrial remodeling [29]. Very recently, Kume et al. showed that pioglitazone reduced inflammatory atrial fibrosis and vulnerability to AF in a pressure overload rat model of AF, possibly via the suppression of MCP-1–mediated inflammatory profibrotic processes [30]. In an in vivo rat model, Xu et al. [31] reported pioglitazone inhibited age-related atrial structural remodeling and AF susceptibility via its antioxidant and anti-apoptotic effects. Gene and protein expression levels of antioxidant molecules such as Mn superoxide dismutase (MnSOD) and heat shock protein (HSP) 70 were significantly enhanced, whereas NADPH oxidase subunits p22phox and gp91phox were significantly reduced in aged rats treated with pioglitazone. Therefore, activation of antioxidant molecules and inhibition of NADPH-derived ROS production may be the mechanisms underlying the favorable effects of TZDs on aging-related atrial remodeling and AF promotion. However, experimental data on the effects rosiglitazone on atrial remodeling in the setting of diabetes is lacking. We have shown that rosiglitazone attenuates atrial structural remodeling reducing the interatrial activation time and the atrial interstitial fibrosis in alloxan-induced diabetic rabbits [31].. Also, rosiglitazone treatment increased plasma antioxidant enzyme superoxide dismutase (SOD) activity and decreased oxidant stress and inflammatory markers including malondialdehyde (MDA), C-reactive protein (CRP), and TNF-α levels. [32]

We have previously described two patients with diabetes who experienced a remarkable improvement in their paroxysmal AF episodes following treatment with rosiglitazone [33]. However, two large RCTs, namely RECORD [34] and PROactive [35] which enrolled high-risk patients with type 2 diabetes failed to demonstrate a significant reduction of AF risk from TZDs compared with controls. The potential explanations were: firstly, AF was not a predefined endpoint and reported as an adverse event; secondly, there was a very low AF incidence in both treatment and control groups (1.5-2%). Also, another case-control study showed that preoperative use of TZDs in diabetic patients undergoing cardiac surgery was associated with a non-statistically significant 20% reduction of POAF [36]. In a prospective cohort study including 150 diabetic patients undergoing catheter ablation for AF, Gu et al. showed that previous pioglitazone use was independently associated with a lower recurrence of atrial tachyarrhythmias during a follow-up period of 23 months [37]. Interestingly, in a recent observational study Chao et al. [38] investigated the possible association between TZDs use and development of new-onset AF in 12,605 patients with Type 2 diabetes. During a follow-up of 5 years, TZDs decreased the risk of new-onset AF by 31% after adjustment for age, underlying diseases and baseline medications. Although growing evidence suggests TZDs use prevents the development and recurrence of AF in diabetic patients, the cardiovascular safety considerations on rosiglitazone recently prompted the European Medicines Agency (EMA) to suspended this drug from the European market and patients taking rosiglitazone were advised to discuss alternative options with their physicians [39]. Since November 18, 2011 the FDA does not allow rosiglitazone to be sold without a prescription from certified doctors. Patients are required to be informed of the risks associated with the use of rosiglitazone. Therefore, it is very hard for rosiglitazone to gain a therapeutic indication for AF in the future [40]. Given the favorable cardiovascular effects of pioglitazone from a recent meta-analysis of 19 RCTs (including PROactive study) enrolling 16,390 patients [41], further large-scale randomized, controlled trials with long-term follow-up or a post hoc analysis from previous trials are still needed to evaluate the potential role of pioglitazone, as an upstream therapy for AF prevention in patients with diabetes [42, 43].

4. N-acetylcysteine

N-acetylcysteine (NAC) is a precursor of l-cysteine and glutathione. As a source of sulfhydryl groups in cells, it may act as a scavenger of free radicals [44]. In clinical practice, NAC is used as an antioxidant, mucolytic agent widely prescribed in chronic pulmonary disease. Carnes et al. [45] showed that atrial myocytes from AF patients incubated with NAC lead to a significant increase in the density of $I_{Ca,L}$. This observation suggests NAC may possibly attenuates atrial electrophysiological remodeling caused by rapid atrial activation. In a randomized study including 115 patients undergoing CABG or valve surgery, Ozaydin et al. [46] demonstrated that NAC markedly reduces the incidence of POAF lasting more than 5 minutes. A previous meta-analysis [47] evaluated potential beneficial effects of perioperative NAC on the prevention of complications after cardiothoracic surgery. In the sub-group analysis of six trials which reported POAF as study endpoints, the use of NAC significantly lowered the risk of developing POAF by 36%. In a more recent meta-analysis, Gu et al. [48] included 8 randomized trials incorporating 578 patients, and indicated that NAC significantly reduces the incidence of POAF by 38% (OR: 0.62, 95% CI: 0.41- 0.93; P =0.021) compared with controls. It is worth mentioning that only one trial [46] included in this meta-analysis had specified POAF as a primary endpoint. The remaining seven studies reported POAF as a secondary endpoint. Therefore, future large-scale randomized studies with an adequate power are urgently in demand.

5. Probucol

Probucol is a lipid-lowering agent with potent anti-oxidant and anti-inflammatory effects. It has been used in clinical practice during the past two decades to decrease atherosclerosis and prevent restenosiss following stent implantation. However, the potential side effects including decreasing serum high-density lipoprotein cholesterol level and QT prolongation have limited the probucol's worldwide clinical use [49, 50]. As a potent antioxidant, it may reduce the production of oxygen free radicals and act as a direct superoxide anion scavenger. In an isolated perfused rat model, probucol increased the expression of an important myocardial antioxidant enzyme, namely glutathione peroxidase, and prevented lipid peroxidation following ischemia reperfusion injury [51]. Moreover, probucol inhibited NADPH oxidase activity in the aorta from cholesterol-fed rabbits [52]. Our previous studies suggested that prophylactic treatment with probucol during the periprocedural period in patients undergoing coronary intervention protects against contrast-induced acute kidney injury [53, 54]. However, experimental studies regarding the possible benefits of probucol on atrial remodeling and AF prevention are lacking. Gong et al. showed that probucol attenuates atrial nerve sprouting and heterogeneous sympathetic hyperinnervation induced by rapid right atrial pacing, and markedly reduces the promotion and maintenance of AF. Also, probucol significantly reduces atrial oxidative stress and increases total antioxidant capacity [55]. A further study from this group suggested that probucol attenuates structural remodeling and preventes atrial apoptosis, decreasing the left atrial MDA content in paced dogs [56]. Very recently, we investigated the effects of probucol on atrial structural and electrical remodeling in alloxan-induced diabetic rabbits [57]. After treatment for 8 weeks, the diabetic rabbits on probucol exhibited alleviation of oxidative stress displayed as decreased plasma MDA and increased plasma SOD levels compared with diabetic controls, while probucol significantly reduced left atrial interstitial fibrosis and AF inducibility [57]. Therefore, it seems reasonable to speculate that the antioxidant effects of probucol may favorably affect atrial autonomic and structural remodeling.

Succinobucol (AGI-1067), a derivative of probucol, is a metabolically stable compound that has greater intracellular antioxidant efficacy in vitro than probucol without causing a significant prolongation of the QT interval [58]. Surprisingly, the ARISE study [59] showed that use of succinobucol was associated with increased incidence of new-onset AF in patients with an acute coronary syndrome. Our previous meta-analysis suggested that increased CRP levels are associated with greater risk of immediate and short-term AF recurrence following electrical cardioversion [60, 61]. In this context, although succinobucol have potent antioxidant effects, its unfavourable influence on CRP levels may be a possible potential explanation for this undesirable effect [62, 63]. Undoubtedly, further studies are needed to elucidate the precise role of probucol and succinobucol in atrial remodeling and their clinical impact on AF.

6. Nitric oxide donors or precursors

Nitric oxide is an important endothelium-derived relaxing factor that plays a pivotal role in the maintenance of vascular tone. NO is synthesized from L-arginine through the effects of endothelial NO synthase (eNOS) with the critical cofactor tetrahydrobrobiopterin (BH_4). BH_4 depletion induces NOS uncoupling which shifts the enzymatic activity from NO production towards superoxide anion (O_2^-) production [64]. Endothelial dysfunction (ED) promotes oxidative stress and inflammation and also impairs NO dependent vaso-relaxation. Endothelial dysfunction with decreased NO production has been implicated on the development of atrial fibrillation [65, 66].

It has been indicated that L-Arginine supplementation, as a NO precursor, increases plasma nitrite levels, decreases MDA release and attenuates ROS mediated myocardial injury [67]. In a canine tachypacing model of heart failure, Nishijima et al. [68] found increased inducible NOS in the left atrium which was associated with BH_4 depletion, NOS2 uncoupling, and increased superoxide anion production. These biochemical changes were associated with atrial electrophysiological changes with increased AF inducibility. BH_4 supplementation reduced atrial oxidative stress and inducibility of atrial fibrillation. Thus, modulation of NOS activity may be an interesting therapeutic approach to prevent AF [69]. At the clinical level, a pilot randomized placebo-controlled study examined the potential role of sodium nitroprusside

(SNP), as a NO donor, in the prevention of POAF [70]. Specifically, 100 consecutive patients undergoing CABG surgery were randomized to receive SNP (0.5 μg /Kg.min) or placebo (dextrose 5% in water) during the rewarming period. The occurrence of AF was significantly lower in the SNP group (P<0.005). Furthermore, the inflammatory biomarker CRP was higher postoperatively in the control group compared to the SNP group (P<0.05). However, a recent study didn't find any association between the use of sodium nitroprusside during cardiothoracic surgery and POAF in a retrospective cohort of 1025 patients undergoing bypass surgery [71]. Therefore, anti-inflammatory and antioxidant effects of NO may have beneficial effects on the prevention of POAF. Further randomized controlled studies are urgently needed to clarify the role of NO and its donor or precursor on the AF prevention.

7. NADPH oxidases inhibitors

NADPH oxidases (NOXs) have been investigated as a key enzymatic source of ROS and seem to play an important role in the pathogenesis of hypertension, atherosclerosis, and heart failure [72-74]. NOXs are multi-subunit transmembrane enzymes that utilize NADPH as an electron donor to reduce oxygen to superoxide anion and hydrogen peroxide. NOX2 and NOX4 are the most abundant NOX subtypes in cardiomyocytes.

Recent evidence indicates that NOX-derived ROS plays a pivotal role in the development and maintenance of AF. Dudley et al. [75] showed reduced NO and increased superoxide production production in the left atrial appendage (LAA), which was related to increased NADPH oxidase activity in an experimental model of atrial tachy-pacing. Of note, the NADPH oxidase inhibitor apocynin reduced the superoxide production by 91%. In addition, Kim et al. [76] investigated the sources of superoxide production from the right atrial appendage (RAA) of patients undergoing cardiac surgery. They indicated that the membrane-bound subunit gp91phox (NOX2) containing NADPH oxidase was the main source of atrial superoxide production in human atrial myocytes during sinus rhythm and AF. Also, NADPH-stimulated superoxide release from RAA homogenates was significantly increased in patients with AF. In a subsequent study, they measured atrial NADPH oxidase activity in RAA samples from 170 consecutive patients undergoing coronary artery bypass surgery. The multivariate analysis showed that atrial NADPH oxidase activity was the strongest independent risk factor for the development of POAF [77]. Remarkably, recent clinical evidence [78] suggests that the behaviour of NADPH oxidase is related to the type of AF. Cangemi et al. demonstrated that NOX2 was upregulated in patients with paroxysmal/persistent AF compared with those with permanent AF and controls [78]. Also, NOX4-derived hydrogen peroxide production is markedly increased in the LAA tissues of AF patients. Moreover, treatment of HL-1 atrial cells with angiotensin II, resulted in upregulation of NOX4 and H_2O_2 production [79]. Bearing in mind the potent NADPH oxidase inhibitors such as NOX2 inhibitors and apocynin [80] may be served as potential candidate for the novel preventive agents on AF.

8. Xanthine oxidase inhibitors

Accumulating evidence suggests that xanthine oxidase (XO) is another important source of ROS and may relate to atrial remodeling and AF [81]. In a pig model of rapid atrial pacing, increased XO activity in LAA and reduced superoxide production by 85% following administration of oxypurinol (a XO inhibitor) was demonstrated [75]. However, no significant effect of oxypurinol on superoxide production in human RAA was demonstrated in another study [76]. A potential explanation for this evident difference is that in the porcine model the increased XO activity was located in the LAA, whereas RAA specimens were examined in the human study. Of note, in a similar porcine model, it was demonstrated that after 1 week of rapid atrial pacing NO expression was decreased in the LAA but not in the RAA, indicating that the oxidative stress was enhanced only in the left atrium [82].

UA is a metabolic product of purine metabolism produced via the action of XO. Therefore, UA represents a marker of oxidative stress and inflammation [83, 84]. There is a positive association between UA levels and AF in different population. In a small observational study, we showed a stepwise increase of UA levels in patients with paroxysmal AF and permanent AF compared to controls [85]. It was also demonstrated that high serum UA levels were independent predictor for AF presence in hypertensive patients [86] and AF recurrence following catheter ablation [87]. In the ARIC study, a large prospective cohort study, elevated serum UA was associated with a greater risk of AF development during the follow-up period [88].

No clinical trial to date has examined the effect of allopurinol administration on AF. Only one observational study reported that patients receiving UA lowering agents had decreased AF prevalence [89]. In a very recent experimental study using a dog model of atrial tachypacing, allopurinol suppressed AF promotion by preventing both electrical and structural remodeling, while it also reduced endothelial NOS protein expression without affecting the left ventricular ejection fraction or LA diameter [90]. Finally, there are no data on the cardiovascular effects of the newly released non-purine XO inhibitor febuxostat.

9. Conclusion

A substantial body of evidence indicates that oxidative stress plays a critical role in the pathophysiology of atrial remodeling. However, the molecular pathways of this pathologic process are complex and depend on different underlying substrates and concomitant diseases. Antioxidant therapy seems to be a promising intervention strategy in the prevention of AF development and perpetuation, at least in the case of POAF. It should be acknowledged that antioxidant substances may be ineffective in many instances since they act at an advanced stage of the oxidative damage cascade. On the other hand, interventions that target early steps of ROS formation seem to be a more promising strategy.

http://dx.doi.org/10.5772/53408

Acknowledgements

This work was supported by grants (30900618, 81270245 to T.L.) from the National Natural Science Foundation of China.

Author details

Tong Liu[1*], Panagiotis Korantzopoulos[2] and Guangping Li[1]

*Address all correspondence to: liutongdoc@yahoo.com.cn

1 Department of Cardiology, Tianjin Institute of Cardiology, Second Hospital of Tianjin Medical University, Tianjin, People's Republic of China

2 Department of Cardiology, University of Ioannina Medical School, Ioannina, Greece

Conflict of interest: None declared

References

[1] Korantzopoulos, P, Kolettis, T. M, Galaris, D, & Goudevenos, J. A. The role of oxidative stress in the pathogenesis and perpetuation of atrial fibrillation. *Int J Cardiol* (2007). , 115, 135-143.

[2] Van Wagoner, D. R. Oxidative stress and inflammation in atrial fibrillation: Role in pathogenesis and potential as a therapeutic target. *J Cardiovasc Pharmacol* (2008). , 52, 306-313.

[3] Huang, C. X, Liu, Y, Xia, W. F, Tang, Y. H, & Huang, H. Oxidative stress: A possible pathogenesis of atrial fibrillation. *Med Hypotheses* (2009). , 72, 466-467.

[4] Negi, S, Sovari, A. A, & Dudley, S. C. Jr. Atrial fibrillation: The emerging role of inflammation and oxidative stress. *Cardiovasc Hematol Disord Drug Targets* (2010). , 10, 262-268.

[5] Jeong, E. M, Liu, M, Sturdy, M, et al. Metabolic stress, reactive oxygen species, and arrhythmia. *J Mol Cell Cardiol* (2012). , 52, 454-463.

[6] Savelieva, I, Kakouros, N, Kourliouros, A, & Camm, A. J. Upstream therapies for management of atrial fibrillation: Review of clinical evidence and implications for european society of cardiology guidelines. Part I: Primary prevention. *Europace* (2011). , 13, 308-328.

[7] Savelieva, I, Kakouros, N, Kourliouros, A, & Camm, A. J. Upstream therapies for management of atrial fibrillation: Review of clinical evidence and implications for

european society of cardiology guidelines. Part II: Secondary prevention. *Europace* (2011)., 13, 610-625.

[8] Sovari, A. A, & Dudley, S. C. Antioxidant therapy for atrial fibrillation: Lost in translation? *Heart* (2012). Aug 15. [Epub ahead of print].

[9] Liu, T, & Li, G. Antioxidant interventions as novel preventive strategies for postoperative atrial fibrillation. *Int J Cardiol* (2010)., 145, 140-142.

[10] Sovari, A. A, & Dudley, S. C. Jr. Reactive oxygen species-targeted therapeutic interventions for atrial fibrillation. *Front Physiol* (2012).

[11] Rasoli, S, Kakouros, N, Harling, L, et al. Antioxidant vitamins in the prevention of atrial fibrillation: What is the evidence? *Cardiol Res Pract* (2011).

[12] Rodrigo, R, Vinay, J, Castillo, R, et al. Use of vitamins c and e as a prophylactic therapy to prevent postoperative atrial fibrillation. *Int J Cardiol* (2010)., 138, 221-228.

[13] Harling, L, Rasoli, S, Vecht, J. A, Ashrafian, H, Kourliouros, A, & Athanasiou, T. Do antioxidant vitamins have an anti-arrhythmic effect following cardiac surgery? A meta-analysis of randomised controlled trials. *Heart* (2011)., 97, 1636-1642.

[14] Rodrigo, R. Prevention of postoperative atrial fibrillation: Novel and safe strategy based on the modulation of the antioxidant system. *Front Physiol* (2012).

[15] Carnes, C. A, Chung, M. K, Nakayama, T, et al. Ascorbate attenuates atrial pacing-induced peroxynitrite formation and electrical remodeling and decreases the incidence of postoperative atrial fibrillation. *Circ Res* (2001). E, 32-38.

[16] Shiroshita-takeshita, A, Schram, G, Lavoie, J, & Nattel, S. Effect of simvastatin and antioxidant vitamins on atrial fibrillation promotion by atrial-tachycardia remodeling in dogs. *Circulation* (2004)., 110, 2313-2319.

[17] Lin, Y. K, Lin, F. Z, Chen, Y. C, et al. Oxidative stress on pulmonary vein and left atrium arrhythmogenesis. *Circ J* (2010)., 74, 1547-1556.

[18] Eslami, M, Badkoubeh, R. S, Mousavi, M, et al. Oral ascorbic acid in combination with beta-blockers is more effective than beta-blockers alone in the prevention of atrial fibrillation after coronary artery bypass grafting. *Tex Heart Inst J* (2007)., 34, 268-274.

[19] Papoulidis, P, Ananiadou, O, Chalvatzoulis, E, et al. The role of ascorbic acid in the prevention of atrial fibrillation after elective on-pump myocardial revascularization surgery: A single-center experience--a pilot study. *Interact Cardiovasc Thorac Surg* (2011)., 12, 121-124.

[20] Rodrigo, R, Gutierrez, R, Fernandez, R, & Guzman, P. Ageing improves the antioxidant response against postoperative atrial fibrillation: A randomized controlled trial. *Interact Cardiovasc Thorac Surg* (2012)., 15, 209-214.

[21] Korantzopoulos, P, Kolettis, T. M, Kountouris, E, et al. Oral vitamin c administration reduces early recurrence rates after electrical cardioversion of persistent atrial fibrillation and attenuates associated inflammation. *Int J Cardiol* (2005). , 102, 321-326.

[22] Ferro, D, Franciosa, P, Cangemi, R, et al. Serum levels of vitamin e are associated with early recurrence of atrial fibrillation after electric cardioversion. *Circ Arrhythm Electrophysiol* (2012). , 5, 327-333.

[23] Palee, S, Chattipakorn, S, Phrommintikul, A, & Chattipakorn, N. Ppargamma activator, rosiglitazone: Is it beneficial or harmful to the cardiovascular system? *World J Cardiol* (2011). , 3, 144-152.

[24] Cariou, B, Charbonnel, B, & Staels, B. Thiazolidinediones and ppargamma agonists: Time for a reassessment. *Trends Endocrinol Metab* (2012). , 23, 205-215.

[25] Giannini, S, Serio, M, & Galli, A. Pleiotropic effects of thiazolidinediones: Taking a look beyond antidiabetic activity. *J Endocrinol Invest* (2004). , 27, 982-991.

[26] Da Ros RAssaloni R, Ceriello A. The preventive anti-oxidant action of thiazolidinediones: A new therapeutic prospect in diabetes and insulin resistance. *Diabet Med* (2004). , 21, 1249-1252.

[27] Ricote, M, Li, A. C, Willson, T. M, Kelly, C. J, & Glass, C. K. The peroxisome proliferator-activated receptor-gamma is a negative regulator of macrophage activation. *Nature* (1998). , 391, 79-82.

[28] Hwang, J, Kleinhenz, D. J, Lassegue, B, Griendling, K. K, Dikalov, S, & Hart, C. M. Peroxisome proliferator-activated receptor-gamma ligands regulate endothelial membrane superoxide production. *Am J Physiol Cell Physiol* (2005). C, 899-905.

[29] Shimano, M, Tsuji, Y, Inden, Y, et al. Pioglitazone, a peroxisome proliferator-activated receptor-gamma activator, attenuates atrial fibrosis and atrial fibrillation promotion in rabbits with congestive heart failure. *Heart Rhythm* (2008). , 5, 451-459.

[30] Kume, O, Takahashi, N, Wakisaka, O, et al. Pioglitazone attenuates inflammatory atrial fibrosis and vulnerability to atrial fibrillation induced by pressure overload in rats. *Heart Rhythm* (2011). , 8, 278-285.

[31] Xu, D, Murakoshi, N, Igarashi, M, et al. Ppar-gamma activator pioglitazone prevents age-related atrial fibrillation susceptibility by improving antioxidant capacity and reducing apoptosis in a rat model. *J Cardiovasc Electrophysiol* (2012). , 23, 209-217.

[32] Liu, T, Zhao, H, Li, J, Korantzopoulos, P, & Li, G. Rosiglitazone attenuates atrial structural remodeling and atrial fibrillation promotion in alloxan-induced diabetic rabbits. *Eur Heart J* (2010).

[33] Korantzopoulos, P, Kokkoris, S, Kountouris, E, Protopsaltis, I, Siogas, K, & Melidonis, A. Regression of paroxysmal atrial fibrillation associated with thiazolidinedione therapy. *Int J Cardiol* (2008). e, 51-53.

[34] Home, P. D, Pocock, S. J, Beck-nielsen, H, et al. Rosiglitazone evaluated for cardiovascular outcomes in oral agent combination therapy for type 2 diabetes (RECORD): A multicentre, randomised, open-label trial. *Lancet* (2009). , 373, 2125-2135.

[35] Dormandy, J. A, Charbonnel, B, Eckland, D. J, et al. Secondary prevention of macrovascular events in patients with type 2 diabetes in the proactive study (prospective pioglitazone clinical trial in macrovascular events): A randomised controlled trial. *Lancet* (2005). , 366, 1279-1289.

[36] Anglade, M. W, Kluger, J, White, C. M, Aberle, J, & Coleman, C. I. Thiazolidinedione use and post-operative atrial fibrillation: A us nested case-control study. *Curr Med Res Opin* (2007). , 23, 2849-2855.

[37] Gu, J, Liu, X, Wang, X, et al. Beneficial effect of pioglitazone on the outcome of catheter ablation in patients with paroxysmal atrial fibrillation and type 2 diabetes mellitus. *Europace* (2011). , 13, 1256-1261.

[38] Chao, T. F, Leu, H. B, Huang, C. C, et al. Thiazolidinediones can prevent new onset atrial fibrillation in patients with non-insulin dependent diabetes. *Int J Cardiol* (2012). , 156, 199-202.

[39] Abbas, A, Blandon, J, Rude, J, Elfar, A, & Mukherjee, D. PPAR-gamma agonist in treatment of diabetes: Cardiovascular safety considerations. *Cardiovasc Hematol Agents Med Chem* (2012). , 10, 124-134.

[40] Raschi, E, Boriani, G, & De Ponti, F. Targeting the arrhythmogenic substrate in atrial fibrillation: Focus on structural remodeling. *Curr Drug Targets* (2011). , 12, 263-286.

[41] Lincoff, A. M, Wolski, K, Nicholls, S. J, & Nissen, S. E. Pioglitazone and risk of cardiovascular events in patients with type 2 diabetes mellitus: A meta-analysis of randomized trials. *JAMA* (2007). , 298, 1180-1188.

[42] Liu, T, Korantzopoulos, P, Li, G, & Li, J. The potential role of thiazolidinediones in atrial fibrillation. *Int J Cardiol* (2008). , 128, 129-130.

[43] Liu, T, & Li, G. Thiazolidinediones as novel upstream therapy for atrial fibrillation in diabetic patients: A review of current evidence. *Int J Cardiol* (2012). , 156, 215-216.

[44] Zafarullah, M, Li, W. Q, Sylvester, J, & Ahmad, M. Molecular mechanisms of n-acetylcysteine actions. *Cell Mol Life Sci* (2003). , 60, 6-20.

[45] Carnes, C. A, Janssen, P. M, Ruehr, M. L, et al. Atrial glutathione content, calcium current, and contractility. *J Biol Chem* (2007). , 282, 28063-28073.

[46] Ozaydin, M, Peker, O, Erdogan, D, et al. N-acetylcysteine for the prevention of postoperative atrial fibrillation: A prospective, randomized, placebo-controlled pilot study. *Eur Heart J* (2008). , 29, 625-631.

[47] Baker, W. L, Anglade, M. W, Baker, E. L, White, C. M, Kluger, J, & Coleman, C. I. Use of n-acetylcysteine to reduce post-cardiothoracic surgery complications: A meta-analysis. *Eur J Cardiothorac Surg* (2009). , 35, 521-527.

[48] Gu, W. J, Wu, Z. J, Wang, P. F, & Aung, L. H. Yin RX. N-acetylcysteine supplementation for the prevention of atrial fibrillation after cardiac surgery: A meta-analysis of eight randomized controlled trials. *BMC Cardiovasc Disord* (2012).

[49] Yamashita, S, & Matsuzawa, Y. Where are we with probucol: A new life for an old drug? *Atherosclerosis* (2009). , 207, 16-23.

[50] Stocker, R. Molecular mechanisms underlying the antiatherosclerotic and antidiabetic effects of probucol, succinobucol, and other probucol analogues. *Curr Opin Lipidol* (2009). , 20, 227-235.

[51] Singla, D. K, Kaur, K, Sharma, A. K, Dhingra, S, & Singal, P. K. Probucol promotes endogenous antioxidant reserve and confers protection against reperfusion injury. *Can J Physiol Pharmacol* (2007). , 85, 439-443.

[52] Umeji, K, Umemoto, S, Itoh, S, et al. Comparative effects of pitavastatin and probucol on oxidative stress, cu/zn superoxide dismutase, ppar-gamma, and aortic stiffness in hypercholesterolemia. *Am J Physiol Heart Circ Physiol* (2006). H, 2522-2532.

[53] Li, G, Yin, L, Liu, T, et al. Role of probucol in preventing contrast-induced acute kidney injury after coronary interventional procedure. *Am J Cardiol* (2009). , 103, 512-514.

[54] Yin, L, Li, G, Liu, T, et al. Probucol for the prevention of cystatin c-based contrast-induced acute kidney injury following primary or urgent angioplasty: A randomized, controlled trial. *Int J Cardiol* (2012).

[55] Gong, Y. T, Li, W. M, Li, Y, et al. Probucol attenuates atrial autonomic remodeling in a canine model of atrial fibrillation produced by prolonged atrial pacing. *Chin Med J (Engl)* (2009). , 122, 74-82.

[56] Li, Y, Sheng, L, Li, W, et al. Probucol attenuates atrial structural remodeling in prolonged pacing-induced atrial fibrillation in dogs. *Biochem Biophys Res Commun* (2009). , 381, 198-203.

[57] Fu, H, Liu, T, Liu, C, et al. Probucol preserves atrial structure and function by attenuates oxidative stress and increases stability of vulnerable atrial fibrillation in alloxan-induced diabetic rabbits. *Cardiology* (2012). suppl1)::48-49.

[58] Midwinter, R. G, Maghzal, G. J, Dennis, J. M, et al. Succinobucol induces apoptosis in vascular smooth muscle cells. *Free Radic Biol Med* (2012). , 52, 871-879.

[59] Tardif, J. C, Mcmurray, J. J, Klug, E, et al. Effects of succinobucol (AGI-1067) after an acute coronary syndrome: A randomised, double-blind, placebo-controlled trial. *Lancet* (2008). , 371, 1761-1768.

[60] Liu, T, Li, G, Li, L, & Korantzopoulos, P. Association between c-reactive protein and recurrence of atrial fibrillation after successful electrical cardioversion: A meta-analysis. *J Am Coll Cardiol* (2007). , 49, 1642-1648.

[61] Liu, T, Li, L, Korantzopoulos, P, Goudevenos, J. A, & Li, G. Meta-analysis of association between c-reactive protein and immediate success of electrical cardioversion in persistent atrial fibrillation. *Am J Cardiol* (2008)., 101, 1749-1752.

[62] Tardif, J. C, Gregoire, J, & Allier, L. PL, et al. Effects of the antioxidant succinobucol (AGI-1067) on human atherosclerosis in a randomized clinical trial. *Atherosclerosis* (2008)., 197, 480-486.

[63] Liu, T, & Li, G. Probucol and succinobucol in atrial fibrillation: Pros and cons. *Int J Cardiol* (2010)., 144, 295-296.

[64] Verma, S, & Anderson, T. J. Fundamentals of endothelial function for the clinical cardiologist. *Circulation* (2002)., 105, 546-549.

[65] Guazzi, M, & Arena, R. Endothelial dysfunction and pathophysiological correlates in atrial fibrillation. *Heart* (2009)., 95, 102-106.

[66] Krishnamoorthy, S, Lim, S. H, & Lip, G. Y. Assessment of endothelial (dys)function in atrial fibrillation. *Ann Med* (2009)., 41, 576-590.

[67] Kiziltepe, U, Tunctan, B, Eyileten, Z. B, et al. Efficiency of l-arginine enriched cardioplegia and non-cardioplegic reperfusion in ischemic hearts. *Int J Cardiol* (2004)., 97, 93-100.

[68] Nishijima, Y, Sridhar, A, Bonilla, I, et al. Tetrahydrobiopterin depletion and nos2 uncoupling contribute to heart failure-induced alterations in atrial electrophysiology. *Cardiovasc Res* (2011)., 91, 71-79.

[69] Bonilla, I. M, Sridhar, A, Gyorke, S, Cardounel, A. J, & Carnes, C. A. Nitric oxide synthases and atrial fibrillation. *Front Physiol* (2012).

[70] Cavolli, R, Kaya, K, Aslan, A, et al. Does sodium nitroprusside decrease the incidence of atrial fibrillation after myocardial revascularization?: A pilot study. *Circulation* (2008)., 118, 476-481.

[71] Bolesta, S, Aungst, T. D, & Kong, F. Effect of sodium nitroprusside on the occurrence of atrial fibrillation after cardiothoracic surgery. *Ann Pharmacother* (2012)., 46, 785-792.

[72] Selemidis, S, Sobey, C. G, Wingler, K, Schmidt, H. H, & Drummond, G. R. Nadph oxidases in the vasculature: Molecular features, roles in disease and pharmacological inhibition. *Pharmacol Ther* (2008)., 120, 254-291.

[73] Zhang, M, Perino, A, Ghigo, A, Hirsch, E, & Shah, A. NADPH oxidases in heart failure: Poachers or gamekeepers? *Antioxid Redox Signal* (2012). Aug 27. [Epub ahead of print]

[74] Octavia, Y. Brunner-La Rocca HP, Moens AL. NADPH oxidase-dependent oxidative stress in the failing heart: From pathogenic roles to therapeutic approach. *Free Radic Biol Med* (2012)., 52, 291-297.

[75] Dudley, S. C. Jr., Hoch NE, McCann LA, et al. Atrial fibrillation increases production of superoxide by the left atrium and left atrial appendage: Role of the nadph and xanthine oxidases. *Circulation* (2005). , 112, 1266-1273.

[76] Kim, Y. M, Guzik, T. J, Zhang, Y. H, et al. A myocardial Nox2 containing NAD(P)H oxidase contributes to oxidative stress in human atrial fibrillation. *Circ Res* (2005). , 97, 629-636.

[77] Kim, Y. M, Kattach, H, Ratnatunga, C, Pillai, R, Channon, K. M, & Casadei, B. Association of atrial nicotinamide adenine dinucleotide phosphate oxidase activity with the development of atrial fibrillation after cardiac surgery. *J Am Coll Cardiol* (2008). , 51, 68-74.

[78] Cangemi, R, Celestini, A, Calvieri, C, et al. Different behaviour of NOX2 activation in patients with paroxysmal/persistent or permanent atrial fibrillation. *Heart* (2012). , 98, 1063-1066.

[79] Zhang, J, Youn, J. Y, Kim, A. Y, et al. Noxdependent hydrogen peroxide overproduction in human atrial fibrillation and hl-1 atrial cells: Relationship to hypertension. *Front Physiol* (2012). , 4.

[80] Sovari, A. A, Morita, N, & Karagueuzian, H. S. Apocynin: A potent nadph oxidase inhibitor for the management of atrial fibrillation. *Redox Rep* (2008). , 13, 242-245.

[81] Korantzopoulos, P, Letsas, K. P, & Liu, T. Xanthine oxidase and uric acid in atrial fibrillation. *Front Physiol* (2012).

[82] Cai, H, Li, Z, Goette, A, et al. Downregulation of endocardial nitric oxide synthase expression and nitric oxide production in atrial fibrillation: Potential mechanisms for atrial thrombosis and stroke. *Circulation* (2002). , 106, 2854-2858.

[83] Strazzullo, P, & Puig, J. G. Uric acid and oxidative stress: Relative impact on cardiovascular risk? *Nutr Metab Cardiovasc Dis* (2007). , 17, 409-414.

[84] Glantzounis, G. K, Tsimoyiannis, E. C, Kappas, A. M, & Galaris, D. A. Uric acid and oxidative stress. *Curr Pharm Des* (2005). , 11, 4145-4151.

[85] Letsas, K. P, Korantzopoulos, P, Filippatos, G. S, et al. Uric acid elevation in atrial fibrillation. *Hellenic J Cardiol* (2010). , 51, 209-213.

[86] Liu, T, Zhang, X, Korantzopoulos, P, Wang, S, & Li, G. Uric acid levels and atrial fibrillation in hypertensive patients. *Intern Med* (2011). , 50, 799-803.

[87] Letsas, K. P, Siklody, C. H, Korantzopoulos, P, et al. The impact of body mass index on the efficacy and safety of catheter ablation of atrial fibrillation. *Int J Cardiol* (2011). Jul 2. [Epub ahead of print].

[88] Tamariz, L, Agarwal, S, Soliman, E. Z, et al. Association of serum uric acid with incident atrial fibrillation (from the atherosclerosis risk in communities [ARIC] study). *Am J Cardiol* (2011). , 108, 1272-1276.

[89] Kuwabara, M, Niwa, K, & Niinuma, H. Hyperuricemia is an independent risk factor of atrial fibrillation due to electrical remodeling through activation of uric acid transporter. *J. Am. Coll. Cardiol* (2012). Suppl.A, A163.

[90] Sakabe, M, Fujiki, A, Sakamoto, T, Nakatani, Y, Mizumaki, K, & Inoue, H. Xanthine oxidase inhibition prevents atrial fibrillation in a canine model of atrial pacing-induced left ventricular dysfunction. *J Cardiovasc Electrophysiol* (2012). Apr 16. [Epub ahead of print].

Chapter 3

Effect of CD3+ T-Lymphocyte and n-3 Polyunsaturated Fatty Acids on the Diagnosis or Treatment of Atrial Fibrillation

Qiang-Sun Zheng, Hong-Tao Wang, Zhong Zhang,
Jun Li, Li Liu and Bo-yuan Fan

Additional information is available at the end of the chapter

http://dx.doi.org/10.5772/54167

1. Introduction

1.1. Review of the relationship between n-3 polyunsaturated fatty acids and the atrial fibrillation

It is well established that the consumption of fish is associated with lower rates of cardiovascular death (Albert CM,et al.,2002; Hu FB, et al.,2002). Dietary fish oil supplementation has been shown to reduce mortality in high-risk groups through a reduction in sudden cardiac death and ventricular tachyarrhythmia. It has been recently reported that atrial fibrillation (AF) is associated with inflammation and inflammatory cytokines, and n-3 polyunsaturated fatty acids (PUFAs) might be of anti-inflammatory effects. Whether PUFAs has some antiarrhythmic effect and can be used in the treatment of AF is still unknown.

1.2. Dietary n-3 PUFA supplementation attenuates the inducibility and maintenance of AF

We established canine sterile pericarditis model and evaluate the anti-inflammatory effect of PUFAs on AF(Zhong Zhang,et al.,2010). Twenty mongrel sex-matched adult dogs were randomly divided into two groups. In the n-3 PUFA group (n=10), oral administration ofeicosapentaenoic+docosahexaenoic acid (EPA+DHA), 2 g/day (Omacor, Solvay Pharmaceuticals GmbH, Hanover, Germany) was started 4 weeks before the baseline study, and was continued until the end of the study. The dogs in the control group (n=10) did not receive n-3 PUFAs or plant oil for 4 weeks. We examined the plasma concentration of the CRP, IL-6, and

TNF-α before the operation and on the second postoperative day in both groups. There were no significant differences in three biomarkers of inflammation between two groups before the operation, and these biomarkers were significantly increased in both groups on the second postoperative day. However, three proinflammatory cytokines were significantly lower in the PUFA group than in the control group respectively (CRP, 7.6±0.5 vs. 11.7± 1.3 mg/dl, Pb0.0001 Fig. 1; IL-6, 112.0±37.3 vs. 142.0±19.6 pg/ml, Pb0.0001 Fig. 2; TNF-α, 83.3±8.5 vs. 112.4±8.2 pg/ml, Pb0.0001 Fig. 3).

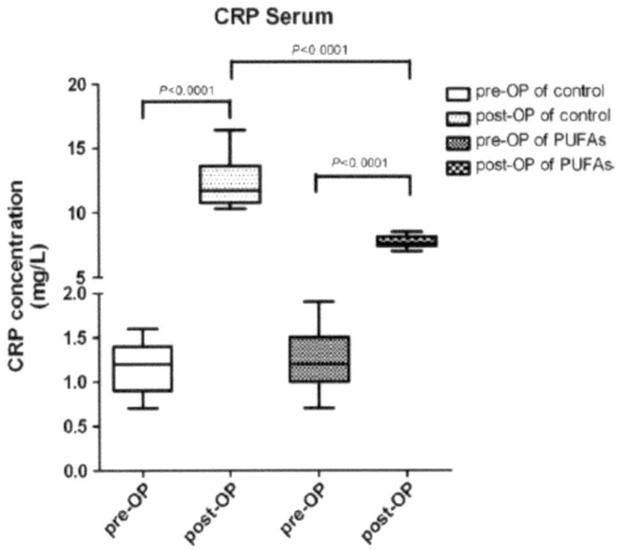

Figure 1. Comparison of CRP levels between the control and PUFA groups before and after operation. Before the operation, there were no significant differences in CRP levels between two groups. On the second postoperative day, CRP was significantly increased in both groups; however, it was significantly lower in the PUFA group than in the control.

The main finding of this study is that EPA and DHA supplementation of the diet can decrease plasma concentration of the CRP, IL-6 and TNF-α in acute inflammation of canine sterile pericarditis, suggesting depression of inflammatory cytokines by n-3 FUFAs may involve in the anti-atrial fibrillation process. The results also showed that the PUFA group had a less AF inducibility and maintenance than the control group (Table1).

Thus we may reasonably conclude that Dietary n-3 PUFA supplementation attenuates the inducibility and maintenance of AF in the sterile pericarditis model by reducing the production of proinflammatory cytokines.

http://dx.doi.org/10.5772/54167

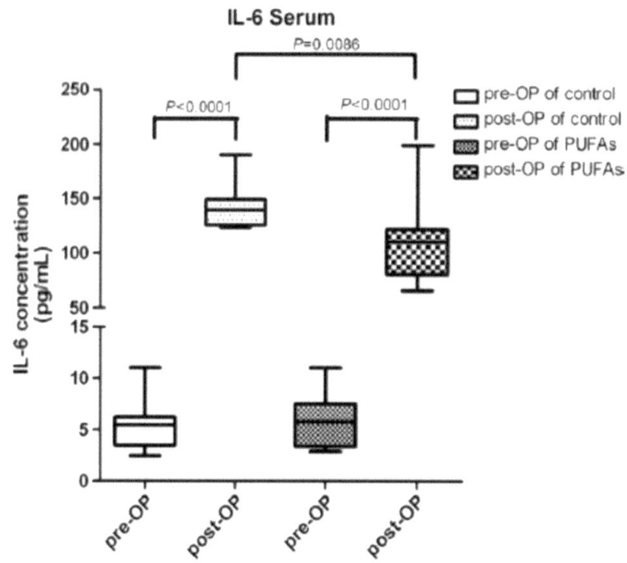

Figure 2. Comparison of IL-6 levels between the control and PUFA groups before and after operation. Before operation, there were no significant differences in IL-6 levels between two groups. On the second postoperative day, IL-6 was significantly increased in both groups; however, it was significantly lower in the PUFA group than in the control.

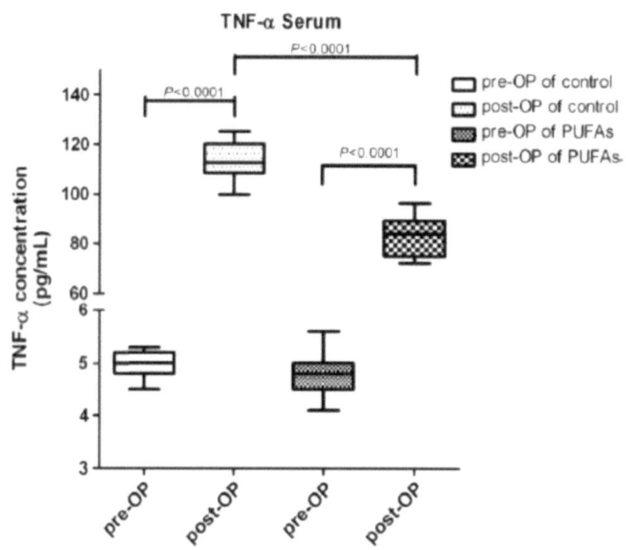

Figure 3. Comparison of TNF-α levels between the control and PUFA groups before and after operation. Before the operation, there were no significant differences in TNF- α levels between two groups. On the second postoperative day, TNF- α was significantly increased in both groups; however, it was significantly lower in PUFA group than in the control.

Comparison of electrophysiological parameters (CT) between the control and PUFA groups before and after operation.

Intra-atrial CT (ms)	Control group ($n=10$)		PUFA group ($n=10$)	
	Before	After	Before	After
RAA-LRA				
200	43.4 ± 2.8	51.9 ± 4.8‡	44.6 ± 5.4	46.6 ± 4.4*
300	44.6 ± 4.6	50.8 ± 4.6‡	45.8 ± 4.5	46.0 ± 4.2*
400	45.2 ± 4.8	51.0 ± 4.3‡	44.6 ± 5.2	47.0 ± 3.4*
RAA-HRA				
200	33.0 ± 3.2	41.2 ± 4.2#	34.0 ± 3.3	36.0 ± 4.6*
300	35.0 ± 5.0	42.0 ± 5.0‡	35.5 ± 4.5	36.8 ± 4.8*
400	36.0 ± 5.4	43.2 ± 4.8†	37.0 ± 4.8	38.4 ± 4.4*
RAA-ARA				
200	26.2 ± 5.5	32.6 ± 5.2†	26.8 ± 4.2	27.4 ± 5.0*
300	25.4 ± 4.6	32.6 ± 4.4‡	27.2 ± 4.7	28.0 ± 4.2*
400	25.6 ± 4.3	33.0 ± 5.0‡	26.4 ± 3.5	28.0 ± 4.0*

CT=conduction time; RAA=right atrial appendage; LRA=low lateral right atrium; HRA=high lateral right atrium; ARA= anterior right atrium.

† $p<0.05$ compared with before the operation

# $p<0.0001$ compared with before the operation

* $P<0.05$ compared with the control group

‡ $p<0.01$ compared with before operation.

Table 1. Comparison of electrophysiological parameters (CT) between the control and PUFA groups before and after operation

1.3. Inflammation and post cardiac surgery AF

Although the pathophysiological mechanism underlying the genesis of post cardiac surgery AF has been the focus of many studies,it only remains partially understood. The inflammatory cascade and catecholamine surge associated with surgery have been thought of playing a prominent role in initiating AF after cardiac surgery. As a prototypic marker of inflammation, CRP has been the focus of many studies, which is driven by the proinflammatory cytokines interleukin (IL)-1, tumor necrosis factor (TNF)-α, and IL-6(Bruins P et al.,1997) found that IL-6 rises initially and peaks at 6 h after cardiac surgery, and CRP levels increases and peaks on the second postoperative day of the cardiac surgery, with complement-CRP complexes levels peaking on the 2nd or 3rd postoperative day. The incidence of atrial arrhythmias similarly peaks on postoperative day 2 or 3. Other researchers have confirmed that IL-6 and CRP increased after cardiac surgery, with the incidence of atrial arrhythmias similarly peaking on the 2nd or 3rd postoperative day [13,14](Ishida K,et al.,2006;Kumagai K,et al., 2004). Many studies have related an increase in CRP and IL-6 in both paroxysmal AF and persistent AF, and concluded that CRP is not only associated with the presence of AF but may also predict an increased risk for future development of AF [15](Aviles RJ,et al.,2003).

Other studies correlated leukocytosis to an increased incidence in AF in postoperative cardiovascular patients [16,17](Abdelhadi RH,et al.,2004;Lamm G,et al.,2006), and found that a more pronounced increase in postoperative WBC count will independently predict development of postoperative AF. Moreover, atrial inflammation of cardiac surgery effects on the electrical properties of atrial tissue, and the degree of atrial inflammation was associated with a proportional increase in the inhomogeneity of atrial conduction and AF duration [18] (Ishii Y, et al.,2005). Administration of anti-inflammatory drugs (dexamethasone or cortisone) significantly decreases the incidence of AF after cardiac surgery [19,20](Yred JP,et al., 2000;Halonen J,et al.,2007), which supports this inflammation-AF

hypothesis. The canine sterile pericarditis model can perfectly simulate inflammatory circumstances of the post cardiac operation, by which AF can be induced and also peaks on the 2nd postoperative day [10](Page PL,et al.,1986). In this model, the multiple unstable reentrant circuits were showed during AF, and it was critical for maintaining AF [10] (Page PL,et al.,1986). According to the multiple-wavelet hypothesis, atrial wavelength determines the number of wavelets, and the atrial wavelength is the product of AERP and the intra-atrial conduction velocity. So, the AERP and the intra-atrial conduction velocity have been thought to be important for the perpetuation of AF. In this canine sterile pericarditis model, we have evaluated CRP, IL-6 and TNF-α level on the baseline and on the 2nd postoperative day, and found that they all significantly increased in both groups. We simultaneously evaluated the role of inflammation on atrial electrophysiological properties, and found that inflammation can shorten AERPs and prolong intra-atrial CT in the canine sterile pericarditis model, which increased the inducibility and stability of AF. Our results are concordant with the previous results. Thus, in this model, elevated CRP, IL-6 and TNF-α were associated with sustained AF, suggesting that electrophysiological changes resulting from inflammation perpetuate AF.

1.4. Other potential mechanisms of antiarrhythmic action of n-3 PUFA administration

The current hypotheses of n-3 PUFAs in preventing AF are based on their inhibiting capacity of some ion channels. Previous studies have demonstrated that n-3 PUFAs have capacity to inhibit fast, voltage dependent sodium currents, L-type calcium currents, the Na /Ca2 exchanger, which might prevent delayed after-depolarizations and triggered activity, as well as their class III antiarrhythmic-like effect on Kv1.5 channel (IKUR current present in the atrium) [36,37](Xial YF,et al.,2004;Honore E,et al.,1994). Other studies found n-3 PUFAs can attenuate atrial structural remodeling not only by activating matrix metalloproteinase-9 mRNA expression and attenuating of collagen turnover [38](Laurent G,et al.,2008), but also by modulating of atrial gap junction protein CX40 and CX43 [39] (Sarrazin JF,et al.,2007). Otherwise, evidence suggests that n-3 fatty acids consumption attenuates oxidative stress in humans, and the underlying mechanisms may lead to suppressed production of reactive oxygen species by leukocytes, inhibition of the prooxidant enzyme phospholipase A2, and induction of antioxidant enzymes [40](Mori TA,et al.,2003).

2. The expression of CD69 and CD3+ T-lymphocytes in the diagnosis or therapy of AF

Recently, the link between inflammation and AF appeals increasing attention. Many studies have demonstrated serum or plasma inflammation biomarkers have a link with the development of AF, which supported chronic inflammatory responses might participate in the development of AF (Chung MK et al.,2006;Hemandez Madrid A et al.,2007;Li J et al.,2010;Psychari SN et al.,2005). Moreover, some other studies reported that activated T-lymphocytes and macrophages infiltrated the endomyocardial of patients with AF, which supported the activation of local T-lymphocytes played a role in the pathogenesis of AF (Chen MC et al., 2008;Nakamura Y et al.,2003;Yamashita T et al.,2010). However, up to now, there are no evidences supporting the link between the activation of peripheral blood T-lymphocytes and AF. As is well-known, CD69 and HLA-DR are markers of activated T-lymphocytes. In other words, they are both specifically expressed on the surface of activated T-lymphocytes.[11, 12](Caruso A et al.,1997;Reddy M et al.,2004) CD69 is known as an early activation marker of T-lymphocytes [13](Sancho D et al.,2005) and HLA-DR is known as a late activation marker of T-lymphocytes.[14] (Geraldes L et al., 2010)They both play a role in the specific immune response to inflammation. [15, 16, 14, 17-19, 13, 20] (Sancho D et al.,2005;Geraldes L et al.,2010;Afeltra A et al.,1993;Ferenczi K et al.,2000;McDonald GB et al.,1987;Miki-Hosokawa T et al.,2009;Oczenski W et al., 2003;Vance BA et al.,2005) To our knowledge, there is little information available about the expression of CD69 and HLA-DR on peripheral blood $CD3^+$ T-lymphocytes in patients with AF.Thus we designed an experiment to investigate the relationship between the activation of peripheral blood CD3+ T-lymphocytes and AF by flow cytometric analysis that we aimed to provide more evidences to support this phenomenon (Liu L, et al., 2012;53(4):221-4.)

Fifty paroxysmal AF patients and fifty-six persistent AF patients, underwent successful electrical cardioversion, were enrolled in this study. Percentage of CD69 and Human leukocyte antigen DR (HLA-DR) positive peripheral blood $CD3^+$ T-lymphocyte, which indicates T-lymphocyte activation, were examined by flow cytometric analysis in the patients and fifty-one healthy controls. Patients groups had higher levels of CD69 and HLA-DR than healthy controls. During three-month follow-up, 37 patients had recurrence of AF (recurrence group) and 50 patients remained in sinus (sinus group).

The results showed that Patients with AF groups had higher levels of CD69 and HLA-DR than healthy controls. The mean value of CD69 was significantly up-regulated in patients with paroxysmal (1.48%±0.42) and persistent AF (1.55%±0.38) compared with healthy individuals (1.07%±0.37; all $p<0.001$). The mean value of HLA-DR was also significantly up-regulated in patients with paroxysmal (35.16%±10.89) and persistent AF (37.73%±10.78) compared with healthy individuals (26.6%±8.41; all $p<0.001$. Figure 4)

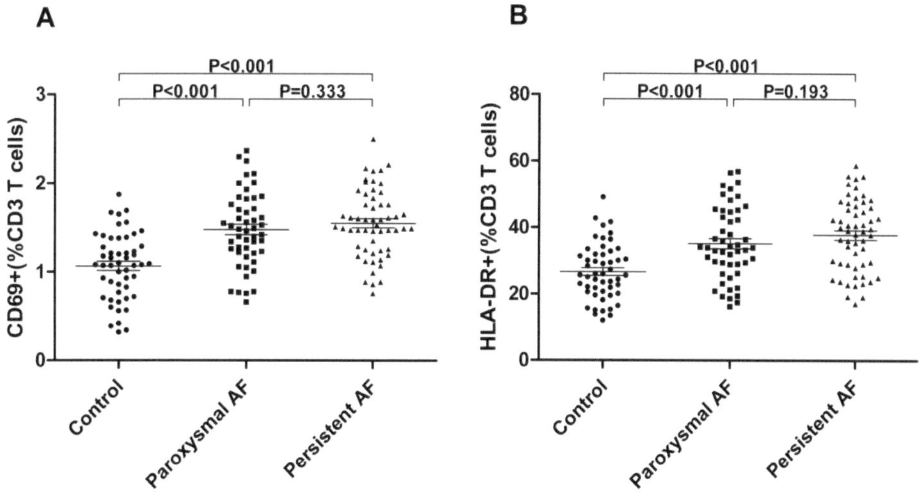

Figure 4. Percentage of $CD3^+CD69^+$ T-lymphocytes (A) and $CD3^+HLA\text{-}DR^+$ T-lymphocytes (B) were shown, respectively.

During three-month follow-up, 37 patients had recurrence of AF (recurrence group) and 50 patients remained in sinus (sinus group). The results demonstrated that the mean values of CD69 and HLA-DR in sinus group at follow-up (1.17%±0.38, 28.71%±8.70) were all significantly down-regulated compared with before cardioversion (1.45%±0.44, 34.71%±9.75; all $p<0.05$). However, there were no statistically significant differences between recurrence group at follow-up (1.57%±0.39, 36.40%±9.32) and before cardioversion (1.60%±0.35, 37.72% ±11.11; $p=0.721$, $p=0.544$. Figure.5)

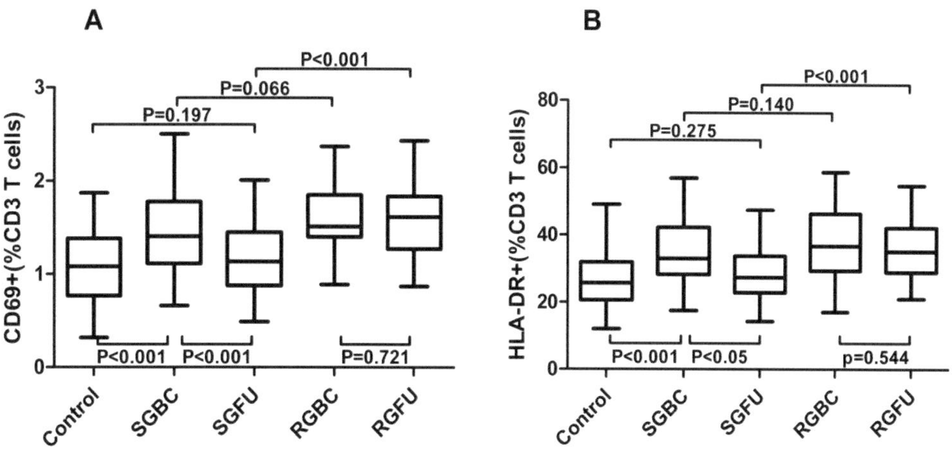

Figure 5. The mean values of $CD3^+CD69^+$ T-lymphocytes (A) and $CD3^+HLA\text{-}DR^+$ T-lymphocytes (B) in the sinus group and recurrence group at follow-up and before cardioversion.

Before we received the result,we conduct the baseline clinical Caracteristics of the Studied Population to ensure facticity of the results (Table 2).

	Control (n=51)	**Paroxysmal AF (n=50)**	**Persistent AF (n=56)**	***p***
Age(yrs)	64.4±8.5	64.3±9.5	67.2±9.7	0.176
Men	31 (61%)	32 (64%)	34 (61%)	0.927
Hypertension	13 (25%)	20 (40%)	25 (45%)	0.106
Hyperlipidemia	11 (22%)	8 (16%)	7 (13%)	0.448
Diabetes	2 (4%)	3 (6%)	5 (9%)	0.566
Drugs:				
ACE-I/ARB	10 (20%)	11 (22%)	21 (38%)	0.074
Statins	8 (16%)	7 (14%)	6 (11%)	0.743
β-blockers	8 (16%)	26 (52%)	30 (54%)	<0.001
CCBs	5 (10%)	12 (24%)	7 (13%)	0.108
WBC count(per uL)	6349±1891	6768±1859	6375±1663	0.819
Lymphocytes(%)	30.9±3.8	32.5±4.3	31.5±4.1	0.147
Monocytes(%)	5.5±1.2	5.8±1.1	5.4±1.1	0.123
CRP(mg/dl)	0.24±0.12	0.48±0.25	0.60±0.22*	<0.001

Table 2. Caracteristics of the Studied Population

ACEI indicates angiotensin-converting enzyme inhibitors; ARB, angiotensin receptor blocking agents; CCBs, calcium channel blockers; WBC, white blood cells; CRP, C-reactive protein; *p*, probability of significance (difference among three groups); and *, $p<0.05$ persistent AF vs paroxysmal AF.

In this study, we found that the respective expression of CD69 and HLA-DR on peripheral blood $CD3^+$ T-lymphocytes in AF patients was significantly higher than control group, which might suggest that high expression of CD69 and HLA-DR was associated with AF. In the subsequent follow-up, we further found that the expression of CD69 and HLA-DR in sinus group at follow-up was significantly down-regulated compared with before cardioversion. However, the expression of CD69 and HLA-DR in recurrence group at follow-up was not significantly down-regulated. It might further support that the CD69 and HLA-DR levels were related with the state of AF.

As demonstrated by the present study, there was a link between high expression of CD69 and HLA-DR and AF. CD69, known as an early activation marker of lymphocytes, is a type II transmembrane glucoprotein and may enhance activation and proliferation/differentiation of T-lymphocytes. (Sancho D et al. 2005;Vance BA et al.,2005;Beeler A et al.,2008;Creeners P et al.,2002) HLA-DR belongs to the MHC class II system which is known as a late activation marker of lymphocytes. It is required for antigen presentation and activation of helper T-lymphocytes. (Geraldes L et al.,2010;Oczenski W et al.,2003;Bobryshev YV et al.,2011)They respectively expressed in some inflammatory infiltrates and played important roles in the pathogenesis of some inflammatory diseases such as allergic airway inflammation, (Miki-Hosokawa T et al.,2009;Wang HY et al.,2006) rheumatoid arthritis, (Afeltra A et al.,1993) psoriasis vulgaris lesional skin active inflammatory bowel disease (McDonald GB et al., 1987). So the increase of CD69 and HLA-DR on $CD3^+$ T-lymphocytes implied there is an activation of peripheral blood $CD3^+$ T-lymphocytes in AF patients.

In fact, the activation of peripheral blood $CD3^+$ T-lymphocytes maybe plays an important role in the pathogenesis of AF. A few studies reported that some inflammatory lymphocytes, such as $CD45^+$ cells, $CD3^+$ T cells, and $CD68^+$ macrophages, infiltrated in the endomyocardial in patients with AF, which supported the local activation of T-lymphocytes played a role in the pathogenesis of AF.(Chen MC et al.,2008;Nakamura Y et al.,2003;Yamashita T et al.,2010) On the other hand, a lot of studies reported that serum or plasma inflammation biomarkers, such as C-reactive protein (CRP), interleukin (IL)-6, IL-8, IL-10, tumor necrosis factor (TNF)-α, monocyte chemotactic protein (MCP)-1, vascular endothelial growth factor (VEGF), et al., increased in AF patients, which supported T-cell-associated chronic inflammatory responses might involve in the pathogenesis of AF. (Chung MK et al.,2001;Hemandez Madrid A et al.,2007;Li J et al.,2010;Psychari SN et al.,2005) In our study, we provided another evidence to support that there is an activation of peripheral blood $CD3^+$ T-lymphocytes in AF patients, demonstrated by the upregulation of CD69 and HLA-DR by flow cytometric analysis.

Generally, our study here further emphasize that activation of T cells is involved in AF. As we all know, T-lymphocytes are the main cells participate in cell-mediated immunity, which is one of the primary ways of human immune. It can be suppressed by many immunosuppressants such as Cyclosporine, Rapamycin, et al. If the activation of peripheral blood T-lymphocytes does participate in the pathogenesis of AF, maybe we can prevent recurrence of AF through suppressing the activation of peripheral blood T-lymphocytes.

As for the underlying mechanisms of activated peripheral blood $CD3^+$ T-lymphocytes participates in the progression of AF, we speculate the following three possibilities. Firstly, the activation of peripheral blood $CD3^+$ T-lymphocytes might cause the upregulation of IL-6 and MCP-1, which could affect the contractility and electrical stability of myocytes inhomogeneously and induce fibroblast activation leading to deposits of extracellular matrix fibrosis. (Ramos-Mondragon R et al.,2008) Secondly, activation of peripheral blood $CD3^+$ T-lymphocytes might promote the local immunologic inflammatory responses in the endomyocardial, and promote infiltrate of inflammatory lymphomononuclear in the endomyocardial in patients with AF. Thirdly, the activation of peripheral blood $CD3^+$ T-lymphocytes could activate the calcineurin-nuclear factor, which involve in the T-lymphocytes signal transduction pathway. (Lin CC et al., 2004)

It is important to note that there are several limitations that need to be addressed regarding this study. Firstly, The results cannot be taken as evidence to support that CD69 and HLA-

DR play a role in the pathogenesis of AF, it only indicate the possible association of CD69 and HLA-DR with AF. Secondly, how CD69 and HLA-DR contribute to the pathogenesis of AF and what is the underlying mechanism need to be further investigated. Thirdly, we did not study the influence of other immune activation-associated molecules (CD25, CD71, and CD122, et al) and co-stimulatory molecules (CD28, CTLA-4, CD80, CD86, et al) during the progression of AF.

3. Summary

The activation of peripheral blood CD3+ T-lymphocytes and immunologic inflammatory responses played a role in the pathogenesis of AF,and might be a diagnostic or therapeutic marker. Dietary n-3 PUFA supplementation attenuates the inducibility and maintenance of AF in the sterile pericarditis model by reducing the production of proinflammatory cytokines.

Author details

Qiang-Sun Zheng, Hong-Tao Wang, Zhong Zhang, Jun Li, Li Liu and Bo-yuan Fan

*Address all correspondence to: qiangsun_tdxn@hotmail.com

Tangdu Hospital, Fourth Military Medical University, Xi' an, China

Hong-Tao Wang and Zhong Zhang contributed equally in this work.

References

[1] Albert CM, Campos H, Stampfer MJ, Ridker PM, Manson JE, Willett WC, Ma J. Blood levels of long-chain n-3 fatty acids and the risk of sudden death. N Engl J Med 2002;346(15):1113-8.

[2] Hu FB, Bronner L, Willett WC, Stampfer MJ, Rexrode KM, Albert CM, Hunter D, Manson JE.Fish and omega-3 fatty acid intake and risk of coronary heart disease in women. JAMA 2002;287(14):1815-21.

[3] Zhang Z, Zhang C, Wang H, Zhao J, Liu L, Lee J, He Y, Zheng Q.n-3 polyunsaturated fatty acids prevents atrial fibrillation by inhibiting inflammation in a canine sterile pericarditis model. Int J Cardiol. 2011;153(1):14-20.

[4] Bruins P, te Velthuis H, Yazdanbakhsh AP, Jansen PG, van Hardevelt FW, de Beaumont EM, Wildevuur CR, Eijsman L, Trouwborst A, Hack CE.Activation of the com-

plement system during and after cardiopulmonary bypass surgery: postsurgery activation involves C-reactive protein and is associated with postoperative arrhythmia. Circulation 1997;96 (10):3542-8.

[5] Chung MK, Martin DO, Sprecher D, Wazni O, Kanderian A, Carnes CA, Bauer JA, Tchou PJ, Niebauer MJ, Natale A, Van Wagoner DR.C-reactive protein elevation in patients with atrial arrhythmias: Inflammatory mechanisms and persistence of atrial fibrillation. Circulation 2001;104:2886-2891.

[6] Hernandez Madrid A, Moro C. Atrial fibrillation and c-reactive protein: Searching for local inflammation. J Am Coll Cardiol 2007;49:1649-1650.

[7] Li J, Solus J, Chen Q, Rho YH, Milne G, Stein CM, Darbar D. Role of inflammation and oxidative stress in atrial fibrillation. Heart Rhythm 2010;7:438-444.

[8] Psychari SN, Apostolou TS, Sinos L, Hamodraka E, Liakos G, Kremastinos DT. Relation of elevated c-reactive protein and interleukin-6 levels to left atrial size and duration of episodes in patients with atrial fibrillation. Am J Cardiol 2005;95:764-767.

[9] Chen MC, Chang JP, Liu WH, Yang CH, Chen YL, Tsai TH, Wang YH, Pan KL. Increased inflammatory cell infiltration in the atrial myocardium of patients with atrial fibrillation. Am J Cardiol 2008;102:861-865.

[10] Nakamura Y, Nakamura K, Fukushima-Kusano K, Ohta K, Matsubara H, Hamuro T, Yutani C, Ohe T.Tissue factor expression in atrial endothelia associated with nonvalvular atrial fibrillation: Possible involvement in intracardiac thrombogenesis. Thromb Res 2003;111:137-142.

[11] Yamashita T, Sekiguchi A, Iwasaki YK, Date T, Sagara K, Tanabe H, Suma H, Sawada H, Aizawa T.Recruitment of immune cells across atrial endocardium in human atrial fibrillation. Circ J 2010;74:262-270.

[12] Caruso A, Licenziati S, Corulli M, Canaris AD, De Francesco MA, Fiorentini S, Peroni L, Fallacara F, Dima F, Balsari A, Turano A.Flow cytometric analysis of activation markers on stimulated t cells and their correlation with cell proliferation. Cytometry 1997;27:71-76.

[13] Reddy M, Eirikis E, Davis C, Davis HM, Prabhakar U. Comparative analysis of lymphocyte activation marker expression and cytokine secretion profile in stimulated human peripheral blood mononuclear cell cultures: An in vitro model to monitor cellular immune function. J Immunol Methods 2004;293:127-142.

[14] Sancho D, Gomez M, Sanchez-Madrid F. Cd69 is an immunoregulatory molecule induced following activation. Trends Immunol 2005;26:136-140.

[15] Geraldes L, Morgado J, Almeida A, Todo-Bom A, Santos P, Paiva A, Cheira C, Pais ML.Expression patterns of hla-dr+ or hla-dr- on cd4+/cd25++/cd127low regulatory t cells in patients with allergy. J Investig Allergol Clin Immunol 2010;20:201-209.

[16] Afeltra A, Galeazzi M, Ferri GM, Amoroso A, De Pità O, Porzio F, Bonomo L. Expression of cd69 antigen on synovial fluid t cells in patients with rheumatoid arthritis and other chronic synovitis. Ann Rheum Dis 1993;52:457-460.

[17] Ferenczi K, Burack L, Pope M, Krueger JG, Austin LM. Cd69, hla-dr and the il-2r identify persistently activated t cells in psoriasis vulgaris lesional skin: Blood and skin comparisons by flow cytometry. J Autoimmun 2000;14:63-78.

[18] McDonald GB, Jewell DP. Class ii antigen (hla-dr) expression by intestinal epithelial cells in inflammatory diseases of colon. J Clin Pathol. 1987;40:312-317

[19] Miki-Hosokawa T, Hasegawa A, Iwamura C, Shinoda K, Tofukuji S, Watanabe Y, Hosokawa H, Motohashi S, Hashimoto K, Shirai M, Yamashita M, Nakayama T.Cd69 controls the pathogenesis of allergic airway inflammation. J Immunol 2009;183:8203-8215.

[20] Oczenski W, Krenn H, Jilch R, Watzka H, Waldenberger F, Köller U, Schwarz S, Fitzgerald RD.Hla-dr as a marker for increased risk for systemic inflammation and septic complications after cardiac surgery. Intensive Care Med 2003;29:1253-1257.

[21] Vance BA, Harley PH, Backlund PS, Ward Y, Phelps TL, Gress RE. Human cd69 associates with an n-terminal fragment of calreticulin at the cell surface. Arch Biochem Biophys 2005;438:11-20.

[22] Liu L, Lee J, Fu G, Liu X, Wang H, Zhang Z, Zheng Q.Activation of Peripheral Blood CD3+ T-lymphocytes in Patients With Atrial Fibrillation. Int Heart J. 2012;53(4):221-4.

[23] Beeler A, Zaccaria L, Kawabata T, Gerber BO, Pichler WJ. Cd69 upregulation on t cells as an in vitro marker for delayed-type drug hypersensitivity. Allergy 2008;63:181-188.

[24] Creemers P, Brink J, Wainwright H, Moore K, Shephard E, Kahn D. Evaluation of peripheral blood cd4 and cd8 lymphocyte subsets, cd69 expression and histologic rejection grade as diagnostic markers for the presence of cardiac allograft rejection. Transpl Immunol 2002;10:285-292.

[25] Bobryshev YV, Moisenovich MM, Pustovalova OL, Agapov, II, Orekhov AN. Widespread distribution of hla-dr-expressing cells in macroscopically undiseased intima of the human aorta: A possible role in surveillance and maintenance of vascular homeostasis. Immunobiology 2011

[26] Wang HY,shen HH,Lee JJ,Lee NA.Cd69 expression on airway eosinophils and airway inflammation in a murine model of asthma.Chin Med J(Engl)2006;119:1983-1990.

Section 2

Mechanisms

Chapter 4

New Candidate Genes in Atrial Fibrillation Polymorphisms of the Alpha 2-Beta-Adrenoceptor and the Endothelial NO Synthase Genes in Atrial Fibrillation of Different Etiological Origins

Svetlana Nikulina, Vladimir Shulman,
Ksenya Dudkina, Anna Chernova and
Oksana Gavrilyuk

Additional information is available at the end of the chapter

http://dx.doi.org/10.5772/53527

1. Introduction

Molecular and genetic bases of atherosclerosis, cardiomyopathy, hypertension are the most studied among cardiovascular diseases. Recently, search for genetic markers associated with various rhythm disorders and conduction attracts researchers. The greatest attention is paid to the genetic aspects of atrial fibrillation as the most frequent and dangerous arrhythmia.

Atrial fibrillation represents the most common type of arrhythmia in clinical practice. The prevalence of atrial fibrillation is 0.4% in the general population and it increases with age [1]. According to the Framingham study atrial fibrillation doubles mortality in cardiac patients and is responsible for 1 \ 3 thromboembolic episodes [2-4]. That's why finding of genealogical and genetic aspects of atrial fibrillation predictors of its occurrence is relevant and offers opportunities for early diagnosis and timely prevention of this pathology.

In most cases, this rhythm disorder is secondary, i.e. it's caused by a disease. But at least in the 1 \ 3 cases etiology of atrial fibrillation cannot be established. Such arrhythmia is known to refer to the terms - idiopathic atrial fibrillation, primary atrial fibrillation, or "isolated atrial fibrillation» (lone atrial fibrillation). It is believed that a significant number of primary atrial fibrillation cases are caused by a hereditary factor [5-10]. However, even in the secondary atrial fibrillation a hereditary component is not excluded in the development of arrhythmia. In the 90s of the 20th century many papers associated with the genealogy of atrial fibrillation described some families whose members had atrial fibrillation and / or atrial flutter [7-9, 11, 12].

Molecular researches of AF are concentrated generally in 2 directions: 1. Identification of genes which mutations lead to arrhythmia (inheritance of such mutations occurs according to the classical Mendel type). 2. Studying of polymorphisms of various genes, so-called genes of susceptibility or genes – candidates.

In this regard, some of the most promising genetic markers are polymorphisms of gene alpha 2-beta-adrenoceptor (ADRA2V). Gene ADRA2V is located on the long arm of chromosome 2 (2q11.2), it has no introns. It encodes a2β-adrenergic receptor [13]. Adrenergic receptors - a class of receptors coupled to G-proteins activated by catecholamines [13, 14]. There are at least four groups of receptors that differ in their mediated effects, localization and affinity for different substances: alpha-1, alpha 2, beta 1 and beta-2 adrenergic receptors [15, 16]. A2 - adrenergic receptors include three subtypes: α2a, a2β and α2c [17].

All these proteins have a similar structure and are associated with G-protein [13]. Receptors of α2 family are important components of vegetative nervous system and provide a physiological response to sympathetic stimulation. A role of the sympathoadrenal stimulation of the atria in the pathogenesis of AF was shown in the works of P. Coumel et al. [18] in 1982.

Molecules of nitric oxide (NO) can play a definite role in the pathogenesis of AF. Nitric oxide in the human body is continuously produced by fermentation from L - arginine and serves as a universal messenger inside and intercellular signaling [19]. The catalyst of this reaction is synthase NO (NO-synthase, or NOS, the enzyme code 1.14.13.39) [19]. Influenced by NO-synthase oxidation of L - arginine and nitric oxide synthesis in endothelial cells of blood vessels take place. Then, getting out of endothelial cells into the smooth muscle cells, nitric oxide activates soluble guanylate cyclase, that leads to increased level of cyclic GMP, activation of cyclic GMP - dependent protein kinases, changes in calcium concentration and sensitivity of conducting cardiac myocytes receptors to the level of catecholamines. In 2005 M. Kim showed that the decrease in the production of NO-synthase can cause oxidative stress and lead to changes in myocardial conduction system, thereby contributing to the development of AF [20]. Polymorphism rs1799983 in exon 7 of the gene NOS3, replacement of G to T in position 894 of the nucleotide sequence leads to the replacement glu298-to-asp (E298D) in the amino acid sequence. So far, the influence of polymorphisms of gene ADRA2B and gene of endothelial NO-synthase on the development of atrial fibrillation has not been investigated.

1.1. Genealogical and genetic aspects of atrial fibrillation

The first familial cases of atrial fibrillation were described in 1943 [21]. In 1950 for the first time Gould pointed out a significant role of heredity in the atrial fibrillation development. He described the family susceptibility to atrial fibrillation, monitored the history of atrial fibrillation in several generations of this family for 36 years [22]. In 1998 T. Tikanoja et al. [23] have published data about the development of familial atrial fibrillation in two fetuses at 23 and 25 weeks of fetal development, and both babies were born with ongoing atrial fibrillation. Researchers have shown particular interest to families that had an accumulation of intraventricular conduction disturbances, combined with a variety of tachyarrhythmias. Families whose members in several generations suffered from atrial fibrillation and/or atrial flutter in a combination with a blockade of various branches of His bundle or atrio-ventricular block [24-27] were described.

C.S. Fox et al. indicated that atrial fibrillation in the parents increases the risk of atrial fibrillation for posterity. Among the examined 2243 patients with atrial fibrillation 681patients (30%) had at least one parent with the registered atrial fibrillation [9]. Postulational piority of the autosomal dominant model atrial fibrillation belongs to J. Girona et al. (1997). They presented two families in which 20 out of 70 members had paroxysmal or persistent atrial fibrillation [28]. A. Gillor, E. Korsch in 1992 [29] described a family case of idiopathic atrial flutter. In this family, two male children were diagnosed with atrial flutter; they were the third and sixth children of seven. Other five children were girls. Two daughters died, the first daughter died at the age of twenty days, parents do not know the cause of death, the fourth - at the age of 5 years, probably from meningitis.

In 1996 French scientists P. Poret, P. Mabo, C. Deplace et al. studied a family with congenital tachyarrhythmia. In three generations five members of the family were diagnosed with idiopathic atrial fibrillation since the young age. The examination of the sick relatives revealed hypertrophy of both atria, mitral and tricuspid regurgitation [27]. In 1997 R. Brugada et al. [30, 31] carried out clinical, electrophysiological and genetic study of three Spanish families with atrial fibrillation.

Genetic analysis revealed that the gene responsible for atrial fibrillation in this family is localized on chromosome 10q in the area 10q22-24. Abnormal gene locus was placed between D10S1694 and D10S1786. The authors supposed that candidate genes of this pathology were genes of beta- adrenoreceptors (ADRB1), alpha- adrenoreceptors (ADRA2) and genes of G-protein coupled receptor-kinase (GPRR5) as localized on the same chromosome 10 in locus 23 - 26. In these families atrial fibrillation was revealed in 21 out of 49 relatives. One of the sick relatives (II-8) died at the age of 68 from stroke. The other relative (III-2) with paroxysmal AF since 20 years' age, died suddenly at the age of 36, but an autopsy was not performed. 18 out of 19 living family members had chronic atrial fibrillation and 1 - paroxysmal atrial fibrillation.

Finally, Chinese scientists H. Yang et al. identified 2 genes responsible for heredity of atrial fibrillation. They appeared to be genes of proteins of potassium channels in myocytes. In particular, H. Yang et al. [32] reported about replacement of arginine to cysteine in position 27 of gene KCNE2 on chromosome 21q22.1-22, encoding the beta subunit of potassium channels. These mutations appeared in 2 out of 28 examined Chinese families with familial atrial fibrillation. H. Yang et al. identified the mutation of (S140G) gene on chromosome 11p15.5, encoding the alpha subunit of the cardiac potassium channel. Atrial fibrillation occurrence in these cases is due to the fact that in these genes function of the corresponding potassium channels increases, leading to the shortening of potential action and atrial effective refractory period. It should be recalled that paroxysmal atrial fibrillation is one of the major phenotypic manifestations of the syndrome of short interval QT, in which the function of potassium channels is increased. Thus, the data of Chinese researchers suggest that certain variants of familial atrial fibrillation can be attributed to channelopathies.

H. Yang et al. [32] in their work also showed an increase in the amount of protein connexin 43 with atrial fibrillation, the highest in the left atrium. Christiansen J. et al. [33] found that mutation in gene 1q21.1, which leads to a decrease in connexin 40, promotes the development of abnormalities of the aortic arch with atrial fibrillation. Somatic mutations in the gene encoding gap - junction protein connexin 40 (GJA5), myocardial protein involved in the coordination of the electrical activity of the atria, can be a cause of idiopathic atrial fibrillation in some cases [34].

"A significant part of patients have no obvious cause for the development of atrial fibrillation and it is possible that 1/3 of these cases actually occurs due to mutations in GJA5 ", Michael R. and H. Gollob wrote (University of Ottawa Heart Institute, Ontario, Canada). The findings, published in New England Journal of Medicine, are based on analysis of GJA5 in cardiac tissue and lymphocytes taken from 15 patients with idiopathic atrial fibrillation. Four out of all these patients had heterozygous mutations in GJA5. Three patients had mutations in heart tissue but not in lymphocytes, that indicates a somatic origin of the defects. The fourth patient's mutation was detected in both types of cells that suggest an embryonic mutation. Dr. H. Gollob believes that connexin 40 may become the object of search for new drugs to treat atrial fibrillation. The findings, according to the authors' opinion, suggest that the so-called idiopathic atrial fibrillation may have a genetic basis in the form of the defect, limited by the sick tissue.

By the present moment a large quantity of data is stored that activity of renin-angiotensin-aldosterone system (RAAS) is of great importance for formation of this peculiar «cardiomyopathies of auricles». A key component of RAAS, significantly affecting its activity through the synthesis of angiotensin - II is a angiotensin-converting enzyme (ACE). ACE gene, located on chromosome 17q23, consists of 26 exons and 25 introns [35, 36]. ACE gene polymorphism concerns a fragment of intron 16 and it is connected with the insertion / deletion of 287 pairs of nucleotides and determines three genotypes - I / I, D / D and I / D. V.I. Tseluyko et al. showed that ACE levels in plasma are significantly higher in patients with genotype D / D than in genotype I / I. Heterozygotes have intermediate levels of ACE [37]. L.O. Minushkina, E.S. Gorshkova et al. (2010) studied association of genes β-adrenoceptors of types 1, 2, and 3 (ADRB1, ADRB2, ADRB3), connexin (CX40) and a voltage - locked potassium channel of type 2 (KCNH2) with the occurrence of atrial fibrillation in patients with hypertension. This study shows that for polymorphic marker Trp64Arg of gene ADRB3 Trp allele frequency was significantly higher and the frequency of the Arg allele was significantly lower in patients with atrial fibrillation. In patients with atrial fibrillation frequency of the homozygous genotypes Arg / Arg appeared to be significantly less [38, 39].

According to the analysis conducted by J.D. Roberts, M.H. Michael, M.H. Gollob [10] at present a connection between atrial fibrillation and gene polymorphism of ion channels subunits KCNQ1 [40], KCNA5 [41], KCNE2, KCNJ2, SCN5A, GJA5, NPPA is established. [10]. Several recent studies have focused on the association between the promoter polymorphisms 786T/C of the endothelial nitric oxide synthase (eNOS) gene and susceptibility to at-

http://dx.doi.org/10.5772/53527

rial fibrillation (AF); however, results have been conflicting. In subgroup analysis, stratified by ethnicity, we observed a positive association between the eNOS 786T/C polymorphism and AF risk among Caucasians but not among mixed populations[42]. Meta-analysis suggests that there is insufficient evidence to demonstrate an association between ACE I/D polymorphism and AF risk. However, there seems to be a significant association between ACE I/D gene polymorphic variation and AF in patients with hypertension [43].

2. Results

2.1. Clinical polymorphism of atrial fibrillation in probands and their relatives

A total of 100 probands with atrial fibrillation and 150 of their relatives of the I st, II nd and III rd degree of relationship were examined. These families composed the study base for our research.

The probands were searched during the course of their in-patient and out-patient treatment in the Cardiological center of the Krasnoyarsk Regional clinical hospital № 20 named after I.S. Berzon. The patients' relatives were examined during doctors' home visits and subsequent check-ups in the Cardiological center. We also studied 91 patients without electrocardiographic manifestations of cardio-vascular diseases (control group).

The families of the probands with atrial fibrillation were divided into two groups according to the atrial fibrillation etiology:

1. Families of the probands with primary atrial fibrillation, in which clinical and instrumental examination revealed no evident cause-effect relation with any cardio-vascular diseases as well as other diseases which may have atrial fibrillation as a complication;

2. Families of the probands with secondary atrial fibrillation, in which the onset of this dysrhythmia was due to specific diseases as ischemic heart disease, arterial hypertension, dilated cardiomyopathy, gastroesophageal hernia and thyrotoxicosis.

The first group (families of the probands with primary atrial fibrillation) included 40 probands (24 males and 16 females) and 79 of their relatives (23 males and 56 females), and the second one (families of the probands with secondary atrial fibrillation) included 60 probands (28 males and 32 females) and 71 of their relatives (20 males and 51 females). Atrial fibrillation was revealed in 5 out of 79 relatives of the first group and in 1 out of 71 relatives of the second group. Differentiated clinical and electrocardiographic characteristics of the patients with primary atrial fibrillation are specified in Table 1.

Paroxysmal atrial fibrillation was revealed in 38 probands with primary atrial fibrillation (95,0±3,4%) and paroxysmal atrial flutter was revealed in 2 persons (5,0±3,4%). Among the sick relatives with primary atrial fibrillation (5 persons) paroxysmal atrial fibrillation was revealed in 5 persons (100%).

Atrial fibrillation type	Probands with primary atrial fibrillation (n=40)		Probands'sick relatives (n=5)	
	Absolute value	%	Absolute value	%
Paroxysmal atrial fibrillation	38	95,0±3,4	5	100
Paroxysmal atrial fibrillation - atrial flutter	2	5,0±3,4	0	0
Paroxysmal atrial fibrillation and atrial fibrillation - atrial flutter summarily	40	100	0	0

Table 1. Differentiated clinical and electrocardiographic characteristics of the patients with primary atrial fibrillation

Atrial fibrillation type	Probands with secondary atrial fibrillation (n=60)		Probands'sick relatives (n=1)	
	Absolute value	%	Absolute value	%
Paroxysmal atrial fibrillation	38	63,3±6,2	1	100
Paroxysmal atrial fibrillation - atrial flutter	6	10,0±3,9	0	0
Paroxysmal atrial fibrillation and atrial fibrillation - atrial flutter summarily	44	73,3±5,7	0	0
Chronic atrial fibrillation	10	16,6±4,8	0	0
Persistent atrial fibrillation	6	10,0±3,9	0	0
Chronic and persistent atrial fibrillation summarily	16	26,6±5,7	0	0

Table 2. Differentiated clinical and electrocardiographic characteristics of the patients with secondary atrial fibrillation

According to Table 2, in the group of probands with secondary atrial fibrillation paroxysmal atrial fibrillation was diagnosed in 38 out of 60 patients (63,3±6,2%), paroxysmal atrial flutter – in 6 persons (10,0±3,9%). In total paroxysmal atrial fibrillation and atrial fibrillation - atrial flutter was observed in 73,3±5,7% of the probands with secondary atrial fibrillation. Chronic atrial fibrillation was revealed in 10 patients (16,6±4,8%), persistent atrial fibrillation – in 6 persons (10,0±3,9%). Due to the small number of persons in these groups, the probands with chronic and persistent atrial fibrillation were integrated into one group (chronic and persistent atrial fibrillation), which included 16 patients (26,6±5,7%).

Cardio-vascular pathology in the probands with idiopathic and secondary atrial fibrillation, as well as other diseases which have atrial fibrillation as a complication, are represented in Table 3. Namely, in 42 probands with secondary atrial fibrillation (70,0±5,9%) we revealed ischemic heart disease (effort angina of II-III functional class) in 29 persons, which made 48,3±7,1% of the total of probands of this group, II nd - III rd functional class effort angina together with the III rd stage hypertension– in 6 probands (10,0±5,4%), postinfarction cardio-

http://dx.doi.org/10.5772/53527

sclerosis – in 7 probands (11,7±5,8%). The II nd stage hypertension from the 1st to the 3rd degree was diagnosed in 12 probands (20,0±5,2%), the III rd stage hypertension from the 2nd to the 3rd degree was diagnosed in 4 persons (6,7±3,2%), gastroesophageal hernia – in 1 person, the 2nd degree nodular goiter with the appearance of euthyroidism as of the time of examination - in 1 person (1,6±1,6%).

In a small number of cases cardio-vascular pathologies were diagnosed in the probands with idiopathic atrial fibrillation: in 7 persons (17,5±6,0%) we diagnosed hypertension: 4 patients (10,0±4,7%) had the Ist stage hypertension of the 1st degree, 3 patients (7,5±4,2%) had the IInd stage hypertension of the 1^{st-} - 2nd degree, 4 probands (10,0±4,7%) had ischemic heart disease (II nd - III rd functional class effort angina). However atrial fibrillation seizures in probands with primary atrial fibrillation were revealed long before the appearance of the first signs of ischemic heart disease and hypertension, therefore atrial fibrillation doesn't seem to be related to the revealed cardio-vascular diseases. As for the probands with secondary atrial fibrillation, they showed temporal relation between the manifestations of the underlying disease and subsequent appearance of atrial fibrillation.

Disorders	Probands with idiopathic atrial fibrillation (n=40)		Probands with the secondary atrial fibrillation (n=60)		p
	Absolute value	%	Absolute value	%	
The Ist stage hypertension.	4	10,0±4,7	0	0	>0,05
The IInd stage hypertension.	3	7,5±4,2	12	20,0±5,2	>0,05
The IIIrd stage hypertension.	0	0	4	6,7±3,2	>0,05
Ischemic heart disease combination (II nd - III rd functional class angina and the IIIrd stage hypertension).	0	0	6	10,0±3,9	>0,05
Ischemic heart disease: postinfarction cardiosclerosis.	0	0	7	11,7±4,1	>0,05
Ischemic heart disease: II nd - III rd functional class angina.	4	10,0±4,7	29	48,3±6,5	<0,005
Gastroesophageal hernia.	0	0	1	1,6±1,6	>0,05
The 2nd degree nodular goiter with the appearance of euthyroidism as of the time of examination.	0	0	1	1,6±1,6	>0,05

Note: Differences in the investigated parameters were calculated using the $\chi 2$ criterion.

Table 3. Cardio-vascular pathology in patients with idiopathic and secondary atrial fibrillation (& other diseases which can cause atrial fibrillation)

Therefore, summarizing the abovementioned, we come to the following conclusion.

In the first group (primary atrial fibrillation) paroxysmal atrial fibrillation was dominant (revealed in all the patients). In probands with secondary atrial fibrillation a significant prevalence of chronic/persistent atrial fibrillation was diagnosed (in 16 out of 60 persons (26,6±5,7%).

In the probands with primary atrial fibrillation paroxysmal atrial fibrillation had been revealed long before any cardio-vascular diseases manifestations appeared.

2.2. Polymorphism of the gene ADRA2B in probands with atrial fibrillation, their healthy relatives and persons of the control group

In our work we investigated polymorphisms of the gene ADRA2B in patients with atrial fibrillation, their healthy relatives and persons from the control group. According to the results of PCR three sorts of genotypes ADRA2B in patients with AF, their healthy relatives and persons from the control group are revealed: I / I - homozygous by the insertion, I / D - heterozygous, D / D - homozygous by the deletion. In patients with atrial fibrillation frequency of the homozygous genotype (D/D) made 8,5±2,7% (9 persons), whereas frequency of the heterozygous genotype (genotype I/D) made 50,9±4,9% (54 persons), frequency of the homozygous genotype in a rare allele (I/I) made 40,6±4,8% (43 persons) (Table 4).

Frequency of the homozygous genotypes among the probands' healthy relatives appeared to be spread as follows: homozygous genotype in a frequent allele (D/D) made 11,8±2,7% (17 persons), heterozygous genotype (I/D) – 50,7±4,2% (73 persons), homozygous genotype in a rare allele (I/I) – 37,5±4,0% (54 persons) (Table 4).

Genotypes	Patients with atrial fibrillation N= 106		Healthy relatives N=144		Control group N=91		p_{1-2}	p_{1-3}	p_{2-3}
	Absolute value	%	Absolute value	%	Absolute value	%			
D/D	9	8,5±2,7	17	11,8±2,7	10	11±3,3	p>0,05	p>0,05	p>0,05
I/D	54	50,9±4,9	73	50,7±4,2	58	63,7±5,0	p>0,05	p>0,05	p>0,05
I/I	43	40,6±4,8	54	37,5±4,0	23	25,3±4,6	p>0,05	p<0,05	p>0,05

Note: Differences in the investigated parameters were calculated using the $\chi 2$ criterion.

Table 4. Frequency of the gene ADRA2B genotypes in probands with atrial fibrillation, their healthy relatives and persons of the control group.

In persons of the control group (D/D) frequency of the homozygous genotype made 11,0±3,3% (10 persons), frequency of the heterozygous genotype (genotype I/D) made 63,7±5,0% (58 persons), frequency of the homozygous genotype in a rare allele (I/I) made 25,3±4,6% (23 persons) (Table 4).

A significant prevalence of homozygous genotype I/I in patients with AF (40,6%) compared with the control group (25,3%) (p = 0,034) was established (Table 4, Fig.1).

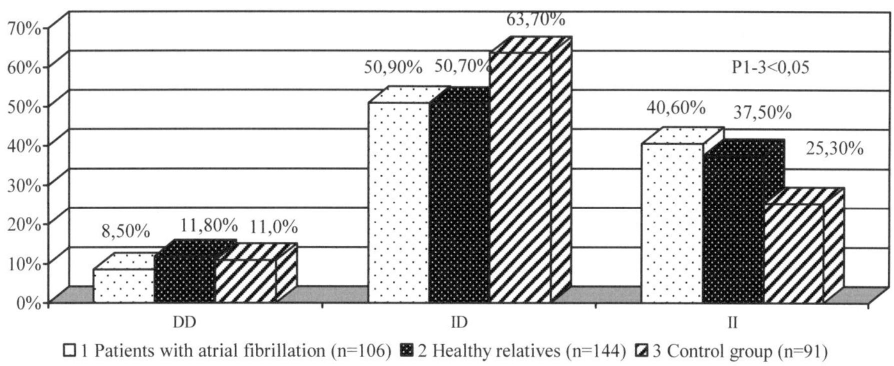

Figure 1. Frequency of the gene ADRA2B genotypes in probands with atrial fibrillation, their healthy relatives and persons of the control group.

In patients with primary atrial fibrillation frequency of the homozygous genotypes (D/D) made 6,7±3,7% (3 persons), frequency of the heterozygous genotype (I/D) made 48,9±7,5% (22 persons), frequency of the homozygous genotype in a rare allele (I/I) made 44,4±7,4% (20 persons) (Table 5). A significant prevalence of homozygous genotype I/I as compared with the control group (25,3%) is established only in patients with primary atrial fibrillation (44,4%) (p = 0,039) (Table 5, Fig. 2).

Genotypes	Patients with primary atrial fibrillation N= 45		Healthy relatives N=144		Control group N=91		p_{1-2}	p_{1-3}	p_{2-3}
	Absolute value	%	Absolute value	%	Absolute value	%			
D/D	3	6,7±3,7	17	11,8±2,7	10	11±3,3	p>0,05	p>0,05	p>0,05
I/D	22	48,9±7,5	73	50,7±4,2	58	63,7±5,0	p>0,05	p>0,05	p>0,05
I/I	20	44,4±7,4	54	37,5±4,0	23	25,3±4,6	p>0,05	p<0,05	p>0,05

Note: Differences in the investigated parameters were calculated using the χ2 criterion.

Table 5. Frequency of the gene ADRA2B genotypes in patients with primary atrial fibrillation, their healthy relatives and persons of the control group.

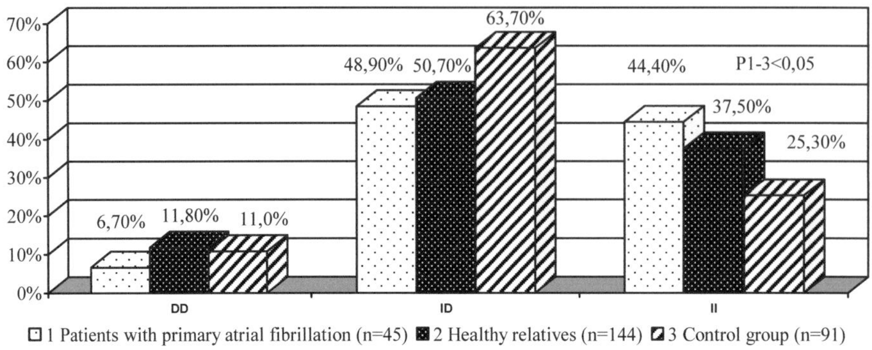

Figure 2. Frequency of the gene ADRA2B genotypes in patients with primary atrial fibrillation, their healthy relatives and persons of the control group.

Among patients with primary atrial fibrillation frequency of the genotypes appeared to be spread as follows: homozygous genotype (D/D) made 9,8±3,8% (6 persons), heterozygous genotype (I/D) – 52,5±6,4% (32 persons), homozygous genotype in a rare allele (genotype I/I) – 37,7±6,2% (23 persons) (Table 6).

No significant differences were established between frequencies of I/D genotypes of the gene ADRA2B in patients with secondary atrial fibrillation, their healthy relatives and persons of the control group. (Table 6, Fig.3).

Genotypes	Patients with secondary atrial fibrillation N= 61		Healthy relatives N=144		Control group N=91		p_{1-2}	p_{1-3}	p_{2-3}
	Absolute value	%	Absolute value	%	Absolute value	%			
D/D	6	9,8±3,8	17	11,8±2,7	10	11±3,3	p>0,05	p>0,05	p>0,05
I/D	32	52,5±6,4	73	50,7±4,2	58	63,7±5.0	p>0,05	p>0,05	p>0,05
I/I	23	37,7±6,2	54	37,5±4,0	23	25,3±4,6	p>0,05	p>0,05	p>0,05

Note: Differences in the investigated parameters were calculated using the χ2 criterion.

Table 6. Frequency of the gene ADRA2B genotypes in patients with secondary atrial fibrillation, their healthy relatives and persons of the control group.

Therefore, summarizing the abovementioned, homozygous genotype I/I of the gene ADRA2B may be regarded as one of the genetic predictors of primary atrial fibrillation onset. The relatives of the probands with primary atrial fibrillation and homozygous genotype I/I compose a high risk group for the appearance of this disorder. The conducted research of the gene ADRA2B polymorphism in patients with primary and secondary atrial fibrillation, can contribute to the decision of the etiological issue of hereditary atrial fibrillation.

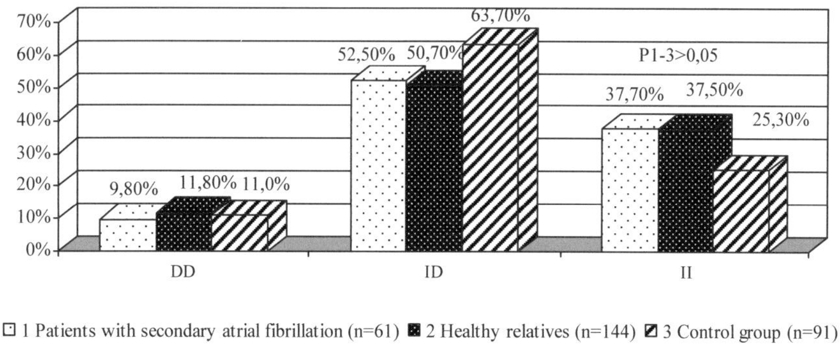

Figure 3. Frequency of the gene ADRA2B genotypes in patients with secondary atrial fibrillation, their healthy relatives and persons of the control group.

2.3. Polymorphism of the endothelial NO synthase (eNOS) gene in probands with atrial fibrillation, their healthy relatives and persons of the control group

In our work we investigated polymorphisms of the endothelial NO synthase (eNOS) gene in patients with atrial fibrillation, their healthy relatives and persons from the control group. According to the results of PCR in patients with atrial fibrillation, their healthy relatives and persons from the control group three sorts of NO synthase genotypes were revealed: G/G – homozygous, G/T – heterozygous, T/T – homozygous.

Homozygous genotype (894 G/G) of the endothelial NO synthase (eNOS) gene in patients with atrial fibrillation was revealed in 58,5±4,8% (62 persons), heterozygous genotype (894 G/T) – in 39,6±4,8% (42 persons). Homozygous genotype in a rare allele (894 T/T) was genotyped in 1,9±1,3% (2 persons) (Table 7).

Among the probands' healthy relatives genotypes appeared to be spread as follows: homozygous genotype (894 G/G) –in 44,4±4,1% (64 persons), heterozygous genotype (894 G/T) – in 52,1±4,2% (75 persons), homozygous genotype in a rare allele (894 T/T) –in 3,5±1,5% (5 persons) (Table 7). As for the control group, homozygous genotype (894 G/G) of the gene of endothelial NO synthase was revealed in 39,6±5,1% (36 persons), heterozygous genotype (894 G/T) – in 50,5±5,2% (46 persons). Homozygous genotype in a rare allele (894 T/T) was genotyped in 9,9±3,1% (9 persons) (Table 7).

A significant prevalence of homozygous genotype G/G in patients with atrial fibrillation (58,5%) as compared with the control group (39,6%) is established; the difference is statistically reliable (p =0,039) (Table 7, Fig. 4).

Genotypes	Patients with atrial fibrillation N= 106		Healthy relatives N=144		Control group N=91		p_{1-2}	p_{1-3}	p_{2-3}
	Absolute value	%	Absolute value	%	Absolute value	%			
G/G	62	58,5±4,8	64	44,4±4,1	36	39,6±5,1	p>0,05	p<0,05	p>0,05
G/T	42	39,6±4,8	75	52,1±4,2	46	50,5±5,2	p>0,05	p>0,05	p>0,05
T/T	2	1,9±1,3	5	3,5±1,5	9	9,9±3,1	p>0,05	P<0,05	p>0,05

Note: Differences in the investigated parameters were calculated using the χ2 criterion.

Table 7. Genotype frequency of the eNOS 894 G/T polymorphism in patients with atrial fibrillation, their healthy relatives and persons of the control group.

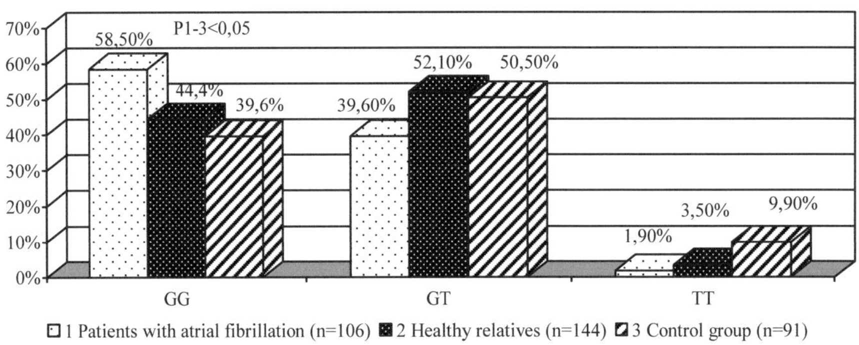

Figure 4. Genotype frequency of the eNOS 894 G/T polymorphism in patients with atrial fibrillation, their healthy relatives and persons of the control group.

In patients with primary atrial fibrillation homozygous genotype (894 G/G) of the endothelial NO synthase (eNOS) gene was revealed in 62,2±7,2% (28 persons), heterozygous genotype (894 G/T) – in 33,3±7,0% (15 persons), homozygous genotype in a rare allele (894 T/T) was genotyped in 4,4±3,1% (2 persons) (Table 8).

A significant prevalence of homozygous genotype G/G as compared with the control group is established only in patients with primary atrial fibrillation, 62,2% и 39,6% respectively; the difference is statistically reliable (p =0,021) (Table 8, Fig. 5).

http://dx.doi.org/10.5772/53527

Genotypes	Patients with primary atrial fibrillation N= 45		Healthy relatives N=144		Control group N=91		p_{1-2}	p_{1-3}	p_{2-3}
	Abs.	%	Abs.	%	Abs.	%			
G/G	28	62,2±7,2	64	44,4±4,1	36	39,6±5,1	p>0,05	p<0,05	p>0,05
G/T	15	33,3±7,0	75	52,1±4,2	46	50,5±5,2	p>0,05	p>0,05	p>0,05
T/T	2	4,4±3,1	5	3,5±1,5	9	9,9±3,1	p>0,05	P>0,05	p>0,05

Note: Differences in the investigated parameters were calculated using the χ2 criterion.

Table 8. Genotype frequency of the eNOS 894 G/T polymorphism in patients with primary atrial fibrillation, their healthy relatives and persons of the control group.

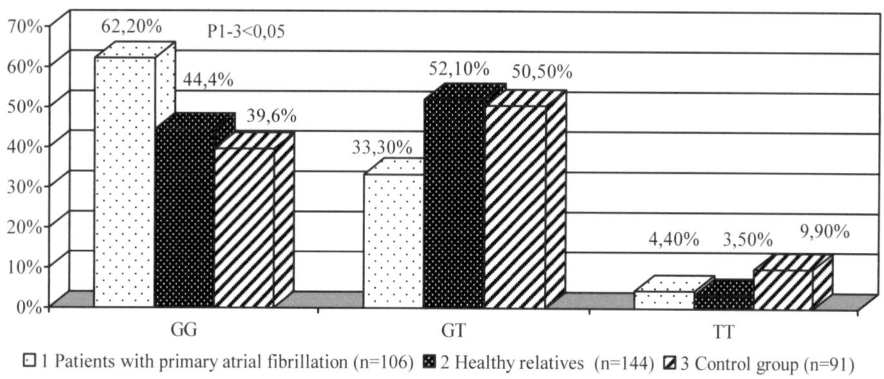

Figure 5. Genotype frequency of the eNOS 894 G/T polymorphism in patients with primary atrial fibrillation, their healthy relatives and persons of the control group.

In patients with secondary atrial fibrillation homozygous genotype (894 G/G) of the endothelial NO synthase (eNOS) gene was revealed in 55,7±6,4% (34 persons), heterozygous genotype (894 G/T) – in 44,3±6,4% (27 persons), homozygous genotype in a rare allele (894 T/T) was not genotyped (Table 9).

No significant differences were established between frequencies of genotypes of the endothelial NO synthase (eNOS) gene in patients with secondary atrial fibrillation, their healthy relatives and persons of the control group (Table 9, Fig. 6).

Genotypes	Patients with secondary atrial fibrillation N= 61		Healthy relatives N=144		Control group N=91		p_{1-2}	p_{1-3}	p_{2-3}
	Absolute value	%	Absolute value	%	Absolute value	%			
G/G	34	55,7±6,4	64	44,4±4,1	36	39,6±5,1	p>0,05	p>0,05	p>0,05
G/T	27	44,3±6,4	75	52,1±4,2	46	50,5±5,2	p>0,05	p>0,05	p>0,05
T/T	0	0	5	3,5±1,5	9	9,9±3,1	p>0,05	P>0,05	p>0,05

Note: Differences in the investigated parameters were calculated using the $\chi 2$ criterion.

Table 9. Genotype frequency of the eNOS 894 G/T polymorphism in patients with secondary atrial fibrillation, their healthy relatives and persons of the control group.

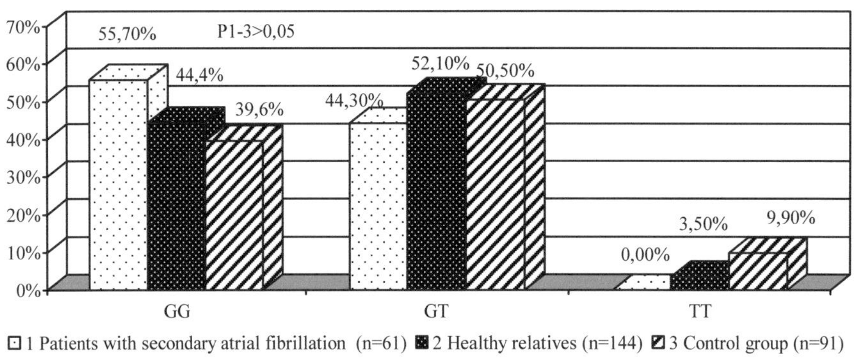

Figure 6. Genotype frequency of the eNOS 894 G/T polymorphism in patients with secondary atrial fibrillation, their healthy relatives and persons of the control group.

As was mentioned above, the decrease in the production of NO-synthase can cause oxidative stress, lead to disturbances in cardiac conduction system and provoke the re-entry mechanism in the atria, thereby contributing to the development of atrial fibrillation [42, 44].

This paper demonstrates a significant prevalence of homozygous genotype G/G of the endothelial NO synthase (eNOS) gene in patients with primary atrial fibrillation. Specifically, polymorphism of the endothelial NO synthase (eNOS) gene causes the decrease in the level of NO and calcium in the cells as well as disturbances in the physiological process of HMF-dependent protein kinases synthesis, all these factors contributing to the development of atrial fibrillation.

The investigated genetic markers may be used in diagnosing of primary atrial fibrillation susceptibility.

3. Conclusion

A significant prevalence of homozygous genotype I/I of the gene ADRA2B in patients with primary atrial fibrillation (44,4%) as compared with the control group (25,3%) is established.

The relatives of the probands with primary atrial fibrillation and homozygous genotype I/I can be subsumed under the risk group for the development of this pathology. Changes in the aminoacid profile of the third intracellular loop of the α2ß- adrenergic receptor due to the polymorphism I/I of the ADRA2B gene disturb the interaction of the receptor with effector proteins (G-protein or receptor protein kinase), which cause changes in receptor activity autoregulation or associated with the activity cAMP processes of intracellular signaling (e.g. migration of the Ca from intracellular stores to the cytosol).

A significant prevalence of homozygous genotype G/G of the endothelial NO synthase (eNOS) gene in patients with primary atrial fibrillation (62,2%) as compared with the control group (39,6%) is shown.

The relatives of the probands with primary atrial fibrillation and homozygous genotype G/G can be subsumed under the risk group for the development of this pathology.

A certain role in atrial fibrillation pathogenesis can be played by nitrogen oxide molecules (NO). Nitrogen oxide is constantly produced in the human organism enzymatically from L – arginine and performs a function of a universal messenger in intracellular signaling [19]. NO synthase (NOS, EC number 1.14.13.39) is a catalyst in this reaction [19]. Under the influence of NOS L – arginine oxidation and nitrogen oxide synthesis takes place in vessel endotheliocytes. Then, going from the endotheliocytes to the smooth muscle cells, NO labilizes soluble guanylate cyclase, thereby contributing to the decrease in the level of the rhythmic hydroxymethylfurfurol (HMF), activation of the rhythmic HMF – dependent protein kinases, changes in Ca concentration, susceptibility of the conducting cardiac myocytes receptors to the level of catecholamines. In case of polymorphism G/G of the endothelial NO synthase (eNOS) gene the level of nitrogen oxide and intracellular Ca decreases, the physiological process of HMF-dependent protein kinases synthesis is disturbed, which contributes to the development of heart rhythm disorders.

We studied the eNOS 894 G/T polymorphism in the group of patients described above.

As was mentioned above, the decrease in the production of NO-synthase can cause oxidative stress and changes in cardiac conduction system, thereby contributing to the development of atrial fibrillation [45].

Continuing the search of candidate genes of the primary and secondary atrial fibrillation and the study of different genes polymorphisms combinations, which are likely to cause the development of atrial fibrillation seems to be necessary.

The final result of these investigations can be genetic identification of the atrial fibrillation risk groups, early diagnostics, ранняя диагностика, specific atrial fibrillation preventive care as well as on-time treatment of this type of arrhythmia.

Acknowledgment We would like to thank Mikhail Voevoda, Vladimir Maksimov and staff of the Research Institute of Therapy, Novosibirsk, Russia for their help in genetic testing and their continued support and assistance in our investigations.

Author details

Svetlana Nikulina[1], Vladimir Shulman[1], Ksenya Dudkina[1], Anna Chernova[1] and Oksana Gavrilyuk[2]

1 Krasnoyarsk State Medical University named after Prof. V.F. Voino-Yasenetsky, Department of internal diseases No. 1, Krasnoyarsk, Russia

2 Krasnoyarsk State Medical University named after Prof. V.F. Voino-Yasenetsky, Department of Latin and foreign languages, Krasnoyarsk, Russia

References

[1] Diagnostika i lechenie fibrilljacii predserdij: Rossiyskie rekomendatsii. Terapevt 2005; (1/2) 11-37.

[2] Benjamin EJ., Wolf PA., Dagostino RB. et al. Impact of atrial fibrillation on the risk of death: the Fremingam Heart Study. Circulation 1998;98(4) 946-952.

[3] Kannel WB., Abbott RD., Savage DD. Epidemiologic faetures of chronic atrial fibrillation: the Framingham study/ N. Engl. J. Med 1982; 306 1018-1022.

[4] Lloid-Jones DM., Wang TJ., Leip E.P.et al. Lifetime risk for development of atrial fibrillation: the Fremingam Heart Study. Circulation 2004;110(5) 1042-1046.

[5] Shulman V.A., Nikulina S.Yu., Ivanitskaya Yu.V. i dr. Idiopaticheskie (pervichnye) zabolevaniya provodyaschey sistemy serdtsa. Kardiologiya 2000;1 89-92.

[6] Lai LP., Tsai CC., Su MJ. et al. Atrial fibrillation is association with accumulation of aging-related common type mytochondrial DNA deletion mutation in human atrial tissue. Chest 2003; 123 539-544.

[7] Christophersen IE., Ravn LS., Budtz-Jooergensen E. et al. Familial aggregation of atrial fibrillation a study in Danish twins. Circ. Arrhythm. Electrophisiol 2009;2(2) 378-383.

[8] Surawicz HJ. Vidaillet M., Lev B. et. al. Familial congenital sinus rhythm anomalies: clinical and pathological correlations. Pacing Clin. Electrophysiol 1992;15(11) 1720-1729.

[9] Fox C.S, Parise H.,. Agostino R.B et al. Parental atrial fibrillation as a risk for atrial fibrillation in offspring. JAMA 2004; 291 2851-2855.

[10] Roberts DJ., Michael H., Gollob M.H. Impact of genetic discoveries on the classification of lone atrial fibrillation. J. Am. Coll. Cardiol 2010;55(8) 705-711.

[11] Bharati S., Surawicz B., Vidaillet HJ. Familial congenital sinus rhythm anomalies: clinical and pathological correlations. PACE 1992; 15 (Pt. 1) 1720-1729.

[12] Wolf L. Familial auricular fibrillation. N. Engl. J. Med 1943; 229 396-397.

[13] Lomasney JW., Lorenz W., Allen LF. et al. Expansion of the α2-Adrenergic Receptor Family: Cloning and characterization of a human α2-adrenergic receptor subtype, the gene for which is located on chromosome 2. Proc. Natl. Acad. Sci. USA 1990; 87 (13) 5094-5098.

[14] Hein L., Altman JD., Kobilka BK. Two functionally distinct alpha2-adrenergic receptors regulate sympathetic neurotransmission. Nature 1999; 402 (6758) 181-184.

[15] Wowern F., Bengtsson K., Lindblad U. et al. Functional variant in the (alpha)2B adrenoceptor gene, a positional candidate on chromosome 2, associates with hypertension. Hypertension 2004;43(3) 231-233.

[16] Hjalmarson A. Heart rate and beta-adrenergic mechanisms in acute myocardial infarction. Basic Res. Cardiol 1990; 85 325-333.

[17] Koch WJ., Lefkowitz J., Rockman HA. Functional consequences of altering myocardial adrenergic receptor signaling. Annu. Rev. Physiol 2000; 62 237-260.

[18] Coumel P. Neurogenic and humoral influences of the autonomic nervous system in the determination of paroxysmal atrial fibrillation. The atrium in health and disease. N. Y.: Futura Publ. Co.; 1982. p213-232.

[19] Pokrovsky VI. Oksid azota, ego fiziologicheskie i patofiziologicheskie svoystva. Terapevt. Arhiv. 2005;1 82-87.

[20] Kim M. Myocardial Nox2 containing NAD(P)H oxidase contributes to oxidative. Stress in human atrial fibrillation. Circ. Res 2005; 97 629-636.

[21] Wolf L. Familial auricular fibrillation. N. Engl. J. Med.; 1943. p396-397.

[22] Dzyak VN. Mercatel'naya aritmiya. Kiev: Zdorovye; 1979.

[23] Tikanoja T. Familial atrial fibrillation with fetal onset. Jpn. Heart J 1998; 79 (2) 195-197.

[24] Boitsov SA. Mercatel'naya aritmiya. SPb: ELBI; 2001.

[25] Zharko KP. O semeynyh formah narusheniya ritma serdtsa i provodimosti. Vracheb. delo 1981;7 67-68.

[26] Zav'yalov AI., Zav'yalov DA. Serdtse i myshechnaya rabota. Aktual'nye voprosy biomedicinskoy i klinicheskoy antropologii: mater. konf. Krasnoyarsk 1997 35-36.

[27] Poret P., Mabo P., Deplace C. Is isolated atrial fibrillation genetically determined? Apropos of a familial history. Arch. Mol. Coeur. Vaiss 1996;89(9) 1197-1203.

[28] Girona J., Domingo A., Albert D. et al. Fibrillation auricular familiar.Rev. Esp. Cardiol 1997;50(8) 548-551.

[29] Gillor A., Korsch E. Familial manifestation of idiopathic atrial flutter. Monatsschr. Kinderheilkd 1992;140(1) 47-50.

[30] Brugada R. Genetic bases of arrhythmias. Rev. Esp. Cardiol 1998; 51 p. 274-285.

[31] Brugada R., Tapscott T. et al. Identification of a genetic locus for familial atrial fibrillation. N. Engl. J. Med; 1997. p905-911.

[32] Yang H., Xia M., Jin Q. Identification of a KCNE2 - gain of function mutation in patients with familial atrial fibrillation. Am. J. Pathol 2004;165(3) 1010-1032.

[33] Christiansen J., Dyck JD., Elyas BG. et al. Chromosome 1q21.1 contiguous gene deletion is associated with congenital heart disease. Circ. Res 2004;94(11) 1249-1435.

[34] Firouzi M., Ramanna H., Kok B. et al. Association of human connexin 40 gene polymorfisms with atrial vulnerability as a risk factor for idiopatic atrial fibrillation. Circ. Res 2004;5 29.

[35] Gensini F., Padeleti L., Fatini C. et al. Angiotensin-converting ensyme and endothelial nitric oxide synthase polymorpisms in patients with atrial fibrillation. Am. J. Cardiol 2003;91 678-683.

[36] Tsai CC., Lai LP., Chang FC. et al. Renin-angiotensin gene polymorphism and atrial fibrillation. Clin. Sci 2004; 653- 659.

[37] Tseluyko VI., Dmitriev SJu. Rol' interstitsial'nogo fibroza kak prediktora vozniknoveniya fibrillyatsii predserdy. Medicina neotlozhnyh sostojany 2007;3 124-126.

[38] Minushkina LO., Zateycshikov DA., Zateycshikova AA. i dr. Polimorfizmy gena endotelial'noj NO – sintazy i gipertrofii miokarda u bol'nyh arterial'noy gipertenziey. Kardiologiya 2002;3 30-34.

[39] Minushkina LO., Gorshkova ES. i dr. Rol' geneticheskih faktorov v razvitii mertsatel'noy aritmii. Kardiologiya 2007;12 57-62.

[40] Otway R., Vandenberg JI., Guo G. et al. Stretch-sensitive KCNQ1 mulation: a link between genetic and environmental factors in the pathogenesis of atrial fibrillation. J. Am. Coll. Cardiol 2007; 49 p. 578-586.

[41] Simard C., Drolet B., Yang P. et al. Polymorphism screening in the cardiac K+ channel gene KCNA5. Clin. Pharmacol. Ther 2005;77 138-141.

[42] Chen H., Chu H., Shi Y. et al. Association between endothelial nitric oxide synthase polymorphisms and atrial fibrillation: a meta-analysis. J Cardiovasc Transl Res 2012;528-534.

[43] Liu T, Korantzopoulos P, Xu G. et al. Association between angiotensin-converting enzyme insertion/deletion gene polymorphism and atrial fibrillation: a meta-analysis. Europace 2011;346-354.

http://dx.doi.org/10.5772/53527

[44] Gurevich MA. Mertsatel'naya aritmiya. Voprosy etiologii, klassifikatsiya i lechenie // Klinich.meditsina 2006;2 7-15.

[45] Daoude E. Effect of atrial fibrillation on atrial refractoriness in humans. Circulation 1996; 94 p.1600 – 1606.

Chapter 5

Voltage-Independent Calcium Channels, Molecular Sources of Supraventricular Arrhythmia

Paul E. Wolkowicz, Patrick K. Umeda,
Ferdinand Urthaler and Oleg F. Sharifov

Additional information is available at the end of the chapter

http://dx.doi.org/10.5772/53649

1. Introduction

Since its identification over one hundred years ago, atrial fibrillation has been shown to occur frequently in the general population and is now recognized as an important medical problem in developed societies. Three major hypotheses to explain cardiac rhythm disorders like atrial fibrillation have been proposed during this time and one of these three, impulse reentry has become predominate. The two other explanations, designated as focal source hypotheses, have been relegated to a secondary role in understanding arrhythmia. Despite widespread acceptance of the reentry hypothesis, however, current non-invasive anti-arrhythmic drugs based on this mechanism poorly prevent or reverse atrial fibrillation or other types of arrhythmia. One interpretation of this paradoxical clinical result is that mechanisms other than reentry initiate arrhythmias like atrial fibrillation in real-life settings. As a consequence, current non-invasive therapeutics may neither target nor effectively suppress important but unrecognized non-reentrant mechanisms that provoke clinical arrhythmia. We have found that challenging isolated non-automatic left atrial muscle, left ventricular papillary muscle, and perfused heart in sinus rhythm with an activator of the voltage-independent Orai calcium channels provokes high frequent tachycardia and fibrillation. Thus the Orais and related voltage-independent calcium channels may be unexpected sources of arrhythmia. This manuscript provides (a) a synopsis of the identification of atrial fibrillation as a clinical entity, (b) an overview of the development of the three current hypotheses for arrhythmia, and (c) our hypothesis that dysregulated voltage-independent calcium channels may be a fourth means to provoke electrical instability in heart muscle.

2. Historical perspective

Atrial fibrillation was first observed as compromised heart mechanical output. By the late 1800s clinicians including Nothnagel, and later MacKenzie and Hering, noted and analyzed abnormal or absent 'a waves' in venous pressure tracings but had not specifically correlated these abnormalities with atrial dysfunction [1,2,3]. Kymographic analyses of the pulse waves of their patients allowed these investigators to report examples of irregularly irregular pulse intervals and pulse heights, a surrogate for ventricular force generation. Towards the end of the nineteenth century physicians also came to realize that these mechanical disturbances often occurred persistently in some patients. Thus by the outset of the twentieth century these types of abnormal pressure wave recordings were grouped into the clinical conditions of *delirium cordis* or the more definitive *pulsus irregularis et inaequalis perpetuus* [4]. Vulpian, Krehl, and Hering were initial proponents of the notion that such irregularities resulted from the defective mechanical output of the atria [5,6,7]. The translational research of Cushny and Edmunds provided the first direct validation of this hypothesis when in 1907 they correlated chance observations of atrial *delirium* made in the dog laboratory with clinical recordings of *pulsus irregularis et inaequalis perpetuus* [8].

In the early 1900s clinical and experimental string galvanometer data formed the basis for the idea that disorganized atrial electrical activity caused both the loss of venous 'a waves' and the appearance of the fine pulsatile activity which define *pulsus irregularis et inaequalis perptuus*. Specifically, string galvanometer tracings published in 1906 by Einthoven [9] and in 1908 by Hering [10] demonstrated that mechanical *pulsus irregularis et inaequalis perpetuus* occurred in humans who lacked p-waves, had F-waves, and had irregularly timed but otherwise normal QRS complexes. These initial reports coupled with the extensive electrocardiographic analyses of Rothberger and Winterberg published in 1909 [11] provided the electrical equivalent of the venous wave data of Cushny and Edwards. That is, the electrocardiographic measurements Rothberger and Winterberg acquired from animals undergoing experimental atrial fibrillation were identical to recordings obtained from patients with *pulsus irregularis et inaequalis perpetuus*. This work together with the earlier report of MacWilliam [12] that faradic stimulation produced atrial fibrillation led to the acceptance of the view that the complete disruption of atrial electrical activity caused the irregular pulse waves that characterize *pulsus irregularis*. Thomas Lewis built on and expanded this work in his elegant electrocardiographic characterization of atrial flutter and fibrillation in humans and in animals [*e.g.*,13]. By 1920 it had been accepted that the organized electrical activity observed using string galvanometers or electrocardiographs sparked rhythmic heart contraction and conversely that disordered electrical activity caused abnormalities like *pulsus irregularis et inaequalis perpetuus*. Importantly, it was accepted that *pulsus irregularis* arose from disturbances that occurred specifically in the atria since hearts in atrial fibrillation often produced normal but irregularly timed QRS complexes.

During the evolution of this explanation for clinical *pulsus irregularis et inaequalis perpetuus* experimentalists developed the initial, non-vitalist explanation for atrial fibrillation and other cardiac rhythm disorders. Engelmann in 1896 [14] and Winterberg in 1906 [15] proposed an original hypothesis centered round the seemingly logical view that a solitary ectopic depolarization occurring spontaneously in a small number of heart cells confined to a specific region of the atria (*or ventricle*) could produce a 'premature' atrial (*or ventricular*) contraction. They reasoned that if such spontaneous electrical activity also could occur repeatedly and at a sufficiently rapid rate then such a 'focus' could likewise produce tachycardia or fibrillation. Variations of this 'focal' hypothesis included multiple 'heterotopic centers' depolarizing at rates sufficient to produce flutter or fibrillation or, as Rothberger proposed [16], a single heterotopic center which depolarized at extremely rapid rates. Several early experimentalists noted that the refractory period of heart muscle must shorten to accommodate rapid ectopic activity and that such abnormal electrical activity might occur at rates fast enough to preclude regular heart muscle contraction [17], foreshadowing the idea of fibrillatory conduction. While these focal source hypotheses were logical, a molecular mechanism through which non-automatic atrial (*or ventricular*) muscle might spontaneously or automatically depolarize was not known at that time. Thus non-focal, that is reentrant hypotheses to explain arrhythmia came to the fore and now dominate this field of inquiry. Nonetheless, the challenge to identify all molecular mechanisms that cause quiescent heart muscle to excite independently of normal sinus rhythm still remains at the center of arrhythmia research today just as it did over one hundred years ago. Thus we seek to *define mechanisms which provoke quiescent heart cells to depolarize (a) independently of normal sinus rhythm, (b) at sporadic or rapid rates, (c) in an organized manner or (d) in an apparently chaotic way, and (e) over inconstant periods of time including apparent perpetuity.* There are three such mechanisms currently known and our data suggest the existence of a fourth one.

3. Mechanism 1: Impulse reentry

Reentry occurs when electrical impulses conduct abnormally through the heart and re-excite quiescent heart muscle (Figure 1, center & right). Multiple experimentalists in the early twentieth century began creating this hypothesis for arrhythmia with the assumption that the mechanisms for normal electrical impulse generation and propagation they were discovering at that time fully explain the production of heart abnormal electrical activity. This hypothesis was formed from experiments Mayer published in 1906 [18] which demonstrated the fundamental event of impulse reentry. He showed that rings of excitable jellyfish tissue exposed to an external electrical impulse would produce recirculating electrical waves when unidirectional impulse block was imposed on these preparations. Subsequently in 1913 and 1914 Mines and Garrey [19,20] published similar results they acquired in heart muscle. Their data provided the initial evidence supporting the view that recirculating electrical impulses produce arrhythmia. Based on this work and their own original observations [17], Lewis, Drury and Ilescu proposed in 1921 [21] that the 'circus movement' of normal electrical activity might explain the five characteristics of atrial fibrillation (*and other arrhythmia*) noted at the end of the preceding paragraph. This simple and elegant circus creation contributed to establishing the impulse reentry hypothesis which has since metamorphosed into the accepted explanation for atrial fibrillation and for other clinically relevant rhythm disorders.

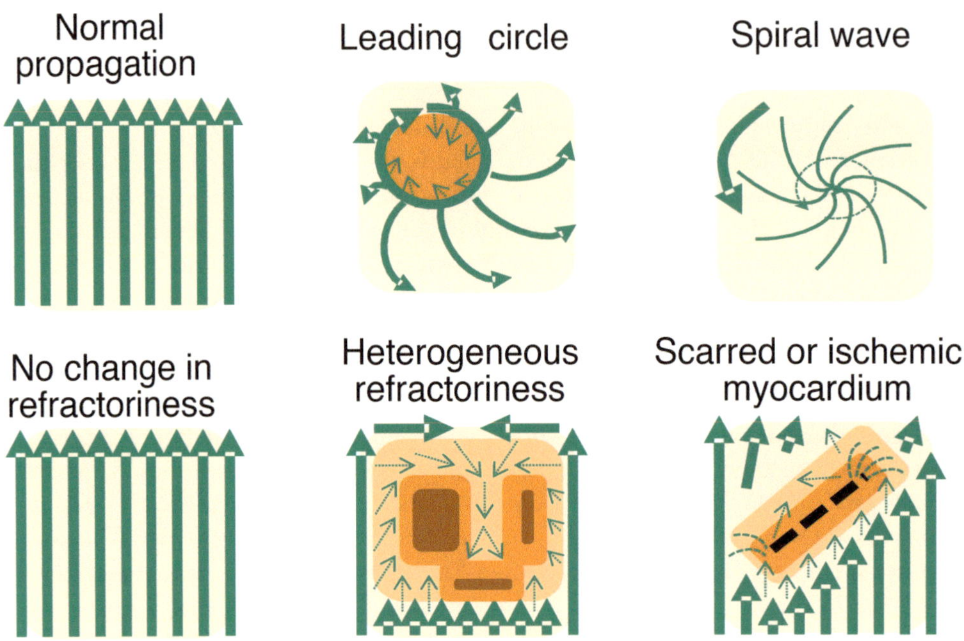

Figure 1. Impulse Reentry. *Left:* Normal heart muscle conduts impulses homogeneously. Uniform fields of excitable and refractory muscle limit impulse recirculation. *Center: Leading circle model:* Inhomogeneous rates of impulse conduction (Small v large arrows) create contiguous regions of excited and quiescent myocardium with altered refractoriness (Light v dark boxes). Electrical activity may recirculate in these regions if unidirectional conduction block were present. *Right: Spiral wave model:* Impulses circulating around scar could encounter local conduction inhomogeneities which cause impulse wavenreak &reentrant rotors.

Lewis realized that variants of the circus hypothesis might arise in pathological settings. In particular he mentioned that the primary arrhythmogenic circuit could fragment to produce secondary or offspring ectopic sources and that local variation in the rate of conduction of ectopic impulses could provoke disorganized fibrillation [17, *see page 591 Figure III and page 592 Figures V & VI*]. Several decades later Moe, Abildskov [22], and others embellished this general circus view of impulse recirculation to explain the persistent nature of fibrillation or other high frequency arrhythmias. Based on his own data and on his careful examination of the earlier high-speed cinematographic work of Wiggers [23], Moe proposed that local variations in impulse conduction induced faradically or arising in diseased heart could cause impulses to fragment and purposelessly but persistently meander through excitable regions of atrial (*or ventricular*) muscle. Moe proposed that such 'wandering wavelets' of impulse reentry were the fundamental cause of atrial fibrillation.

This 'wandering wavelet' hypothesis has been modified or superseded during the 50 years since it was first proposed. Work published by Allessie in 1977 [24] demonstrated that local variations in the refractory period of heart muscle can produce 'leading circle' reentry. In his model, impulses circulate like a pinwheel around a small region of refractory, non-excitable myocardium, producing vortices of electrical activity that emanate from a central inexcitable

http://dx.doi.org/10.5772/53649

core. In this view recirculating abnormal electrical emanations disrupt normal electrical activity and cause arrhythmia. Allessie indeed observed 'leading circle' or 'functional' reentry under experimental conditions in which acetylcholine markedly shortened atrial action potential duration and either bursts of high frequency stimulation or ectopic impulses administered during so-called 'vulnerable periods' induced a type of atrial fibrillation. This hypothesis of 'leading circle reentry' has evolved since 1977 and variants of it are now the dominant means to explain arrhythmia [25]. In particular, one current 'state-of-the-art' view proposes that the interaction of normal or ectopic impulses with refractory objects of an appropriate size leads to impulse fractionation and impulse reentry (Figure 1, right). This type of 'wavebreak' allows for impulse recirculation to occur around fixed anatomical sites like papillary muscles, around scar tissue or around myocardium that poorly conducts electricity. These rotors of fractionated impulse can remain fixed in or meander through heart muscle. Elegant imaging methodologies produced from decades of engineering coupled with mathematical-biophysical modeling have theorized, searched for and characterized wavebreak. The high frequency pin-wheel rotors of electrical activity that this model posits have sometimes been directly observed in the aftermath of high frequency burst stimulation. Their direct observation has been reported less frequently in myocardial pathologies like ischemia where arrhythmia arises 'naturally' in the absence of either burst pacing or exquisitely timed ectopic stimulations. Regardless, the intellectual flexibility and elegance of the wavebreak construct allowed for the development of multiple concepts espoused as fundamental mechanisms for arrhythmia including atrial fibrillation [25].

The current iteration of the impulse reentry hypothesis thus proposes that arrhythmia is the response of contiguous regions of discontinuously excitable and non- or poorly excitable heart muscle to an external depolarizing influence (Figure 1). That is, reentry requires (a) extremely localized inhomogeneity in the conduction properties of heart muscle such as might occur in the border between scar tissue and viable myocardium, (b) pathological conditions that affect the biophysical properties of the voltage-dependent sodium or potassium channels or (c) decreasing the activity of proteins like connexins which would impose conduction heterogeneities on the heart. This dominant hypothesis to explain atrial fibrillation or other arrhythmia views these disorders from a vantage point developed in the early twentieth century. Arrhythmia in this view begins primarily as a disturbance in heart electrical activity. The fact that faradic methods like burst-pacing or stimulation during an 'electrically vulnerable period' remain mainstays in inducing arrhythmia and that arrhythmia is assessed by the electrocardiograph or by other devices that measure myocyte electrical activity sustains the opinion that rhythm disorders are mainly or solely electrical problems. An alternate view might ask whether the voltage-dependent ion channels that produce heart electrical activity are themselves regulated by voltage-independent cell signaling events. Might such cell signaling events drive arrhythmia? That is, *can cardiac non-electrical sources cause heart electrical problems*?

The creative hypothesis proposed by Engelmann to explain arrhythmia emphasized that changes or defects in small regions of heart muscle might generate sporadic or high frequency focal ectopic impulses. The inability to identify a candidate mechanism for focal ectopy at the turn of the twentieth century, the identification of impulse reentry in jellyfish, and its ascendance as a facile, malleable explanation for arrhythmia caused the focal view to fall into disfavor. By the middle of the twentieth century only few proponents supported it, in particular investigators like Rothberger, Scherf, and Kisch [16,26,27]. They continued to present data which showed that focal (*or cellular*) sites of spontaneous depolarization could provoke arrhythmia just as well as impulse reentry. From the 1920s through the 1950s Scherf repeatedly reported that focal administration of toxins like aconitine or alkaloids like veratradine incite cardiac rhythm disturbances that mimic atrial (*or ventricular*) fibrillation and atrial flutter. It is important to note that these pharmacological agents initiate arrhythmia by modifying sodium channel gating properties to disrupt this gatekeeper of the action potential. Jervell and Lange-Nielsen published a groundbreaking report in 1957 [28] which first documented the long QT syndrome and laid the foundation for research on the genetic basis for arrhythmia. Dessertenne [29] and others greatly developed the appreciation that genetic mutation can alter the biophysical properties of voltage-dependent sodium and potassium channels in a manner analogous to the pharmacological approach of Scherf. Consequently, in addition to changes in the gross electrical properties of heart muscle proposed to underlie wavebreak and impulse reentry, pharmacological or genetic modification of ion channels came to be accepted as potential sources of clinical arrhythmia. But this toxin and genetic view have at least three critical limitations when used as evidence to support a cell-based focal hypothesis of arrhythmia

Toxins and alkaloids modify the biophysical properties of the sodium channel to provoke arrhythmic activity. These changes in channel properties at the site of toxin administration may provoke conditions that favor impulse reentry. Thus these pharmacological approaches might incite arrhythmia in a reentrant manner analogous to faradic sources.

Mutations of voltage-dependent ion channels also might create conditions for functional or anatomic impulse reentry. Indeed reentry is invoked to explain genetically-linked arrhythmia including the long QT syndromes [30].

Even if toxin-induced arrhythmia were purely a focal event, this approach to induce arrhythmia does not identify the cellular process which might alter the biophysical properties of the sodium or other voltage-dependent ion channels to recapitulate the arrhythmogenic effects of aconitine or veratradine.

The development of a robust focal explanation for arrhythmia requires the identification of cellular mechanisms that destabilize quiescent atrium (*or ventricle*) to produce sporadic, tachycardic or fibrillatory ectopic electrical activity. There are two mechanisms now accepted to generate such abnormal electrical impulses.

4. Mechanism 2: Triggered afterdepolarization

The first is afterdepolarization or triggered activity. This ectopic event (a) arises within stressed or failing atrial (*or ventricular*) myocytes, (b) appears to require specific changes in intracellular signaling and post-translational protein modification including phosphorylation, (c) is hypothesized to depend on changes in intracellular calcium homeostasis, and (d) needs a preceding action potential as a triggering event.

The groundbreaking work of Arvanataki in 1939 [31] provided the initial evidence for afterdepolarization. This series of papers demonstrated that spontaneous electrical activity occurred in a wide range of excitable cells including snail muscle when these preparations were stimulated at extremely rapid rates and the pacing stimulus then was abruptly stopped. Studies reported by Bozler in 1943 [32] expanded on this breakthrough work, demonstrating that cardiac muscle also can afterdepolarize. The two types of afterdepolarization are designated as early or delayed events.

Early afterdepolarization occurs either during the Phase II plateau or during Phase III repolarization of a prolonged action potential. Increased late sodium current [33] or decreased potassium channel activity, lowered 'repolarization reserve' [34], may prolong the duration of the action potential. Numerous studies show that early afterdepolarization occurs more readily with increased late sodium current compared to decreased repolarization reserve even though action potential durations are similarly prolonged. Interesting to a focal view of arrhythmia described later on, stimulating Gαq receptors greatly increases the frequency at which early afterdepolarization occurs in muscles with decreased repolarization reserve. The molecular basis for this curious effect has not been conclusively established. Early afterdepolarization occurs most often at low rates of muscle stimulation and materializes much less frequently as the stimulation rate increases toward normal. Thus arrhythmia that arises in settings of bradycardia or in conditions where heart rate is highly variable is often ascribed to early afterdepolarization. In addition, early afterdepolarization is a likely source for premature atrial (*or ventricular*) contraction and more complex arrhythmia when genetic mutation or pharmacological intervention prolongs the myocardial QT interval.

Delayed afterdepolarization is the second type of triggered activity. By contrast to early afterdepolarization, muscle or myocytes with normal action potentials that have returned to their Phase IV resting potential generate this type of abnormal impulse. Delayed afterdepolarization usually arises following high frequency burst stimulation of heart or myocytes or when heart calcium stores are greatly increased. Depending on the precise experimental condition, afterdepolarization can occur as a solitary event, as a few afterdepolarizations or as ectopy that lasts for seconds or longer. This latter type of event has been termed 'sustained triggered activity' [33]. Hypotheses for afterdepolarization must explain isolated events, sustained activity, and the transition between the two. That is, how can a single isolated ectopic event lead to sustained tachycardic or fibrillary activity?

Schmitt and Erlanger initially explained premature contraction of intact muscle using the impulse reentry hypothesis [35]. In their view, electrical impulses might recirculate through junctions in the Purkinje system or around a region of the heart if both somehow came to possess unidirectional impulse block and altered conduction properties. They envisioned a scenario wherein recirculation could occur once or in a sustained manner depending on the electrical characteristics of the recirculating loop. The observation of afterdepolarization in isolated myocytes indicated that mechanisms besides the gross physiological ones of reentry might also initiate triggered activity. January and others [36] proposed voltage-dependent sodium or calcium channel window currents as potential mediators of early afterdepolarization. In their view, the biophysical properties of these voltage-dependent ion channels favor channel reopening during their prolonged exposure to the membrane potentials of the action potential plateau phase. For a wide range of reasons reviewed by Salama and others [37,38], neither of these purely electrical explanations adequately explain the production or the properties of early afterdepolarizations. Window currents also appear to be a less likely explanation for delayed afterdepolarizations which occur from resting potentials. Pogwizd among others [39] hypothesized that decreased activity of the inwardly rectifying potassium channel could sensitize heart muscle to depolarizing influences during diastole. This enhanced sensitivity would favor myocyte delayed afterdepolarization during Phase IV. All of these explanations, however, view afterdepolarization as essentially an electrical phenomenon. That is, they hold that the voltage-dependent ion channels which produce normal electrical activity are the sole cause for the ectopic electrical instability of afterdepolarization. An alternate view of afterdepolarization began to evolve from data first reported in 2000 [40,41] which proposed that abnormalities in the calcium homeostasis responsible for muscle contraction might cause afterdepolarization.

The mechanism which couples myocyte excitation and contraction remained unresolved into the 1970s [42]. The experiments of Fabiato established that the passage of small amounts of calcium across the myocyte plasma membrane initiated the rapid release of a much larger myocyte calcium store sequestered within the lumen of the sarcoplasmic reticulum (SR) [43]. This calcium release causes the rapid elevation of cytosolic free calcium which induces myofilaments to shorten. The subsequent accumulation of this free cytosolic calcium back into the SR lumen promotes muscle relaxation. This process of calcium-induced calcium release is the mechanism through which myocyte electrical depolarization promotes contraction. Particularly important details of this process were provided by the molecular and electrophysiological studies of the voltage-dependent slow calcium channel by Fleckenstein and others [44], the SR ryanodine receptor calcium release channel by Fleischer and others [45], and the SR calcium ATPase by MacLennan, Katz, Tada, and others [46-49].

Beta-adrenergic receptor stimulation provokes the phosphorylation of several myocyte proteins critical for excitation-contraction coupling including SR phospholamban. Phosphorylation of phospholamban dissociates it from the SR calcium ATPase which activates this transporter and enhances the sequestration of cytosolic calcium into the SR lumen [48]. As a result, SR calcium stores increase which contributes both to the positive inotropic effect of beta-adrenergic stimulation and to the production of delayed afterdepolarizations. Myocyte calcium stores likewise increase in response to increased cytosolic sodium, for example following exposure to the Na/K-ATPase inhibitor ouabain. Excess sodium exits myocytes via the plasma membrane sodium-calcium exchange transporter leading to myocyte calcium loading. As first quantitated by Pitts and by Reeves [50,51], this transporter facilitates the electrogenic exchange of three sodium ions for one calcium ion.

Fleischer [45] and others defined the mechanism through which calcium egresses from the SR. They demonstrated that the alkaloid ryanodine binds with high affinity to an SR calci-

http://dx.doi.org/10.5772/53649

um release channel, locks it into an open state, and permits the leakage of SR calcium. Using ryanodine binding as a molecular probe, they identified and purified the ryanodine receptor calcium release channel and demonstrated its central role in calcium-induced calcium release. The development of reporter molecules that measure intracellular free calcium, molecules such as aequorin by Blinks [52] and fura-2 by Grynkiewicz and Tsien [53], allowed the interrogation of the intracellular calcium dynamics of cardiac calcium-induced calcium release.

This myocyte calcium-handling system also offers a cell-based mechanism for triggered activity. Marks [40] and then others [41,54,55], proposed that slow leakage of SR calcium through dysfunctional ryanodine receptors might incite afterdepolarization especially delayed afterdepolarization. This 'calcium leak' hypothesis for triggered arrhythmia (Figure 2) takes advantage of the localization of the ventricular SR ryanodine receptor calcium release channel in SR terminal cisternae near the myocyte T-tubule. It posits that SR calcium leak stimulates calcium efflux on the electrogenic sodium-calcium exchanger which would depolarize myocytes during diastole. Thus conditions that (a) increase the content of myocyte calcium stores, (b) create a steady-state leak of SR calcium or (c) create a preferential leak of calcium during diastole would raise myocyte resting membrane potential to more positive values and reach threshold. Delayed aftedepolarization would result. To some degree this general model may also hold in atrial myocytes that lack well developed T-tubules. Here junctional ryanodine receptors appose the atrial myocyte plasma membranes [54]. Increases in ryanodine receptor calcium leak have been reported in experimentally and pathologically challenged atrial myocytes, indicating that calcium leak might be a generally applicable cause for delayed afterdepolarization. How the disruption of calcium homeostasis generates early afterdepolarization remains under active investigation.

'Hyperphosphorylation' of the ryanodine receptor is proposed to incite its leakiness. Using experimental systems as diverse as lipid bilayers and failing hearts the inventive work of Marks [40] and others supported protein kinase A as the agent that hyperphosphorylates the ryanodine receptor and causes leakiness. Work from the laboratory of Bers [41] and others [54,55] highlighted isoforms of calmodulin-dependent protein kinase II (CaMKII) as a second potential initiator of ryanodine receptor hyperphosphorylation/leakiness. The ryanodine receptor is a large protein critical to the normal function of heart muscle. Thus it is not unexpected that many cell factors regulate its properties including its leakiness; redox stress and the interactions between the FKBP12.6 protein and the ryanodine receptor are two such factors [40,56].

5. Germane questions about 'calcium leak' & afterdepolarization

Several questions arise about the logical & widely accepted calcium-leak hypothesis for triggered arrhythmia.

Does the accepted axis of [SR calcium leakage→electrogenic calcium efflux] describe the entire mechanism for afterdepolarization or does afterdepolarization result from more compli-

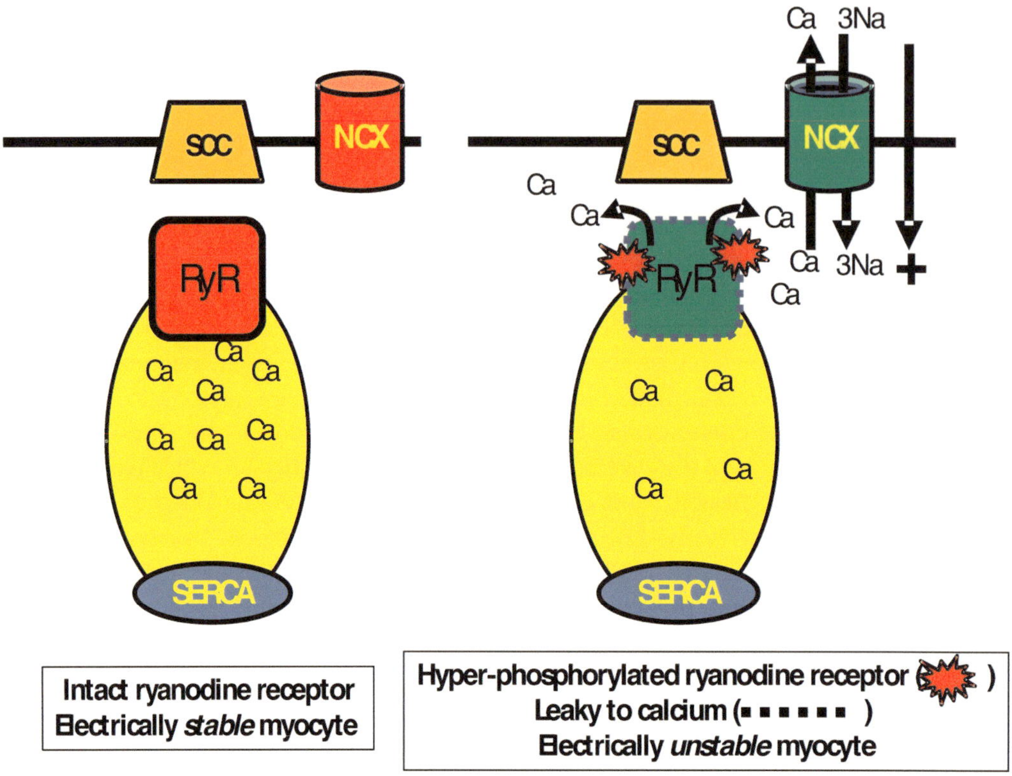

Figure 2. Model for 'Calcium Leak' Afterdepolarization. *Left:* Ryanodine receptors (RyR) are impermeant to calcium except during the action potential when 'trigger calcium' enters myocytes via the voltage-dependent calcium channel (*SCC*). *Right:* Hyper-phosphorylated ryanodine receptors are leaky to calcium. This depletes SR stores. Leaked calcium leaves myocytes on the sodium calcium exchanger (*NCX*). Electrogenic calcium efflux drives positive charges into the myocyte which acts as a depolarizing influence. At impulse threshold, afterdepolarization would occur.

cated molecular pathways? Numerous observations in the literature support the latter view. For example, Ben-David and Zipes [57] showed that reduced repolarization reserve effectively prolongs the action potential duration of intact heart but does not produce a high incidence of arrhythmia. By contrast, alpha-adrenergic agonists provoke fulminant early afterdepolarization and complex arrhythmia in intact hearts with low repolarization reserve. Beta-adrenergic stimulation of these hearts does not provoke arrhythmia. Both Kimura and co -authors and Molina-Viamonte and colleagues [58,59] reported that alpha-adrenergic stimulation provoked delayed afterdepolarization in calcium loaded or ischemic Purkinje fibers. These authors concluded that a specific alpha 1-adrenergic pathway is involved in inducing triggered activity in the setting of ischemia and reperfusion. Finally Lo and coauthors [60] among others report that alpha- and beta-adrenergic receptor stimulation provokes afterdepolarization in intact pulmonary veins and that CaMKII inhibitors block this triggered activity. While SR calcium leak might account for these results, one or more events specific to alpha-adrenergic receptor stimulation/Gαq signaling might also exacerbate afterdepolarization in hearts with reduced repolarization reserve.

- Can the stimulation of Gαq-coupled signaling by means other than the alpha-1 receptor enhance afterdepolarization in isolated pulmonary veins or in hearts with reduced repolarization reserve? There is evidence indicating this is the case [61]. Pharmacological and molecular dissection of the interaction between voltage-independent Gαq-coupled signaling and early- or delayed-afterdepolarization might reveal new mechanisms for arrhythmia.

- Does alpha-adrenergic stimulation of Purkinje fibers, isolated pulmonary veins, and normal heart muscle with reduced repolarization reserve 'hyperphosphorylate' ryanodine receptors compared to normal preparations. If 'hyperphosphorylation' were not to occur, then additional molecular mechanisms contribute to afterdepolarization.

- In the particular case of the pulmonary veins, does calcium loading by approaches other than beta-adrenergic stimulation, approaches like slow calcium channel activation, provoke spontaneous ectopic activity?

- Does 'arrhythmogenic' calcium activate afterdepolarization solely as a charge carrier or as a signaling intermediate that accelerates ryanodine receptor calcium leak? Anderson and co-authors reported in 1998 [62] that CaMKII inhibitors prevent afterdepolarization in intact and isolated cardiac preparations, a result since widely validated [63]. Whether CaMKII acts by hyperphosphorylating the ryanodine receptor or whether it has multiple arrhythmogenic targets remains open to investigation.

- What source of calcium activates CaMKII to provoke triggered activity? Is this source calcium leaked from the SR or might alternate mean exist to activate arrhythmogenic calmodulin and CaMKII?

Triggered afterdepolarization often begins as an isolated event but evolves into more robust and continuous ectopy, so-called sustained triggered activity. This transition depends on the duration of high-frequency burst pacing, the dose of pharmacological activators of the late sodium current, or the apparent timing of R-on-T phenomena. How does the transition from afterdepolarization to complex arrhythmia like tachycardia or fibrillation actually occur? It is now generally accepted that these transitions arise from abnormalities in impulse conduction. In this view, ectopic afterdepolarization triggers reentry in arrhythmogenic 'substrate,' heart muscle that conducts impulses heterogeneously. This facile explanation, however, may not address all potential causes for the transition from isolated to complex ectopy. Might afterdepolarization and sustained activity be manifestations of a common cell arrhythmogenic signaling pathway?

Do both 'isolated' and 'sustained' triggered activities require CaMKII signaling? That is, could myocytes or Purkinje cells express an arrhythmogenic pathway in which CaMKII and afterdepolarization lie upstream of a second calcium-linked mechanism whose stimulation elicits CaMKII-independent 'sustained' ectopic activity?

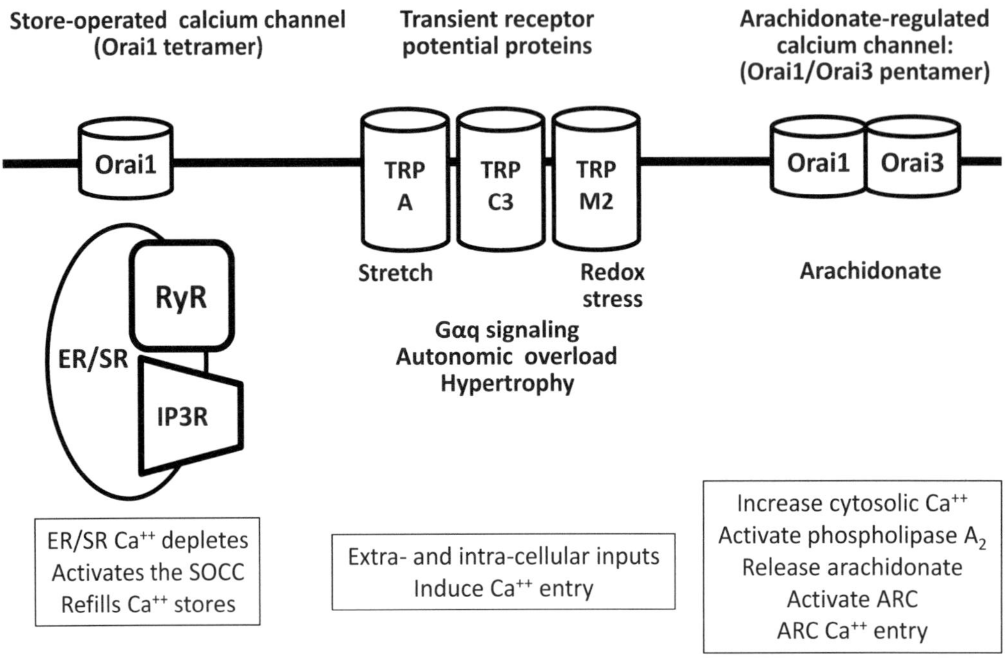

Figure 3. Four Families of Voltage-Independent Calcium Channels. *Left:* IP3Rs allow calcium release from intracellular ER/SR stores. This generates intracellular signals. ER store depletion activates calcium entry via the Orail a/o Orai1/TRPC1 store-operated calcium channel (*Left box*). *Center:* The transient receptor potential channels permit calcium entry into cells in response to a wide range of influences pertinent to atrial fibrillation (*Middle box*). These calcium signals mediate the phenotypic response of atria to stretch or to autonomic signaling. *Right:* Orail and Orai3 create an arachidonate-sensitive calcium channel. This channel permits calcium entry in response to stress signals that activate eicosanoid metabolism (*Right box*).

The well-documented role of calcium in arrhythmogenesis and the central role of SR calcium in heart muscle contraction focused the 'calcium leak' hypothesis on the SR ryanodine receptor as the source of arrhythmogenic calcium. At the time of its formulation only the ryanodine receptor, the voltage-dependent slow calcium channel, and the sodium-calcium exchanger were accepted to greatly affect cytosolic calcium in atrial or ventricular myocytes and Purkinje cells. Now extensive work in non-excitable cells has established the voltage-independent inositol-tris-phosphate receptors (IP3R), the transient receptor potential protein (TRP) channels and the Orai channels are the predominant means to generate cell calcium signals (Figure 3).

Stating our proposition succinctly, do after depolarization and complex arrhythmia arise from cell processes other than those which produce excitation and the ECG (voltage-dependent ion channels) or myocyte contraction (calcium-induced SR calcium release)? Might myocardial non-electrical, voltage-independent processes provoke myocardial electrical instability including after depolarization?

Reports in the literature and our data suggest they do. Myocytes and Purkinje cells express the cellular calcium transporters, kinases, lipases and other proteins that initiate and regulate voltage-independent calcium entry and calcium signaling. These include the IP3Rs, the

TRP channels, the Orai channels, and Stim1. This signaling system normally regulates the Gαq-coupled growth response, stress responses, and other events in all cells including myocytes. Our data and that of others lead to an initial hypothesis that voltage-independent calcium signaling assumes an additional, apparently untoward task in cells like myocytes or Purkinje cells that highly express voltage-dependent ion channels. This task is the activation of a calcium-dependent arrhythmogenic signaling pathway. This putative pathway is normally silent until appropriate arrhythmogenic stimuli or pharmacological activators rouse it into action. Depending on the intensity of the activation challenge, we believe this complex pathway can co-opt the activity of voltage-dependent ion channels to produce isolated afterdepolarization, afterdepolarization that leads to sustained activity, and high frequency sustained ectopic activity. In this view, solitary afterdepolarizations are focal events that result from the activation of one part of a broader calcium-dependent arrhythmogenic pathway. The activation of an interrelated downstream part of this pathway provokes high-frequency focal tachycardia or fibrillation. The two parts of this putative pathway functionally interact which allows the transition between afterdepolarization and complex arrhythmia. This interaction might transpire in a manner analogous to that described by Shuttleworth [64] for the sequential activation of voltage-independent calcium signaling and calcium entry pathways in non-excitable cells. In heart the putative calcium signaling events that cause afterdepolarization would gradually deplete cell voltage-independent calcium stores specific for calcium signaling. This depletion stimulates voltage-independent calcium entry via the Orai channels. We suggest that this type of calcium entry activates sustained ectopic activity.

6. Mechanism 3: Typical abnormal automaticity

Abnormal automaticity occurs when ectopic sites in the atria (*or ventricle*) spontaneously depolarize independently of normal sinus rhythm or without a preceding triggering event. Investigators like Vassalle [65] have made important contributions to our current understanding of this type of ectopy. Typical abnormal automaticity occurs during hypoxia and ischemia when myocytes partially depolarize from their resting potential of ~-85 to about -65mV. An additional mechanism for abnormal automaticity takes advantage of the fact that the hyperpolarization-activated 'funny currents', which contribute to normal automaticity, are expressed throughout the heart [66]. The activation of atrial or ventricular funny currents might induce spontaneous depolarization akin to the sinoatrial pacemaker but the properties of these ectopic channels indicate that they are inactive in normal myocytes. How ectopically expressed funny channels might spring to life to provoke focal abnormal automaticity is unresolved.

Several reports suggest the existence of alternate, atypical forms of abnormal automaticity and that atypical automaticity may be an unrecognized contributor to arrhythmogenesis. For example, in 1999 Nuss and co-workers [67] reported that myocytes isolated from failing hearts produced sporadic, spontaneous depolarizations while normal myocytes did not. These ectopic depolarizations occurred from normal resting potentials, did not require a preceding external stimulation, and occurred independently of any significant change in intracellular calcium homeostasis. Furthermore, the spontaneous action potentials these 'failing' cells produced showed no Phase 4 depolarization which might occur if cell funny currents had somehow become active. One interpretation of this provocative report is that pathological conditions like failure change the fundamental properties of ventricular myocytes, transforming normal, non-automatic myocytes into cells that are capable of an atypical automatic activity. This change survives cell isolation indicating it is reasonably permanent and possibly acutely reversible. Nuss did not define a mechanism to transform non-automatic (*normal*) myocytes to sporadically or rapidly automatic (*failing*) ones. The voltage-independent arrhythmogenic pathway we describe in some detail below is one candidate mechanism.

Robichaux and others [68] assessed the arrhythmogenic mechanisms that underlie experimental fibrillation and reported that reentry does not predominant either soon after the induction of faradic fibrillation or several minutes after the start of fibrillation. Rather they showed that organized sources of relatively regular high frequency ectopic activity drives long-duration ventricular fibrillation. Others also have reported that focal sources of non-reentrant activity predominate during experimental ventricular fibrillation [69]. Automatic activity was among the proposed explanations for both sets of data. It is possible that an atypical form of automaticity underlies these results and affords an unrecognized means to produce sporadic or high frequency myocardial electrical instability.

7. Summary of the mechanisms for arrhythmia

The three current mechanisms for arrhythmia assume that abnormalities in (a) the well-defined process of normal cardiac excitation-contraction coupling, (b) the propagation of electrical waves through the heart or (c) the electrical response of heart muscle to enormous faradic insults circumscribe all the properties of the myocardium needed to fully explain clinical arrhythmia including atrial fibrillation. In other words, all other non-electrical cell processes are by-standers in arrhythmogenesis and they little influence heart muscle electrical stability. None of these three theories is a true focal hypothesis for arrhythmia as envisioned by Engelman and championed by Scherf and others.

Our fourth view of arrhythmia proposes that non-electrical cell signaling events can destabilize the electrical activity of myocytes and conduction system cells. Such destabilization produces isolated focal ectopic events or high frequency focal tachycardia or fibrillation. Thus our unconventional hypothesis for arrhythmia proposes that heart muscle can produce electromechanical activity in two ways. First is by the well-defined pathway of sinus rhythm and impulse conduction. This pathway for normal heart electromechanical activity integrates heart function with systemic physiology. Second, the activation of a cellular 'arrhythmogenic' signaling pathway can transform non-automatic myocytes into cells that spontaneously produce sporadic or high frequency electrical activity independent of external regulators like sinus rhythm or systemic physiology. Aberrant or exuberant myocyte or Purkinje cell voltage-independent calcium homeostasis is one means we have identified to

http://dx.doi.org/10.5772/53649

activate this cryptic arrhythmogenic signaling pathway. The novel fourth mechanism outlined below satisfies the requirements for a purely focal hypothesis for arrhythmia.

8. Mechanism 4: Relevant overview of voltage-independent calcium homeostasis

Cell calcium entry and cell calcium homeostasis are divided operationally into voltage-independent and voltage-dependent domains. Voltage-independent calcium homeostasis regulates non-excitable and excitable cell signaling events that are critical to cell growth, survival, and death. Four families of proteins control the generation and propagation of these calcium signals thereby allowing cells to respond appropriately to challenges or changes in their environment. Two families of plasma membrane calcium transporters permit voltage-independent calcium entry in response to extra- or intra-cellular signals. While cell membrane potential influences these carriers, they are not voltage-gated proteins. A third family of intracellular calcium release channels interacts functionally with these transporters. A fourth family maintains the cell calcium stores used to continually generate calcium signals, a task critical for cell viability. None of these families of voltage-independent proteins is now widely believed to greatly influence heart excitability. Our data and that of others directly challenge this view. They propose that deranged voltage-independent calcium homeostasis and we suggest the dysregulated activity of one family of voltage-independent calcium channels can provoke heart muscle electrical instability.

The first family is the well-characterized Gαq-coupled receptor proteins (Figure 4). A broad range of agonists including bioactive peptides like angiotensin II, bioactive lipids like prostaglandins, and hormones like norepinephrine stimulate this family of receptors. Agonist binding to a specific Gαq-coupled receptor activates a plasma membrane phosphatidylinositoyl-specific phospholipase C. This lipase generates two active intermediates for voltage-independent calcium signaling. Water-soluble inositol-1,4,5-trisphosphate is the first intermediate as defined in the elegant work of Berridge in the 1970s [70]. The second is the membrane-bound lipid diacylglycerol. A highly complex interaction among G-protein regulators, inositol phosphate kinases and phosphatases, and diacylglycerol kinases and lipases set the rate of production and the steady-state levels of these signaling intermediates.

Inositol-1,4,5-trisphosphate diffuses from the environ of the cytosolic face of the plasma membrane and binds with high affinity to the IP3Rs, the second family of proteins central to voltage-independent calcium homeostasis. The ~300kDa IP3Rs are membrane proteins inserted into the endoplasmic reticulum of non-excitable cells and the SR of excitable cells, and are active as tetramers. IP3Rs are calcium release channels that regulate the egress of pools of calcium stored within the lumen of the endoplasmic reticulum or the SR. The IP3R calcium release process is highly regulated and depends on factors including lumen calcium content, cytosolic free calcium, the post-translational modification of the receptor, and the binding of regulator proteins like bcl-2 [71]. IP3R calcium release contributes to cytosolic calcium signaling events through the information encoded in the amplitude of released calci-

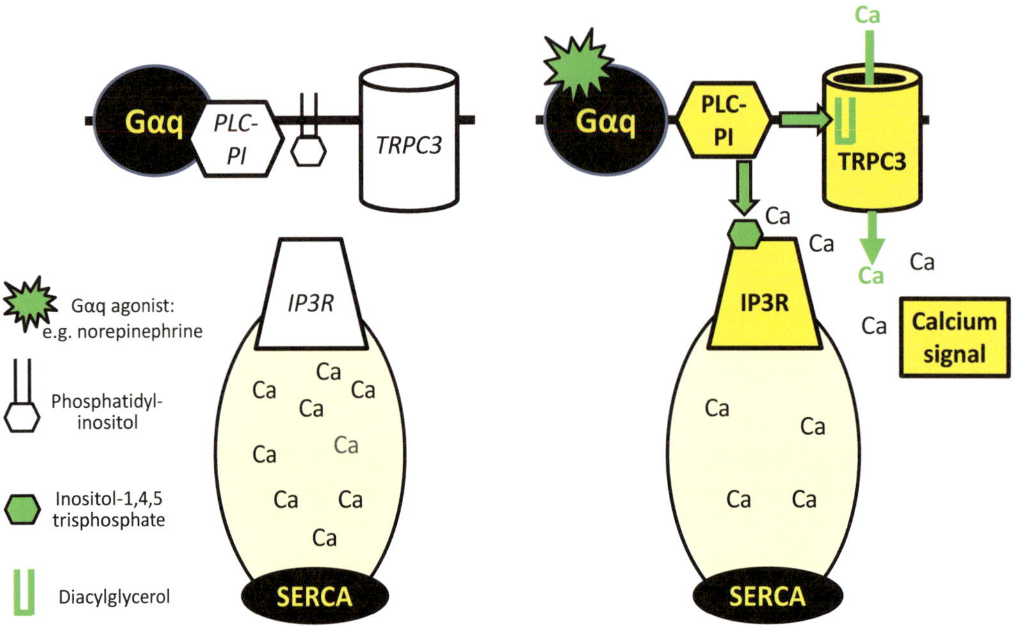

Figure 4. Model of Gag Signaling. Agonist occupation of specific Gαq receptor proteins activate a phosphatidylinositol specific phospholipase C (PLC-PI). Active lipase hydrolyzes plasma membrane phosphatidylinositol. This produces diacylglycerol and inositol-1,4,5-trisphosphate. Both intermediates activate calcium signaling: the former via plasma membrane TRPC3, the latter by binding to the IP3R which initiates SR/ER calcium release.

um and the frequency at which release occurs. Whether the IP3Rs and the ryanodine receptor access identical calcium stores in excitable cells remains an actively investigated question.

Diacylglycerol the second signaling intermediate is hydrophobic so it remains intercalated in membranes following its release from plasma membrane phosphatidylinositol. Diacylglycerol first was believed to signal by activating a protein kinase C. Subsequent work has shown that it also activates members of the third family of voltage-independent calcium signaling proteins which may be germane to arrhythmia, the TRPC family of calcium channels [72,73].

The TRP channels were first identified in drosophila where they play a central role in vision transduction [74]. Subsequent work from the laboratories of Birnbaumer [75], Montell [76], and others identified multiple families of mammalian TRP channels including the classical (TRPC), the melatonin, the vallinoid, and the ankyrin repeat forms. TRP channels contain six transmembrane domains and an ion pore domain which selects calcium over sodium under most conditions. Diacylglycerol released following Gαq receptor stimulation binds to TRPC3 and TRPC6, activates these channels, and permits cell calcium entry. The TRPC1 channel may participate in cell signaling as a subunit of the store-operated calcium channel (SOCC) which maintains cell calcium stores [75]. The TRPM3 &TRPA channels appear to activate when cells are stretched while TRPM2 responds to increased oxidant stress [75]. Calcium entering cells through the TRP channels spark downstream signaling responses to receptor stimulation or to environmental challenges. As muscle stretch and oxidant stress contribute to the pathophysiology of atrial fibrillation [77], calcium entry linked to TRP channels may contribute to the hypertrophy and fibrosis that accompany atrial fibrillation.

In 1986 Putney raised a critically important question about voltage-independent calcium homeostasis [78]. He noted that calcium release events initiated by inositol-1,4,5-trisphosphate could deplete intracellular calcium stores. This depletion would disrupt continued calcium signaling. Putney proposed that cells must contain a mechanism to sense the calcium content of their stores and promote calcium entry in response to store depletion. This logical proposition was widely accepted. Electrophysiological and calcium imaging protocols clearly demonstrate that depleting cell calcium stores in calcium-free media provokes a dramatic calcium entry when external calcium is restored to these cells. That is, calcium store depletion activates a cell mechanism to replenish these stores. The initial hypotheses to explain SOCC calcium entry included a calcium-inducible factor, a direct-coupling mechanism between the store and the channel involving the actin cytoskeleton, and an indirect coupling mechanism [79]. In 2005, however, the elegant molecular mechanism for SOCC calcium entry came into focus. Dziadek and colleagues [80] identified stromal interaction molecule 1 (Stim1) which subsequently was shown to be a sensor for the lumenal calcium of the endoplasmic reticulum. Stim1 resides mainly in the endoplasmic reticulum, contains a single transmembrane domain, and has a calcium-binding EF-hand domain positioned within the lumen of the endoplasmic reticulum. In unstimulated cells, Stim1 distributes throughout the endoplasmic reticulum membrane. Depletion of calcium from the endoplasmic reticulum lumen by any mechanism including calcium release through the IP3R causes Stim1 to translocate to plasma membrane-endoplasmic reticulum junctions. Here Stim1 docks with plasma membrane SOCCs and activates SOCC calcium entry which repletes cell calcium stores [81].

Controversy exists about the exact molecular constituents of the SOCC. In one current paradigm plasma membrane Orai1 proteins constitute the SOCC. This model proposes that Orai1 distributes throughout the plasma membrane of cells with full calcium stores, calcium replete cells, and is inactive. Calcium store depletion causes Stim1 to translocate to endoplasmic reticulum-plasma membrane junctions. Stim1 there binds and activates Orai1 to allow calcium entry. In this model the active channel is an Orai1 tetramer [82]. An alternate model posits a complex of Orai1 and TRPC1 or other isoforms of TRPC as the active calcium channel which responds to cell store-depletion but not to extracellular depolarizing influences [75]. Regardless of this debate, the Orai proteins are the fourth family of proteins critical to voltage-independent calcium homeostasis whose tightly regulated function allows continued physiological calcium signaling.

How might this general SOCC pathway relate to current views of arrhythmia? As one example, SR calcium store depletion through 'leaky' ryanodine receptor might initiate [Stim1-Orai1/TRPC1] voltage-independent calcium entry in an effort to maintain SR or other myocyte calcium stores. This type of calcium entry may exacerbate the driving force for afterdepolarization posited by Marks and others(Figure 5). It also might provoke more serious unexpected forms of electrical instability which we outline below.

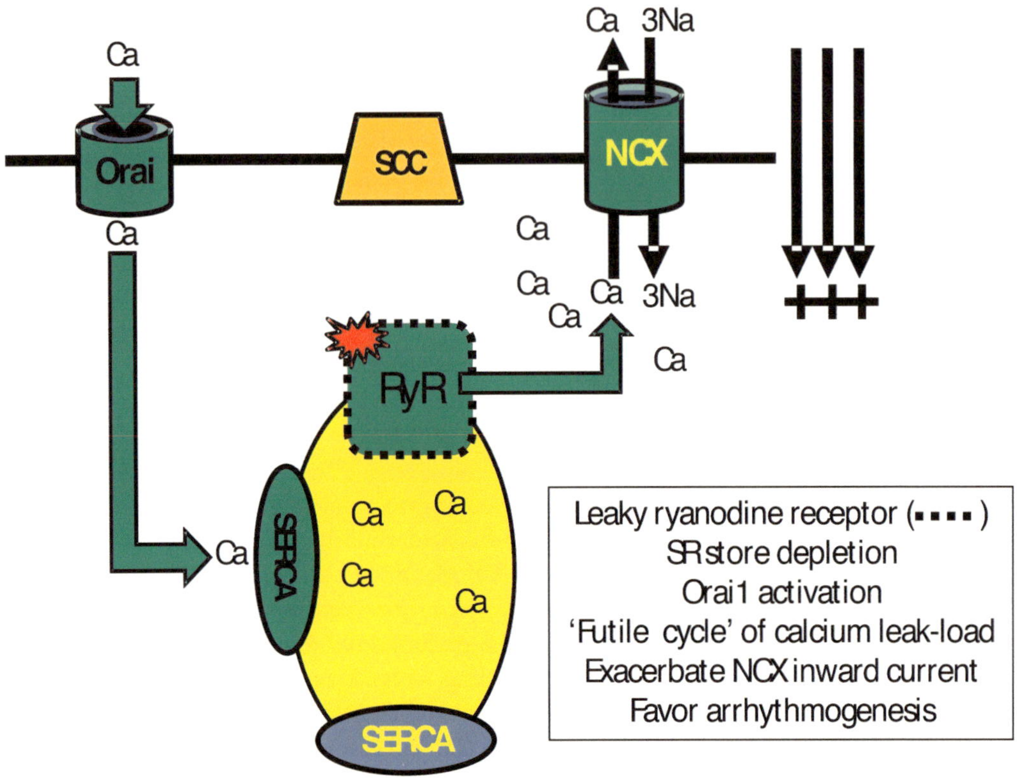

Figure 5. Potential Interaction between Orai Calcium Entry and Arrhythmogenic SR Calcium Leak. Calcium leak through the ryanodine receptor. (*RyR & right green arrow*) depletes SR calcium. This depletion may activate Orai1-linked calcium entry (*Left green arrow*) to maintain E-C patency & muscle function. A futile cycle of calcium entry-leak may exacerbate NCX-linked calcium efflux and cell depolarization, driving it more frequently or more quickly toward threshold (*Rightmost black arrows*).

Orai2 and Orai3 are the remaining members of this fourth family. Orai2 is a pseudogene and has garnered some interest. By contrast, Shuttleworth first demonstrated that Orai3 is an important participant in voltage-independent calcium signaling [64]. Elegant work from his lab group shows that pentamers of Orai3 and Orai1 form an arachidonate regulated calcium channel (ARC). Arachidonate binding to ARC causes channel activation and permits voltage-independent calcium entry. Like the SOCC, ARC also requires Stim1 but it uses the small pool of Stim1 present in the plasma membrane. The arachidonate which activates ARC can arise from several sources. In cell culture experiments it is usually added exogenously. Calcium-dependent cytosolic phospholipase A_2 is a key source of cellular free arachidonate in physiological settings. Importantly, the arachidonate arising from the action of calcium-dependent cytosolic phospholipase A_2 on cell phospholipids is a key source for inflammatory prostaglandins and leukotrienes. CaMKII phosphorylates and activates this phospholipase [83]. Thus two possibilities emerge. First, myocyte calcium loading may activate CaMKII which then phosphorylates cytosolic calcium-dependent phospholipase A_2;

second, the arachidonate this lipase produces may activate ARC, voltage-independent calcium entry, the production of inflammatory molecules, and possibly ectopic activity.

The past 50 years of research in heart calcium and arrhythmogenesis have focused principally on voltage-dependent calcium homeostasis. Indeed there are only few reports which identify atrial, ventricular, sinoatrial or Purkinje cell expression of the molecular constituents of voltage-independent calcium homeostasis. Even fewer of these reports detail the unique intracellular distribution of these proteins in the different types of heart cells or study how this pattern of distribution might contribute to arrhythmogenesis.

Bootman and co-authors [84] provide convincing evidence that atrial myocytes contain predominately the type 2 IP3R. They show that atrial myocytes express about 10-fold more IP3R than do ventricular myocytes. An impressive observation they and others report is that this calcium release channel distributes mainly in the junctional SR near to the sarcolemmal membrane and that these IP3Rs associate with the junctional ryanodine receptors that encircle each atrial myocyte. Bootman and others suggest that these IP3Rs sensitize ryanodine receptor calcium release and may participate in the response of atria to inotropic $G\alpha q$ receptor agonists.

Only little is known about the expression of the TRP channels, the Orai channels, and the Stim proteins in normal atrial muscle and pulmonary veins. To our knowledge how pathological situations like paroxysmal or sustained atrial fibrillation affect the expression of these calcium channels and channel regulators has not been investigated. This is important information as these families of proteins control the induction of hypertrophy, the response to stretch, fibrosis, and the intrinsic pathway for apoptosis. A complete evaluation of these signaling proteins in normal and diseased atria would dissect the molecular mechanisms through which atria responds to clinically relevant stressors and how these responses may favor dysfunction including electrical instability like atrial fibrillation.

Ventricular myocytes contain much lower levels of the IP3Rs relative to atria. Of interest Mohler [85] and others report that ventricular IP3Rs preferentially associate with the parajunctional SR of the T-tubule. The purpose or consequence of the specific localization of these calcium release channels is actively investigated. The responsiveness of heart muscle to $G\alpha q$ stimulation increases during hypertrophy and heart failure. These results are in keeping with reports that the expression of ventricular IP3Rs increases in these diseases. Using probes specific for the type 1 IP3R, Marks [86] showed that the ventricular content of these channels nearly triples in failing heart while characteristically the content of the ryanodine receptor decreases by a factor of at least two. Little is known about the expression or functional properties of ventricular TRP channels, Orai channels, and Stim proteins either in normal or diseased heart.

By comparison with the paucity of work in ventricular myocytes, in 1994 Volpe [87] provided the first evidence that IP3Rs are highly expressed in the conduction system. Subsequent elegant and thorough analyses by Boyden, ter Keurs and colleagues demonstrated an intricate distribution of the IP3Rs and the ryanodine receptors in the Purkinje cells of the conduction system [88]. Much like atrial myocytes, the IP3Rs distribute at the periphery of

Purkinje cells. Here they associate with ryanodine receptors within specific regions of the cytoplasm just below the Purkinje plasma membrane. Boyden, ter Keurs and co-authors speculate that this striking arrangement plays a role in the arrhythmogenic potential of the conduction system. Establishing this critically important conclusion is a clear priority in arrhythmia research. Little is known about Purkinje cell expression of the TRP channels, the Orai channels or Stims. One could speculate that Stim1, Orai1 and TRPC1 might be highly expressed in the conduction system as they are functionally related to the IP3Rs. One question of potential importance is whether the marked increase in IP3R expression reported in failing heart occurs in the Purkinje system, in myocytes or in both. Furthermore, it would be useful to determine whether the expression of Orai1, Stim1, and TRPC1 respond similarly to 'failure' as do the IP3Rs. If the expression of these three IP3R partners were to increase, then the activity or hyperactivity of voltage-independent calcium signaling may contribute to the increased arrhythmogenicity seen in heart failure, as Boyden and ter Keurs speculate [88].

Ju and co-authors [89] and Demion and co-authors [90] reported that the sinoatrial node expresses the TRP channels which play a role in normal automaticity. A more detailed analysis of the expression of other voltage-independent calcium signaling proteins and how they contribute to normal automaticity is clearly required. To our knowledge nothing is known of the expression or activity of voltage-independent calcium signaling proteins in the muscular sleeves of the pulmonary or other supraventricular vessels. Since alpha-adrenergic agonists induce afterdepolarization and automatic activity in these anatomical structures, characterizing 'muscular sleeve' TRP channel, Orai channel, Stim, and IP3R expression should aid in establishing whether these channels contribute to paroxysmal atrial fibrillation.

9. Is voltage-independent calcium signaling a focal source of arrhythmia?

Experimental evidence acquired in intact animals, in intact heart muscle, and intact pulmonary veins coupled with clinical studies of human arrhythmia strongly suggest that $G\alpha q$-coupled receptor stimulation and by inference voltage-independent calcium signaling can initiate afterdepolarization and more complex arrhythmia. However, no attempt was made in these intact preparations to positively connect the calcium signaling linked to IP3Rs, the TRP channels or the Orai channels to atrial electrical instability.

Bootman and Blatter [84,91] acquired such evidence in isolated atrial myocytes. They demonstrated that $G\alpha q$ agonists like endothelin-1 and pharmacological activators of the IP3Rs provoke ectopic calcium sparks, calcium waves, spontaneous calcium transients, and calcium alternans in atrial myocytes. Both groups concluded that exuberant calcium release from IP3Rs sensitizes the junctional ryanodine receptors of atrial myocytes, increasing their susceptibility to spontaneous calcium release events. Importantly, low concentrations of 2APB that block both the IP3Rs and the TRP channels suppress abnormal atrial myocyte calcium release. Blatter then showed [92] that the genetic ablation of the atrial myocyte type 2 IP3R suppresses 'arrhythmogenic' calcium release in atrial myocytes treated with endothelin-1.

Together these data support and extend earlier intact animal studies and provide striking evidence that voltage-independent calcium homeostasis contributes to atrial arrhythmogenic calcium signaling.

The depletion of inositol-1,4,5-trisphosphate sensitive calcium stores which likely occurs with high levels of Gαq stimulation provokes SOCC calcium entry [64,78,81,82]. Thus while disturbed inositol-1,4,5-trisphosphate-linked calcium signaling is arrhythmogenic, it remains open to question whether (a) calcium release through IP3Rs, (b) the attendant increase in SOCC calcium entry or (c) both provoke ectopy. Furthermore whether these ectopic calcium release events produce myocyte depolarization in a 1:1 manner remains to be established as well as the mechanism through which ectopic depolarization might occur. It is also important to define whether the cause for abnormal depolarization in these myocytes is solely or mainly calcium efflux on the sodium-calcium exchanger or if other calcium signaling events are involved.

Hirose and co-authors [93] used transgenesis to obtain molecular and pharmacological evidence that dysregulated Gαq-coupled calcium signaling profoundly disrupts atrial and ventricular electrical stability. They employed a mouse model developed by Mende [94] which transiently overexpresses constitutively active Gαq in a heart-specific manner. The atria of these genetically modified mice are grossly enlarged and exhibit paroxysmal or persistent fibrillation. To establish that deranged diacylglycerol metabolism caused these atrial abnormalities, Hirose created a second mouse which overexpresses both Gαq and diacylglycerol kinase ζ. Such a double transgenic would accelerate diacylglycerol phosphorylation to phosphatidic acid, reduce heart content of diacylglycerol, and thus TRPC3 signaling. Mice harboring both transgenes had essentially normal atrial anatomy and electrical activity. The current reentry hypothesis for atrial fibrillation would propose that the electrical instability observed in the atria of Gαq overexpressors results from atrial enlargement and from the high levels of fibrosis observed in these muscles. In this electrocentric view, transgenically increasing diacylglycerol kinase activity would suppress atrial fibrillation by restoring normal atrial size and by reducing arrhythmogenic atrial scarring/abnormal conduction. Curiously, reentry also proposes electrical abnormalities like fibrillation should not occur in muscles as small as mouse atria (*or ventricle*) [20,22,24]. Vaidya and authors [95] first reported a similar egregious violation of Garrey's 'critical mass' tenet for reentry when they reported the occurrence of faradic fibrillation in mouse heart. They postulated unusual forms of wavebreak to account for this unexpected result.

Hirose and co-authors addressed this possible interpretation of their data in a follow-on paper [96]. Here they investigated how Gαq overexpression affected ventricular electrical stability and heart failure. They observed that mice which overexpress constitutively active Gαq exhibit heart failure and sustained or paroxysmal ventricular tachycardia and fibrillation. Some of the ventricular arrhythmia recorded in these transgenic mice may result from the irregularly irregular electrical activity produced by fibrillating atria but much of this ectopy appeared to originate in the ventricles themselves. Importantly, they reported that the acute administration of SKF-96365, a TRP and Orai channel inhibitor [97], reverses ventricular fibrillation and restores sinus rhythm in Gαq transgenic mice. This result could only occur if SKF-96365 also effectively suppressed atrial fibrillation in these animals. It is vital to remember that the atria of these transgenic mice treated acutely with SKF-96365 remained grossly enlarged and fibrotic. This single result, obtained in a model which mimics the high autonomic drive associated with atrial fibrillation, dissociates fibrillation from atrial enlargement and fibrosis.

Hirose's data argue that a focal, non-reentrant mechanism can produce atrial and ventricular fibrillation. Specifically, the genetic activation of Gαq-coupled signaling promotes cardiac hypertrophy which would enlarge the atria in Gαq transgenic mice. Atrial fibrosis may result from enhanced Gαq signaling or from the activation of specific gene programs. This transgenic intervention enhances heart diacylglycerol content and consequently the activity of TRPC3/6. Exuberant Gαq stimulation, voltage-independent calcium entry and signaling might deplete or disrupt voltage-independent calcium stores initiating compensatory SOCC calcium entry. The acute administration of SKF-96365 would block calcium entry via TRPC3/6 and/or the Orai1/3 channels. Thus calcium entry via voltage-independent calcium channels or arrhythmogenic signaling events downstream of these channels may cause atrial and ventricular fibrillation in this model.

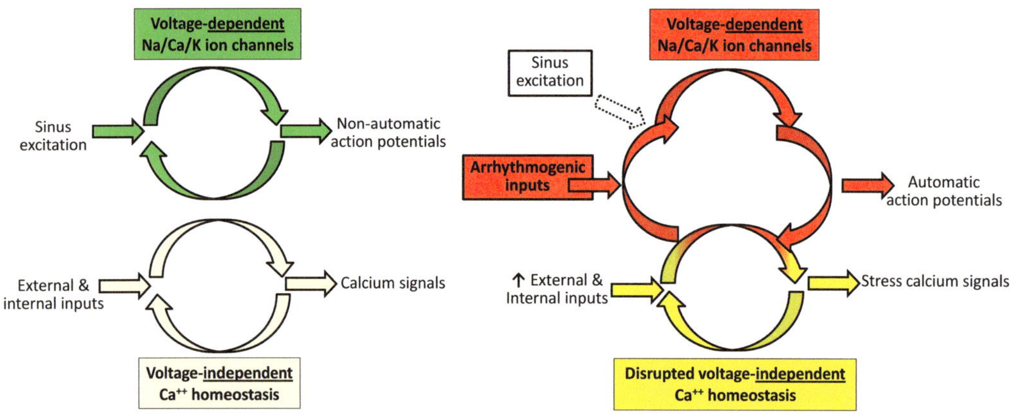

Figure 6. General Model for a Voltage-Independent Mechanism for Arrhythmia. *Left:* **Normal:** - Voltage-dependent ion channels regulate excitation-contraction coupling in normal cells while voltage-independent calcium signaling controls growth and apoptosis. *Right:* **Arrhythmogenic**: In stressed cells, voltage-independent calcium signaling subserves a novel, untoward function. It co-opts voltage-dependent ion channels to act independently of external electrical impulses and produce high frequency ectopic depolarizations. These arrhythmogenic foci of myocytes electrically capture the heart, subvert organized sinus rhythm & cause arrhythmia.

The reentry hypothesis would propose that rhythm disturbances in Gαq overexpressing mice occur because hypertrophy and fibrosis provide an 'arrhythmogenic substrate' that inhomogeneously conducts electrical impulses. In a reentrant view fibrosis, hypertrophy, and arrhythmia cannot be completely dissociated. By contrast, a focal view proposes that arrhythmia arises from cell signaling events that may be functionally distinct from those that produce fibrosis or hypertrophy; these three events may be dissociable. Hirose's SKF-96365 data support a focal view. If the atrial and ventricular fibrillation in these mice were self-

http://dx.doi.org/10.5772/53649

sustaining and provoked by atrial enlargement and fibrotic substrate, they should not have reversed abruptly or at all. That they did suggests that cell events may indeed drive this arrhythmic activity.

These data in humans, intact animals, preparations of pulmonary vascular tissue, and in isolated myocytes pinpoint voltage-independent calcium homeostasis as an underappreciated source of arrhythmia (Figure 6). That is, these types of signaling events when regulated and occurring at normal levels allow hearts to increase mass in response to hypertrophic stimuli. By contrast, the dysregulation or hyperactivity of one or more aspects of voltage-independent calcium entry or downstream signaling appears to elicit spontaneous sporadic or high frequency ectopic depolarizations in intact atria and ventricle. Consequently some arrhythmia might be purely a cell's response to extra- or intra-cellular conditions that disrupt voltage-independent calcium homeostasis. Note that in contrast to 'calcium leak' models which often require burst pacing to induce atrial (*or ventricular*) arrhythmia [40,54,55], the disruption of voltage-independent calcium homeostasis results in intact heart muscle spontaneously producing profound complex arrhythmia.

While provocative these evidences for a focal mechanism for arrhythmia leave unanswered at least four questions.

- Which part or parts of voltage-independent calcium homeostasis underlie this arrhythmic activity, (a) calcium release through the IP3R, (b) calcium entry via one of more of the TRP channels, (c) calcium entry via the Orai channels and/or (d) calcium signaling downstream of these channels?
- Can this novel mechanism for arrhythmia account for the gamut of ectopic activities from sporadic depolarization to paroxysmal or sustained tachycardia to fibrillation?
- How might pathological stimuli or high autonomic activity favor the activation of this arrhythmogenic mechanism?
- What is the final molecular initiator of this putative focal mechanism for arrhythmia?

Work from our laboratory has begun to address these questions using the following rationale.

Lewis [98,99], Putney [78], Shuttleworth [64] and others identify voltage-independent calcium homeostasis as a dynamic process that depends on the inter-relationship between multiple families of calcium channels and the filling state of intracellular calcium stores. In this model Gαq agonists provoke calcium entry via TRPC3 as well as the release of calcium from internal stores regulated by IP3Rs. These calcium entry and release events sum to generate intracellular signals which are then terminated by re-accumulation of calcium into the endoplasmic reticulum lumen. The net flux of calcium out of the reticular lumen is a sum of all inputs experienced by a cell under any particular physiological or pathophysiological conditions. As one or more of these agonist signals increases in intensity, the local or the net calcium content of the reticular calcium stores begins to decrease. As stores deplete, the [Stim1-Orai1/TRPC1] channel complex activates to refill them, permitting continued calcium signaling. Excessive or continual calcium store depletion initiates a strong SOCC calcium entry response. Earlier studies suggest a potent arrhythmic effect associates with excessive or

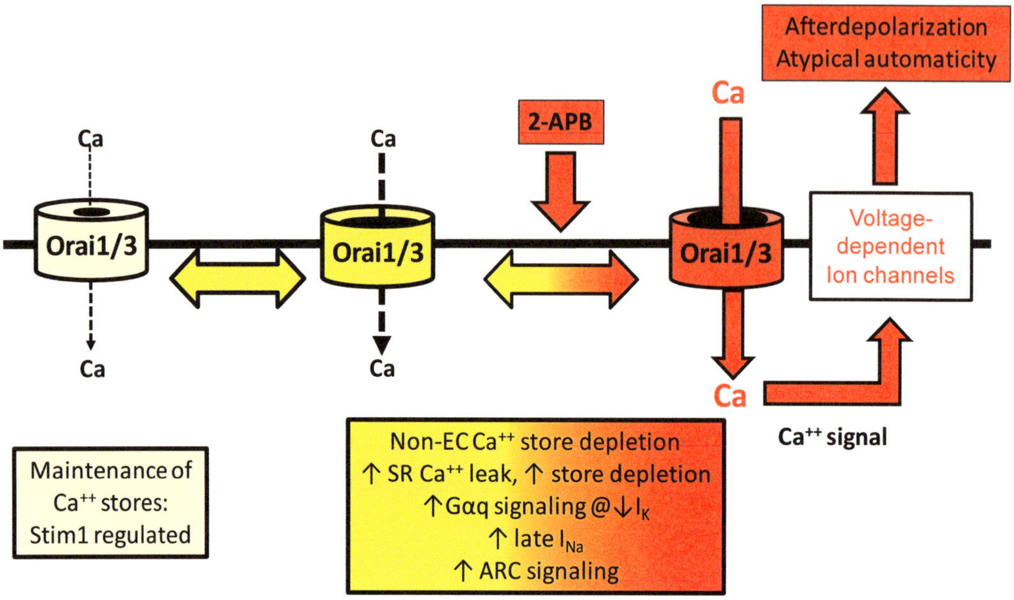

Figure 7. Model for Orai Arrhythmogenesis. *Left:* Under normal conditions Orais are tightly regulated and not arrhythmogenic. *Center*: Low level dysregulation (or activation) of Orais by numerous factors (*Lower right box*) will produce a progressive arrhythmic effect. At intermediate levels the calcium signal will provoke afterdepolarization. *Right*: At high levels of Orai opening the calcium signal co-opts myocyte voltage-dependent ion channels to provoke ~20Hz atypical automaticity and fibrillation. 2APB causes automatic tachycardia and fibrillation in this manner.

dysregulated activation of this overall pathway [57-61]. The interpretation of this data focused on calcium release through the IP3R and showed that pharmacological blockade or genetic ablation of this protein suppresses ectopic electromechanical activity. However, (a) Gαq stimulation, (b) voltage-independent calcium release from the IP3Rs, and (c) Orai-linked SOCC calcium entry are interrelated events [64,98]. Thus exuberant arrhythmogenic Gαq stimulation [96] or IP3R calcium release [91,92] will activate Orai-linked calcium entry (Figure 7). Previous experiments did not fully address whether the first two of these voltage-independent events or the third one, Orai-linked calcium entry, might drive arrhythmic activity. Thus we wished to test whether increased Orai channel opening might be an unrecognized arrhythmic principle (Figure 7). This requires a means to activate the Orais.

Putney reported [100] that 2-aminoethoxydiphenyl borate (2APB) activates calcium entry in non-excitable cells apparently by a store-operated mechanism. Subsequent work [101-102] conclusively demonstrated that 2APB pharmacologically opens Orai1 with an EC_{50} of 20μM and Orai3 with an EC_{50} of 13μM. 2APB also alters the ion conduction properties of these channels to enhance sodium transport. We took advantage of this Orai channel opener to interrogate in a crude manner whether activating voltage-independent calcium channels might underlie a focal mechanism for arrhythmia.

We found that 2APB provokes a novel type of arrhythmic activity [103-106] which appears to satisfy the demands of the focal source hypothesis of Engelmann and Scherf. In particular,

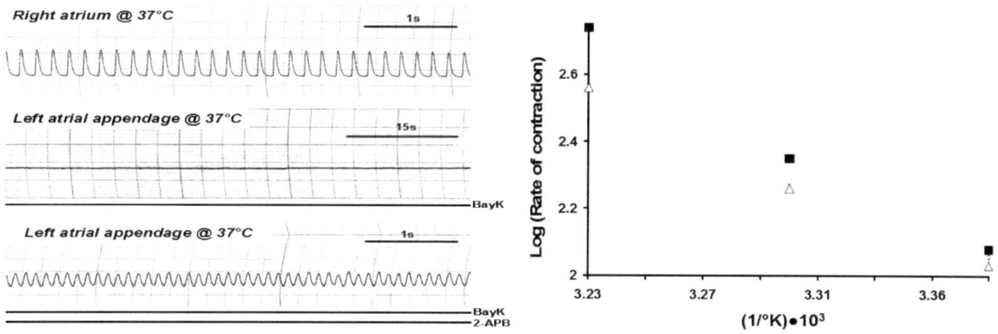

Figure 8. 2APB Activation of 10Hz Atypical Automaticity in Superfused Rat Left Atria.*Left. Upper:* The mechanical function of an unpaced rat right atrium superfused at 37°C. Spontaneous sinoatrial node-driven normal automaticity occurs at −6Hz in this muscle. *Middle:* An unpaced rat left atrial appendage superfused with 300nM Bayk at 37°C. This left atrium and all others do not contract under this condition. *Bottom.* An unpaced rat left atrium superfused with 300nM BayK and 20μM 2APB. This muscle produces spontaneous mechanical activity at 10Hz. *Right.* Summary of groups of unpaced right atria (Δ; n=7) superfused at 23, 30, and 37°C and unpaced left atria superfused with BayK and 20μM 2APB (■; n=9) at 23, 30, and 37°C. Left atria treated with BayK and 2APB perfused at 37°C spontaneously contract at rates of 543±13 contractions/minute.

intact, superfused normal rat left atria and rat left ventricular papillary muscles begin to spontaneously contact when they are challenged with 2APB at concentrations greater than 10μM. This ectopic activity takes several minutes to arise following muscle exposure to 2APB but once initiated it occurs persistently until this borinate is removed from the superfusate. Increasing muscle calcium by several disparate means including slow channel activation and ouabain markedly increases the rate of this ectopic activity [104 *see Table I*]. Under well-defined conditions isolated left atria and left ventricular papillaries can produce persistent ectopic activity at rates of at least 10 to 12 Hz at 37°C (Figure 8). These rates are similar to those reported for arrhythmic drivers of clinical and experimental arrhythmia [107]. Reentrant mechanisms are usually invoked to explain such drivers but cell-based focal means may also exist to provoke persistent high frequency ectopy. The disruption of heart muscle electromechanical stability by 2APB is not self-sustaining as this high frequency ectopy stops immediately after the removal of this molecule from the superfusate. One implication from this reversible destabilization is that a cell-based voltage-independent mechanism for arrhythmia would produce electrical instability only as long as it remains stimulated. Paroxysmal or persistent arrhythmia thus might result if the pathological disturbance of voltage-independent calcium homeostasis were ephemeral or unrelenting in nature regardless of the presence or absence of arrhythmogenic 'substrate.' Hirose's work and our data in fibrillating hearts discussed in a following section substantiate this speculation.

2APB induces a unique atypical automaticity in non-automatic heart muscle. Specifically, 2APB provokes high frequency ectopic action potentials and muscle contraction even when added to the superfusate of quiescent left atria or left ventricular papillary muscles [105 *see Figure 3*]. That is, non-automatic heart muscle which normally requires external stimulation to produce action potentials and contract will do both spontaneously, at high-frequency, and in the absence of a triggering depolarizing stimulus if these quiescent muscles are exposed to 2APB. The action potentials produced by these spontaneously contracting muscles are identical to those produced by electrically paced untreated muscles [105 *see Figure 2 & Table I*]. That is, exposing non-automatic normal left atria and papillary muscles to >10μM 2APB causes them to produce spontaneous normal action potentials and muscle contractions at extremely high frequency in the absence of an external electrical stimulus. Under all other conditions, these muscles require an external electrical stimulus to generate an action potential and contract (Figure 8 Left; *middle panel*). These ectopic action potentials also occur from normal resting potentials and have no visible Phase 4-type depolarization. These criteria rule that 2APB induces neither a triggered activity nor typical abnormal automaticity as defined earlier. Heart muscle thus may contain a cryptic pathway whose activation transforms non-automatic tissue to a fully automatic state.

Several pharmacological studies assessed whether 2APB provokes atypical automaticity through the activation of Orai channels. SKF-96365, an inhibitor of calcium entry via the TRP and the Orai channels, completely prevents or reverses 2APB-linked atypical automaticity [105 *see Figure 3 & 5*]. Importantly, if paced left atria or papillary muscles are exposed to 2APB, they produce electromechanical activity independently of the pacing stimulus. That is, they produce both paced and 'spontaneous' electromechanical events. SKF-96365 added to the superfusate stops only the spontaneous ectopy which occurs independently of pacing. These isolated muscles then follow the pacing stimulus faithfully, requiring external pacing to contract or produce action potentials [105 *see e.g. Figure 5*]. ML-7, a congener of a second inhibitor of Orai-linked calcium entry [108], also suppresses this high frequency atypical automaticity as do two calmodulin inhibitors [105 *see Figure 6*]. These data suggest that the Orai channels and cell calcium signaling participate in converting non-automatic muscles to an automatic state. These atrial and papillary muscles weighed 3 to 5mg wet-weight. Thus they were unlikely to support reentry based on the criteria of Garrey and Moe. The high frequency automaticity they produced following the presumed activation of the Orai channels could, however, form focal sites of paroxysmal or permanent electrical instability in intact heart muscle.

Some current hypotheses for focal arrhythmia require high levels of SR calcium (SR calcium load) to drive afterdepolarization or more complex arrhythmia [40, 41,55]. In support of this view, increased muscle calcium has long been known to favor arrhythmogenesis. However, SR calcium load decreases in heart failure, a condition that also exhibits high rates of arrhythmia. Thus muscle calcium load appears to not always associate with ectopic activity. Despite this paradoxical complication, a great deal of exquisite experimental expertise has defined SR calcium leak rates in relation to SR calcium load with an eye toward explaining arrhythmogenic activity in failing heart [109]. Rates of 2APB atypical automaticity increase with increases in muscle calcium, so we wished to test whether SR calcium stores were, in fact, critical to the persistence of atypical automaticity. Left atria were challenged with BayK 8644 to increase their calcium content and then with 2APB to provoke high frequency atypical automaticity. These unpaced muscles produced persistent action potentials and contractions at a very fast rate (Figures 9A & 9B). Treating these muscles with 800nM ryanodine greatly reduces their force of contraction, evidence for ryanodine receptor opening and near complete SR calcium store depletion (Figure 9C). Interestingly, these muscles continue to produce spontaneous action potentials at a high rate (Figure 9D) with no discernible difference in their characteristics compared to action potentials produced in 'calcium loaded' muscles (cp. Figures 9B & 9D). Treating these spontaneously contracting muscles with SKF-96365 abolished any residual automatic contractions (Figure 9E), and these muscle now required pacing to produce action potentials (Figure 9F, *cp. Rest with 3Hz pacing*).

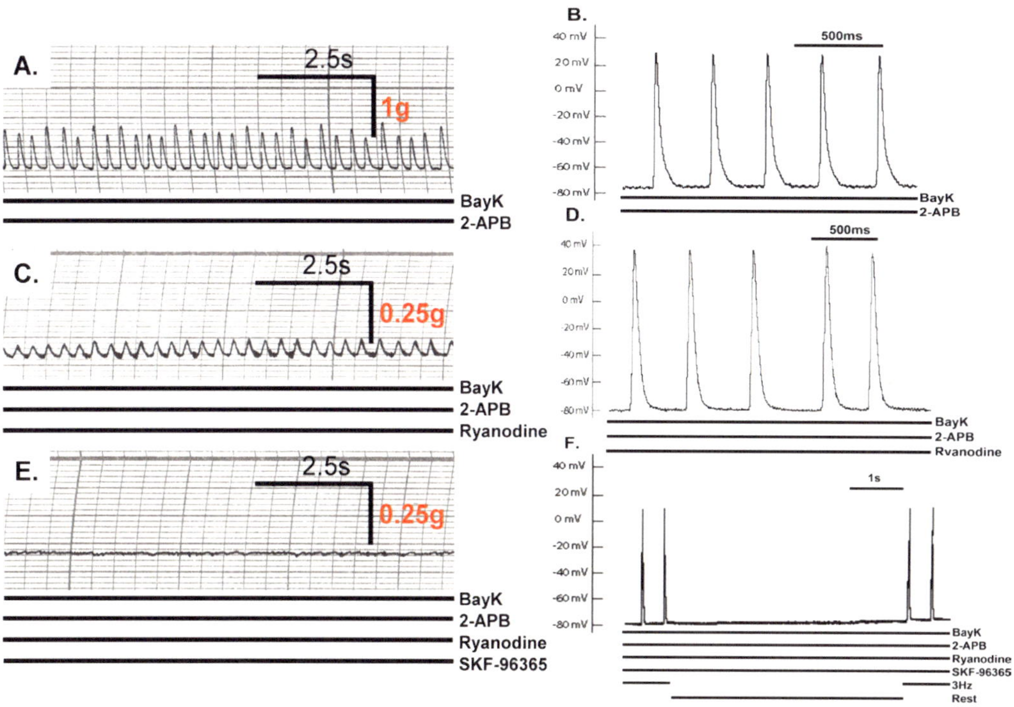

Figure 9. Ryanodine Depletion of Left Atrial SR Calcium Does Not Affect 2APB Atypical Automaticity. (A) Mechanical function of an *unpaced* left atrium treated with 300nM BayK 8644 (BayK) and 22μM 2APB (2APB). Atypical mechanical automaticity is observed. **(B)** Action potentials from an *unpaced* left atrium treated as in (A). Spontaneous, automatic action potentials are recorded. **(C)** Mechanical function of a left atrium treated as in (A), ~8min after exposure to 800nM ryanodine (*Ryanodine*). Ryanodine depresses mechanical function by opening the ryanodine channel which leaks SR calcium (*N.B.* force scales on right of (A) & (C)). Automatic mechanical activity persists but at low levels. **(D)** Electrical activity of a left atrium treated as in (C). Spontaneous electrical activity continues unabated. **(E)** Mechanical function of an atrium treated as in (C) followed by SKF-96365 (*SKF-96365: 50μM*). SKF-96365 blocks spontaneous mechanical activity. **(F)** Electrical activity of a left atrium treated as in (E) in the absence (*Rest*) or presence (3Hz) of 3Hz pacing. No action potentials are recorded in the presence of SKF-96365; it blocks spontaneous ectopy. Pacing is required to generate action potentials (3Hz).

We then compared how an alternate calcium efflux enhancer, caffeine affected the rate of atypical automaticity. In these experiments left atria were not 'loaded' with calcium before they were exposed to 2APB; loading was avoided to assess how the disruption of normal calcium stores affected automaticity.

Impressively, 10mM caffeine markedly increased the rate of left atrial spontaneous contraction from 106±25 to 362±38 contractions per minute (Figure 10). This significant increase in the rate of atypical automaticity was transient as after 3 to 5 minutes of exposure to these conditions the rates of automaticity decrease to 10±7 per minute. Normal paced mechanical function remained intact albeit at lower forces of contraction because of caffeine treatment (Data not shown).

This notable result leads to four interesting speculations. First, the rates of atypical automaticity measured in caffeine-treated muscles at 30°C are about 50% faster than those measured for 'calcium loaded' atria at the same temperature [104-105]. Thus calcium loading does not produce the most rapid rates of automaticity, caffeine a calcium efflux agent does. Second, the rate of atypical automaticity does not greatly slow with the depletion of ryanodine-sensitive SR calcium. Thus a distinction must exist between ryanodine and caffeine in their interaction with the source of atypical automaticity. Third, if the rate of automatic activity observed with caffeine treatment exhibits identical Q_{10}s as our earlier data (Figure 8), then this type of atypical automaticity might reach rates of ~15Hz at 37°C. Fourth, ryanodine calcium stores do not appear to greatly influence atypical automaticity indicating that this form of ectopic activity may occur readily at low and at high muscle calcium loads.

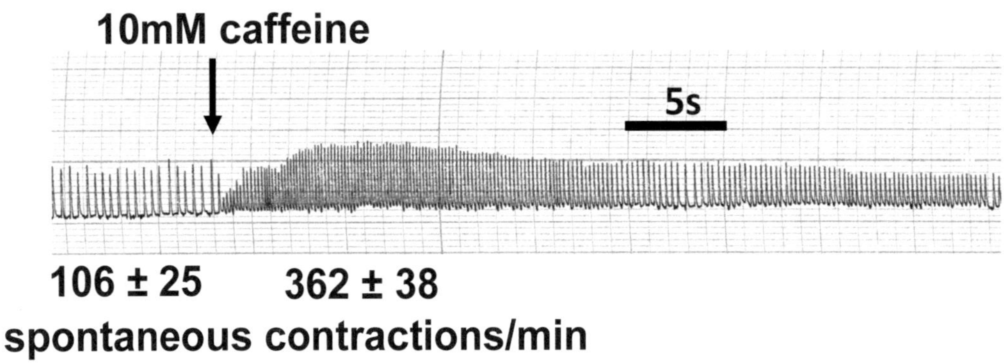

Figure 10. Caffeine Transiently Accelerates the Rate of Atypical Automaticity. Rat left atria (n=6) were exposed to 30μM 2APB in the absence of calcium loading agent. These muscles spontaneously contracted sporadically at a rate shown at the left of the figure. Muscles then were rapidly exposed to superfusate containing 30μM 2APB and 10mM caffeine. This treatment greatly increased the rate of atypical automatic activity to over 350 contractions per minute. After 3-5 minutes under these conditions, the rate of automaticity decreased to 10 contractions per minute.

The literature contains one possible explanation for the difference between the ryanodine and the caffeine responses observed in automatically contracting left atria. Corda noted that while ryanodine affects calcium leak from internal stores it does not activate a voltage-independent store-operated response [110]. By contrast, caffeine does. That is, in their experimental system, exposing cultured cells to caffeine provoked a prominent entry of calcium presumably through the Orai-linked store-operated channel. This result supports a contention that voltage-independent calcium entry and downstream signaling are the source for atypical automaticity (Figure 11). Many more experiments are needed to establish this possibility.

http://dx.doi.org/10.5772/53649

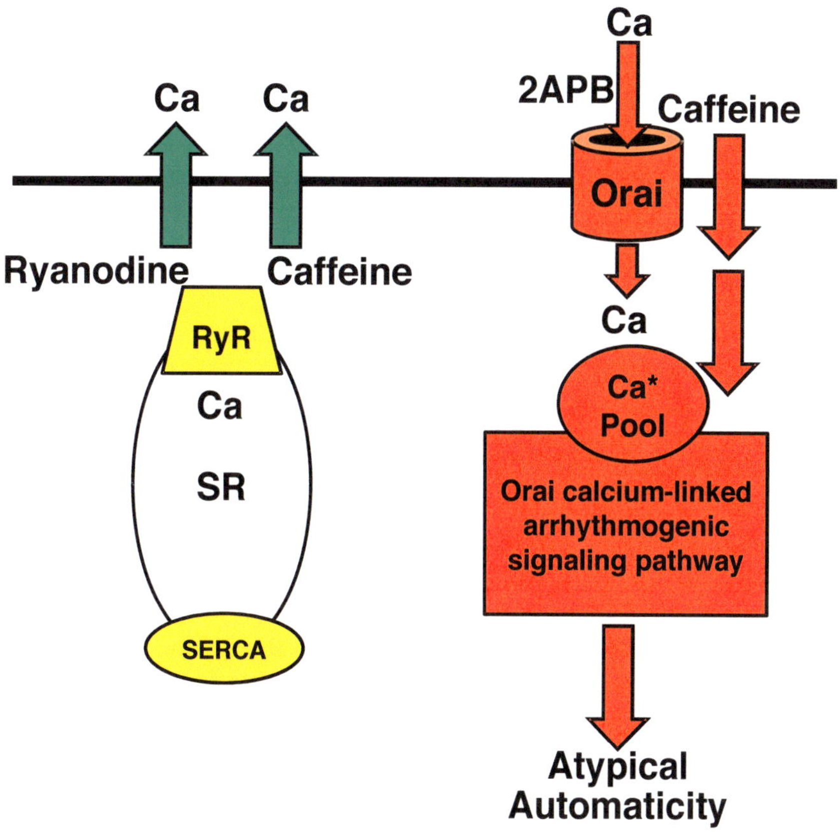

Figure 11. Interpretation of Ryanodine-Caffeine Effects on Atypical Automaticity.*Left.* Both ryanodine and caffeine deplete SR calcium stores. *Right.* Caffeine accelerates store-operated calcium entry in some experimental settings [110]. We suggest this latter effect of caffeine enhances the rates of automaticity (Figure 10).

Thus heart may possess two ways to produce action potentials that provoke contraction. First is the well-known and long-studied pathway whereby an external input derived either from the sinoatrial node or from a pacing stimulus causes myocyte depolarization. Second, an activator of the voltage-independent Orai channels appears to uncover a pathway whose activation allows non-automatic muscles to produce normal action potentials and muscle contraction independent of an external stimulus. This atypical automaticity can occur sporadically or at high frequency depending on the calcium loading of isolated muscles.

All of these experiments were performed in intact superfused muscles. Consequently, we harbored concern that conditions like hypoxia might influence our results. To address this point rat hearts were perfused in the Langendorff mode to test how 2APB affects well-oxygenated muscle. These perfusions also assessed (a) whether high frequency 2APB-induced automaticity requires muscle calcium loading and (b) how 2APB affects hearts with an intact conduction system in sinus rhythm. The first point arises because the isolation of atria or papillary muscles might unload unique cell calcium pools that are critical for instigating atypical automaticity. Hence the effect of the calcium loading of isolated muscles to increase the rate of 2APB automaticity [104] might be mistaken to reflect loading of the SR pool involved in contraction rather than the concurrent loading of a pool central to atypical automaticity. The second point addresses questions by Boyden and ter Keurs [88].

Perfused hearts yield several important and impressive results. First, the perfusion of hearts with 5μM 2APB generates spontaneous, sporadic electrical activity from multiple sites, a conclusion based on the morphology of these ectopic depolarizations [106 see Figure 2]. Increasing the perfusate 2APB concentration produces striking changes in the electromechanical activity of these hearts [http://www.dom.uab.edu/pwolkowicz/IPH_Fibrillation2-APB.mov]. After a few minutes of perfusion with 22μM 2APB hearts begin to produce spontaneous but broad QRS complexes and contract at rates that increase from sinus rhythm (~5Hz) to upwards of 12Hz [106 *see Figures 3 & 4*]. Heart mechanical function briefly follows this ectopic electrical activity but electro-mechanical dissociation occurs as ectopic electrical activity continues to steadily increase in rate to apparent values of ~20Hz. These hearts lose the ability to generate organized mechanical activity which may reflect a form of fibrillatory conduction originating from high frequency focal sources [25,111]. A brief but impressive increase in diastolic pressure from 5mm to ~60mmHg accompanies electromechanical dissociation. A minute or so later fibrillating hearts reach and then maintain a resting tension of 30mmHg [106 *see Figures 3 & 4*]. Coronary flow remains normal during fibrillation and persistent contracture lessening the possibility that ischemia occurs in these preparations.

The Orai and TRP channel inhibitor SKF-96365 reverses this ventricular fibrillation in an intriguing way [106 *see Figure 5*] [http://www.dom.uab.edu/pwolkowicz/IPH_SKF-96365-Reversal.mov]. After a few minutes of perfusion with 2APB and 20μM SKF-96365, the electrical disorganization recorded by our bipolar electrodes begins to resolve. The resolution of electrical fibrillation occurs quickly over about one second but at first it is only a transient event as electrical instability reappears immediately after this initial flash of stability. As the time of perfusion with SKF-96365 increases, periods of stable electrical activity get longer until sinus rhythm is restored. In all cases, the temporal interface between fibrillation and electrical quiescence produce a rapid decrease in resting tension from 30mmm to about 8mmHg, mechanical quiescence, and then normal, potentiated mechanical contractions [106 *see Figure 5*]. This very rapid restoration of normal diastolic pressure and electro-mechanical quiescence most likely are not caused by a decrease in bulk cytosolic calcium throughout the heart. We suspect this change likely reflects the interdiction by SKF-96365 of signaling events initiated by 2APB. Note that 2APB remains in the perfusate throughout these experiments. These electrical results remarkably mimic those reported by Hirose for Gαq overexpressing mice [96]. Together these data indicate that SKF-96365 suppresses fibrillation caused by genetic enhancement of the initiation site for voltage-independent calcium signaling [96], the Gαq receptor, and by perfusion with a pharmacological activator of Orai channel calcium entry, which might occur in Gαq transgenic mice for reasons stated earlier. The concentrations of 2APB used in our work inhibit both the IP3Rs and many of the relevant TRPC channels. Thus the voltage-independent Orai channels, either Orai1 or Orai3, appear as a likely source of arrhythmia. If the model for the functional inter-relationship of voltage-independent calcium channels and calcium pools proposed by Shuttleworth [64], Lewis [98] and others is correct, then (a) inputs which excessively stimulate the Orai channels or (b) a yet-to-be-identified cell signaling system which mirrors the action of 2APB on the Orai channels might create focal sources of high frequency atypical automaticity in muscle as small or smaller than 3mg wet-weight. The duration of this automaticity would depend on the presence of input signals that stimulate voltage-independent calcium entry.

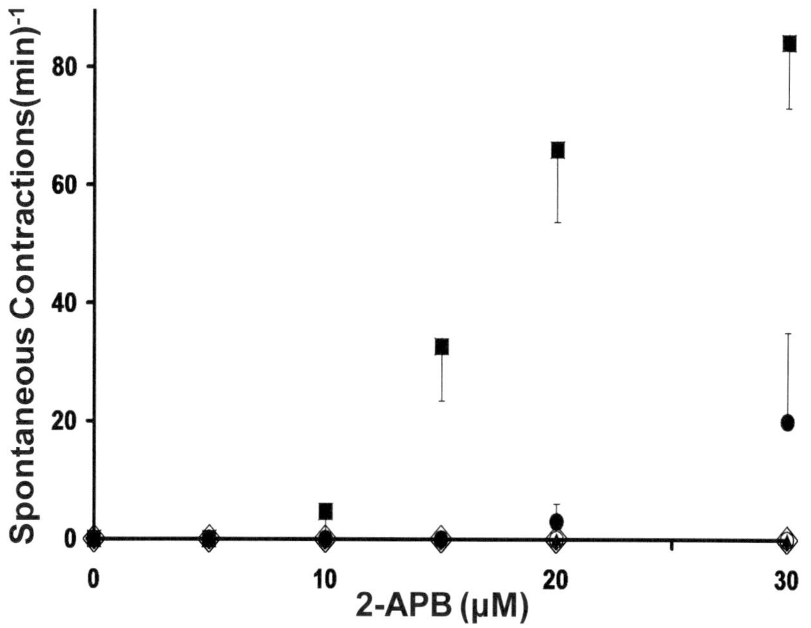

Figure 12. Bcl2 Antagonists Block 2APB Atypical Automaticity. Rat left atria (n=5 per group) were superfused and paced [105]. Atria were left untreated (▪) or were pre-incubated with 80µM methoxy-antimycin A3 (•) 80 µM HA-14-1 (◊), 30 µM EGCG (o), or 30 µM gossypol (x). Increasing concentrations of 2APB were added to the superfusate for 3min at each concentration. The pacing stimulus then was stopped and the rate of spontaneous atrial contraction was recorded. All four bcl2 antagonists suppressed 2APB automaticity.

If voltage-independent calcium entry via the Orai channels initiates atrial and ventricular electrical instability *in vivo*, then this putative fourth mechanism would offer (a) a dynamic means to explain arrhythmia and (b) a mechanism which extends the three current hypotheses to explain these disorders. Dynamism arises because a multitude of physiological and pathophysiological inputs directly stimulate or indirectly activate the Orai channels [64,75,98]. The apparent arrhythmogenicity of calcium entry via the Orai channels may extend the 'calcium leak' hypothesis for arrhythmia (Figure 5). Specifically, certain types of SR calcium leak may favor the compensatory activation of voltage-independent calcium entry [112]. Thus coupling SR calcium leak and voltage-independent calcium entry may increase the depolarizing influence which calcium leak exerts on compromised myocytes. This could contribute to the increased propensity for arrhythmia observed in 'leaky' failing hearts.

With respect to 'abnormal' automaticity, exuberant Orai channel activation might produce automatic foci under conditions that do not require partial myocyte depolarization. Regarding reentry, if dysregulated Orai channels were *in vivo* sources of >10Hz atypical automaticity, then they could lead to ectopy at rates that promote atrial (*and ventricular*) fibrillatory conduction which begins at 6Hz [111]. Finally, if this fourth mechanism of voltage-independent arrhythmogenesis were to hold in Purkinje cells, it might explain some types of idiopathic ventricular fibrillation [113].

We are cognizant that the available data allow for only the barest of frameworks for the hypothesis that voltage-independent calcium entry and signaling are important sources of focal arrhythmia. Undoubtedly multiple unexpected cellular signaling intermediates participate in this pathway and they may provide new targets for anti-arrhythmics. For example, bcl-2 is a small protein that regulates the intrinsic pathway for apoptosis through its interaction with mitochondria. By contrast, Distelhorst [114] has championed the concept that bcl-2 binding to the IP3R suppresses calcium signals related to apoptosis while enhancing signals related to cell survival. Sub-sets of bcl-2 bind to the endoplasmic reticulum and the plasma membrane [115]. Thus bcl-2 might play a role in the atypical automaticity which 2APB induces. To test this possibility rat left atria were superfused and paced at 0.1Hz as previously described [105]. Left atria (n=5 per group) were then left untreated or were pretreated with 80μM HA14-1 and methoxyantimycin A, two cell permeable inhibitors of bcl-2, or with 30μM of two naturally occurring bcl-2 inhibitors EGCG and gossypol [116-119]. Increasing concentrations of 2APB from 0 to 30μM were added to the superfusate and the rate of spontaneous activity was recorded after three minute incubation at any concentration. All four bcl-2 inhibitors significantly or completely prevented atypical automatic activity (Figure 12). EGCG and gossypol were tested for their ability to reverse high frequency atypical automaticity in left atria treated with BayK 8644 and 20μM 2APB. Both naturally occurring bcl-2 inhibitors reversed this automatic activity but did not affect normal paced muscle contraction (Figure 13). Thus bcl-2 may play a role in this type of ectopy but these provocative data require significant follow-on experiments to more firmly establish this conclusion.

The evidence summarized in this review suggests the existence of a cell mechanism to generate focal arrhythmia. Some limitations must be addressed to afford a more sound footing for the concept that focal, cellular sources of arrhythmia arise from the activation of voltage-independent calcium channels.

- How does the activation of voltage-independent calcium channels produce electromechanical instability in intact heart muscles (Figure 7, Calcium signal)? Does voltage-independent calcium entry *per se*, that is calcium acting as a charge carrier, activate this high frequency ectopy? Or, do calcium signaling events specific to this type of channel lead non-automatic heart muscle to become automatic? We favor the latter view. Supporting this possibility calmodulin inhibitors suppress atypical automaticity in heart muscles treated with 2APB [105]. By contrast CaMKII inhibitors do not [105]. Thus calmodulin targets other than CaMKII may be involved in this automatic activity.
- What molecular entities lie between voltage-independent calcium signaling and automatic depolarization at rates of 10-12Hz? While a current view would favor calcium ions themselves as the arrhythmogenic principle, we have preliminary data that will be pub-

http://dx.doi.org/10.5772/53649

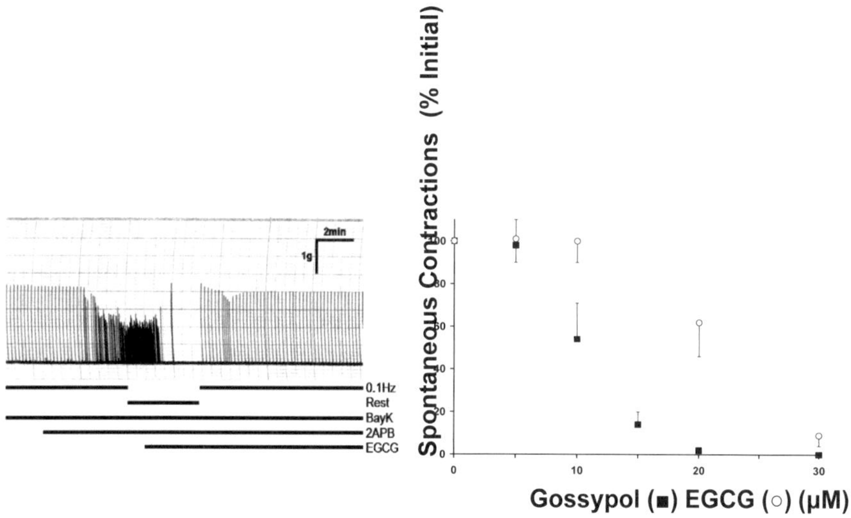

Figure 13. Naturally Occurring bcl2 Antagonists Suppress 2APB Atypical Automaticity.*Left.* Rat let atrium was superfused, paced at 0.1Hz, and treated with 300nM BayK 8644 [105]. 2APB (22μM) was added where indicated (2APB). After two to three minutes this atrium began to spontaneously contract at a high rate (*dark area in center of trace*). The pacing stimulus then was stopped. (*Rest*). Atypical automatic activity persists unabated. EGCG (30μM) was added where indicated (EGCG). Shortly thereafter, atypical automaticity ceased and this *now* **unpaced** muscle became quiescent. The 0.1Hz pacing stimulus then was reinstated and the left atrium faithfully followed it (*Right 0.1Hz*). *Right.* Average of exeriments like the one shown to the left where increasing concentrations of gossypol and EGCG were used to staunch atypical automaticity. Gossypol induced a 50% reduction at 10μM while EGCG required 25μM.

lished under separate auspices which demonstrate that these signaling events profoundly change the fundamental characteristics of heart voltage-dependent ion channels. We believe these fundamental changes underlie the fourth mechanism for arrhythmia we propose here.

- Can this voltage-independent mechanism provide a connection between afterdepolarization and sustained triggered activity/high frequency atypical automaticity? To test this possibility we investigated whether voltage-independent calcium channels also participate in the triggered activity that occurs with increased late sodium current. We find that atria treated with appropriate concentrations of sea anemone toxin type II [33] produce triggered early afterdepolarization in a steady-state manner. Our preliminary data to be published elsewhere show that (a) the ARC channel inhibitor LOE-908, (b) an antibody that binds plasma membrane Stim1 which is required for ARC channel activity, (c) the Orai inhibitor SKF-96365, (d) the CaMKII inhibitor KN-93, and (e) several inhibitors of the calcium-dependent cytosolic phospholipase A_2 all suppress late sodium current-induced triggered activity. Importantly, we assessed whether SKF-96365 shortens action potential duration in atria treated with sea anemone toxin. It does not. Also neither LOE-908 nor KN-93 suppresses the high frequency automaticity which 2APB induces.

Thus related panels of voltage-independent calcium signaling inhibitors suppress early afterdepolarization and/or 2APB automaticity. We propose that the calcium loading which occurs with increased late sodium current stimulates cytosolic phospholipase A_2 to produce the arachidonate ligand for ARC (Figure 14). Calcium entry through the voltage-independent ARC calcium channel may activate CaMKII which participates in provoking early afterdepolarization. Conditions in which calcium stores begin to deplete would stimulate voltage-independent calcium entry through Orai1 [64]. Greater store depletion resulting from exuberant ARC channel activity would lead to fulminant voltage-independent calcium entry through the Orai1 calcium channel [64] and possibly a 'sustained triggered activity' which resembles 2APB-linked automaticity.

Are there intracellular, naturally occurring activators of Orai1 or Orai3 that mimic 2APB? At present none are known but such Orai-activators would link cell signaling with focal arrhythmogenesis. The interrelationship between ARC and store-operated voltage-independent calcium entry [64] may be one such link.

The following four figures outline a putative mechanism through which voltage-independent calcium signaling might induce afterdepolarization, sporadic and high-frequency atypical automaticity.

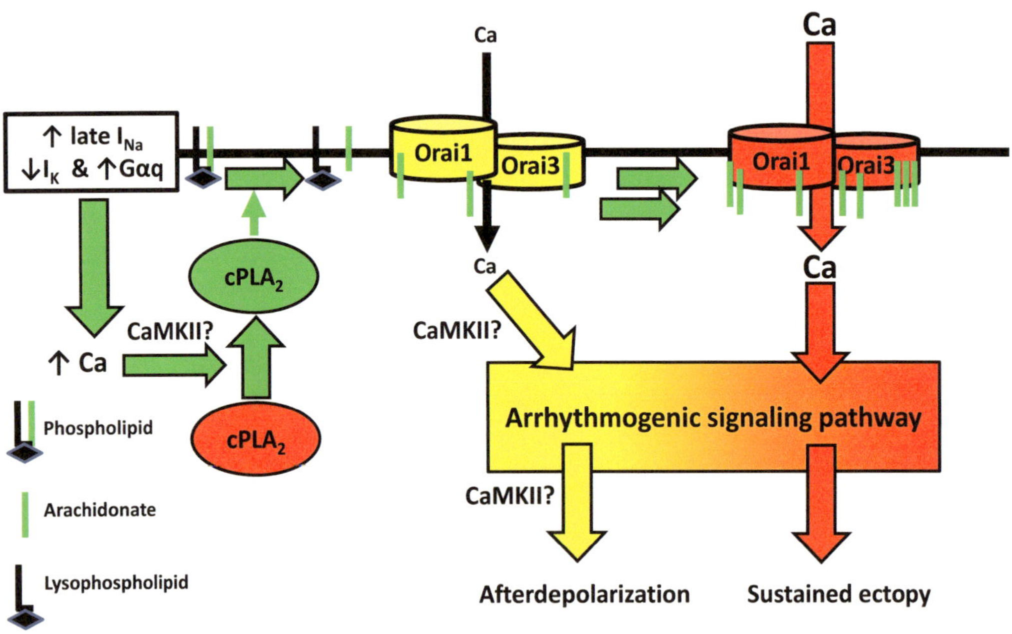

Figure 14. Model linking voltage-independent ARC channel and late sodium current early afterdepolarization.*Left*. Late sodium current loads myocytes first with sodium and then with calcium [33]. This loading activates cytosolic phospholipase A_2 ($cPLA_2$) to hydrolyze membrane phospholipids and release free arachidonate. *Right*. This eicosonoid activates the Orail/Orai3 pentamer ARC channel which permits calcium entry into myocytes. This also disturbs intracellular calcium stores [64]. CaMKII may participate in this pathway by phosphorylating $cPLA_2$ or elsewhere. Low level ARC activity leads to afterdepolarization. More intense ARC activity depletes myocyte calcium stores, opens Orais and provokes high frequency sustained triggered activity. Both events require the co-opting of cardiac voltage-dependent ion channels to produce spontaneous depolarization.

http://dx.doi.org/10.5772/53649

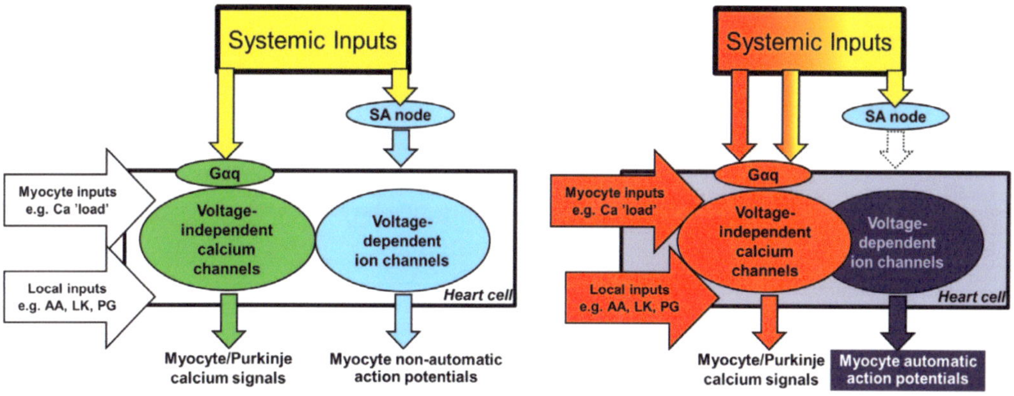

Figure 15. A Putative Mechanism for Focal Ectopy.*Left.* In excitable cells, voltage-independent & voltage-dependent ion channels co-exist. Both sets of channels respond to common or distinct inputs to produce (a) calcium signals for cell homeostasis and (b) action potentials. These two events are generally considered as separate and non-interacting entities [22,25,55,64,75,76]. *Right.* A wide range of systemic, myocyte, and local inputs may provoke the 'inappropriate' interaction of these two systems. This results in voltage-independent signaling events co-opting myocyte voltage-dependent ion channels. Myocytes transform from a non-automatic to an automatic state. This change can occur for an inconstant time period and it is reversible. AA=arachidonate; LK=leukotrienes; PG=prostaglandins

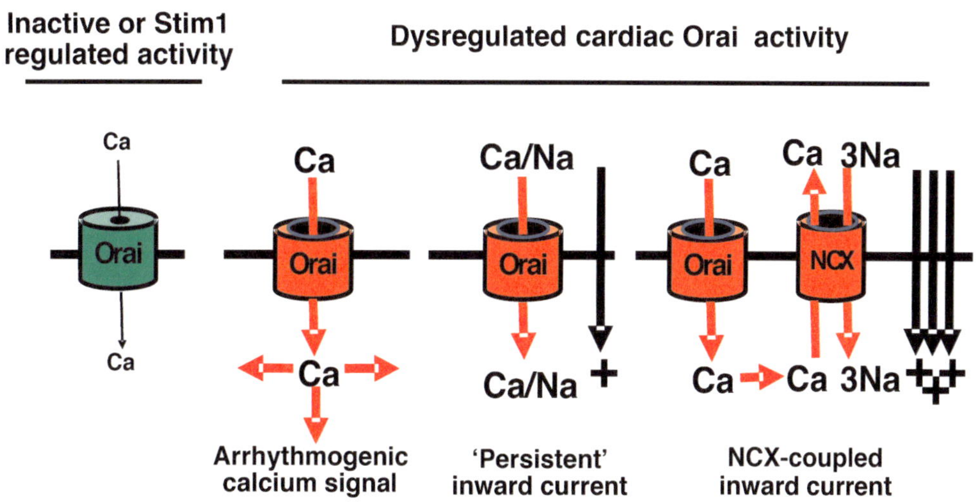

Figure 16. Potential Arrhythmogenic Mechanisms for Dysfunctional Orai Channels. Our data suggest dysfunctional Orais may be a source of focal arrhythmia. *Left.* These proteins normally are well-regulated by the Stim1 calcium sensing system & faithfully fulfill their function of refilling cell calcium stores. *Second from left.* Dysregulated Orals will enhance calcium transport which might activate a cryptic arrhychmogenic calcium signaling pathway. **We favor this view.** *Second from Right & Right*. Dysregulated Oral calcium transport may generate a persistent inward current which acts independent of changes in membrane potential associated with the action potential or Orai calcium entry may couple with the sodium-calcium exchanger (NCX) to create a futile calcium cycle that drives myocyte depolarization. Such a general type of mechanism is similar to that proposed by Huo to explain 2APB ectopy [120].

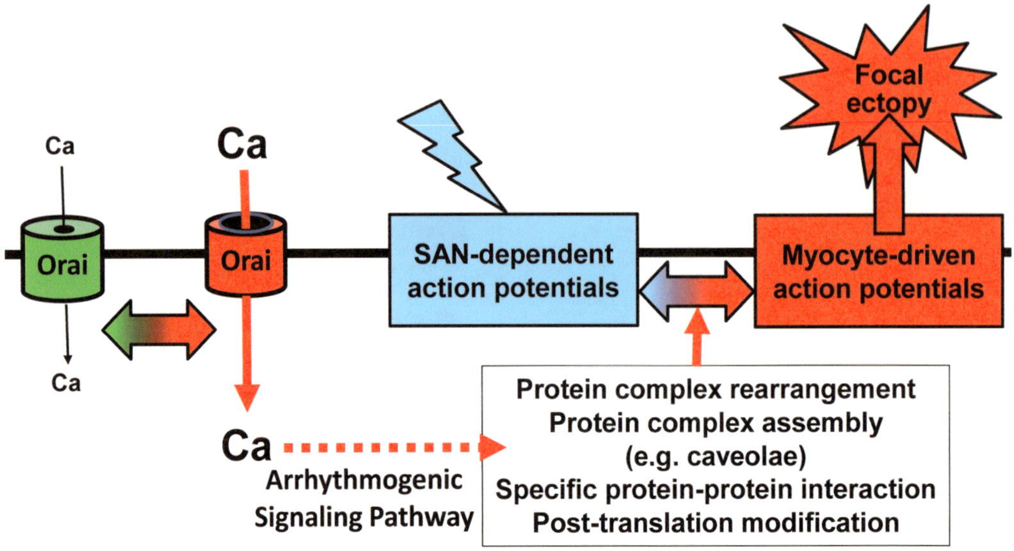

Figure 17. Potential Cellular Mechanism for Orai Atypical Automaticity. Our preliminary data favor a mechanism for Orai atypical automaticity in which calcium entry activates a signaling pathway that modifies the properties of the voltage-dependent ion channels critical to myocyte excitation. We do not have a preferred view as to how this modification occurs but the lower open box notes four possibilities we are now investigating

10. Conclusions

Atrial (*and ventricular*) arrhythmias are disturbances in electrical activity that disrupt the regular, rhythmic contraction of the upper (*or lower*) heart chambers. These electrical instabilities arise from normal or dysfunctional heart muscle, from the heart specialized conduction system or from the 'muscular sleeves' of major supraventricular vessels. Because arrhythmia is recorded as abnormal electrical activity and since experimental faradic stimulation can initiate arrhythmia, it is viewed as having a purely electrical origin. Indeed the dominant explanations for arrhythmia hypothesize it originates from (a) changes in the electrical properties of heart muscle that alter electrical impulse conduction, (b) changes in the properties of the voltage-dependent ion channels responsible for normal electrical activity which alter impulse conduction, (c) changes in the myocytic milieu that permit normal voltage-dependent ion channels to spontaneously generate electrical impulses or (d) changes in myocyte calcium homeostasis that alter heart resting membrane potential or otherwise indirectly enhance muscle excitability.

During the past fifty years, however, it has become clear that all cells contain a staggering array of interrelated signaling pathways and processes which regulate normal and 'abnormal' cell functions. Like all other cells, heart cells, too, express voltage-independent calcium signaling pathways which underlie cardiac processes like inotropy and diseases like hypertrophy or atherosclerosis. The three earlier hypotheses for arrhythmia noted above ignore

http://dx.doi.org/10.5772/53649

the importance of voltage-independent cell signaling in heart ectopy. That is, they assume that voltage-independent cell signaling does not influence cardiac voltage-dependent ion channels or affect arrhythmia. One corollary of this dominant electrocentric view of arrhythmia is that the fundamental biophysical properties of voltage-dependent ion channels measured in normal muscle are the only properties these proteins can evince, that these ion channels are essentially immutable activities. However, clinical and experimental data suggest that one or more signaling events greatly influence the electrical properties of heart muscle and somehow increase its ability to generate ectopic electrical impulses.

Our data demonstrate that a recognized activator of the voltage-independent Orai calcium channels provokes persistent or paroxysmal tachycardia at rates of up to 12Hz in non-automatic rat left atrial or left ventricular papillary muscles. This activator also induces a reversible type of fibrillation in intact perfused rat hearts. These data lead to the hypothesis outlined here that calcium entry through voltage-independent ion channels, specifically through the Orai channels, and/or calcium signaling events downstream of these channels elicit ectopic electrical activity in atrial (*and ventricular*) muscle. This hypothesis implies that a wide range of extracellular and intracellular signals may disrupt heart muscle electrical stability through their actions on voltage-independent calcium homeostasis that enhance voltage-independent calcium channel activity. This hypothesis provides a framework for future experimental tests of whether voltage-independent calcium signaling related to autonomic activity, to stress or to calcium store filling state are key molecular sources for arrhythmia. Importantly, our data to be published elsewhere indicate that dysregulated voltage-independent calcium signaling alter the fundamental characteristics of voltage-dependent ion channels, transforming them from non-automatic activities that require an external depolarizing influence to automatic activities that spontaneously depolarize heart muscle. If rigorously validated, this fourth putative arrhythmogenic mechanism would satisfy the 'focal source' hypothesis for arrhythmia.

Acknowledgements

The authors gratefully acknowledge the help of Dr. Pei Pei Wang in conducting the perfused heart studies described here. PEW appreciatively thanks Dr. David D. Ku of the UAB Department of Pharmacology for unfettered access to lab space and equipment during the course of much of this work. PEW thanks Dr. Jian Huang of the UAB Department of Medicine for performing microelectrode measurements of left atrial action potential mentioned in the text. He also gratefully acknowledges the assistance of Drs. Hernan E. Grenett, Edlue Tabengwa, and John C. Chatham of UAB at various points along this journey. He also would like to thank Dr. Neal Kay of UAB for his interest in this endeavor. PEW is the President and Chief Scientific Officer of KOR Therapies, LLC which seeks to develop the technology discussed in this paper. This technology is now controlled by the University of Alabama Research Foundation and under patent review.

Author details

Paul E. Wolkowicz[1*], Patrick K. Umeda[2], Ferdinand Urthaler[2] and Oleg F. Sharifov[2]

*Address all correspondence to: Kor.cures@gmail.com

1 KOR Therapies, LLC, Drive, Hoover, Alabama, USA

2 The Department of Medicine, The Division of Cardiovascular Diseases, The University of Alabama at Birmingham, Birmingham, Alabama, USA

References

[1] Nothnagel H. Ueber arythmische Hersthatigkeit. Deutsches Archiv fur Klinische Medizin 1876;17: 190-220

[2] MacKenzie J. The inception of the rhythm of the heart by the ventricle. British Medical Journal 1904;1: 529-536.

[3] Hering HE. Ueber die haufige Kombination von Kammervenenpul mit Pulsus irregularis perpetuus. Deutsche Medizinische Wochenschrift 1906;32: 213-215.

[4] Flegel KM. From Delirium Cordis to atrial fibrillation: Historical development of a disease concept. Annals Internal Medicine 1995;122(11): 867-873.

[5] Vulpian A. Note sur les effets de la faradization directe des ventricules du Coeur chez le chien. Archives Physiologie Normale et Pathologique 1874;6: 975-881.

[6] Krehl l, Rohmber E. Ueber des Bedeuting des Herzmuskels und der Herzganglien fur die Herzhatigkeit des Saugethiers. Archiv fur Experimentelle Pathologie und Pharmakologie 1892;30: 49-92.

[7] Hering HE. Analyses des pulsus irregularis perpetuus. Prager medizinsche Wochenschrift 1903;28: 377-381.

[8] Cushny AR, Edmunds CW. Paroxysmal irregularity of the heart and auricular fibrillation. American Journal of Medical Science 1907;133: 66-77.

[9] Einthoven W. Le telecardiogramme. Archives Internationales de Physiologie 1906;4: 132-164

[10] Hering HE. Das electrocardiogram des irregularis perpetuus. Deutsches Archi fur Klinische Medizin 1908;94: 205-208.

[11] Rothberger CJ, Winterberg H. Vorhofflimmern und arrhythmia perpetua. Wiener Klinische Wochenschrift 1909;22: 839-844.

[12] MacWilliam JA. Fibrillar contraction of the heart. Journal of Physiology 1887;8: 296-310.

[13] Lewis T, Feil HS, Stroud WD. Observations upon flutter, fibrillation, II: the nature of auricular flutter. Heart 1920;7: 191-233.

[14] Engelmann TW. Ueber den einfluss der systole auf der motorische leitung in der herzkammer, mit bemerkungen zur theorie allorhythmischer herzstorungen. Archivs fur die Gesamte Physiologie 1896;62: 543-566.

[15] Winterberg H. Ueber herzflimmern und siene beeinflussung durch kampher. Zeitschrift fur Experimentelle Pathologie und Therapie 1906;3: 182-208.

[16] Rothberger CJ. Neue theorien ueber flimmern und flattern. Klinische Woschenschrift 1922;8: 82-94.

[17] Lewis T. The nature of flutter and fibrillation of the auricle. British Medical Journal 1921;1 (April 16): 551-555 & 590-593

[18] Mayer AG. Rhythmical pulsations in Sychphomedusae. Washington D.C.: Carnegie Institute of Washington 1906;47: 1-61.

[19] Mines GR. On dynamic equilibrium in the heart. Journal of Physiology 1913;46: 349-383.

[20] Garrey WE. The nature of fibrillary contraction of the heart: Its relation to tissue mass and form. American Journal Physiology 1914;33: 397-414.

[21] Lewis T, Drury AN, Iliescu CC. A demonstration of circus movement in clinical flutter of the auricles. Heart 1921;8: 361-369.

[22] Moe GK, Ablidskov JA. Atrial fibrillation as a self-sustaining arrhythmia independent of focal discharge. American Heart Journal 1959;58: 59-70.

[23] Wiggers CJ. Studies on ventricular fibrillation produced by electric shock. II Cinematographic and electrocardiographic observations on the natural process in the dog's heart. American Heart Journal 1930;5: 351-374. Moe GK, Harris AS, Wiggers CJ. Analysis of the initiation of fibrillation by electrocardiographic studies American Journal of Physiology 1941;134: 473-491.

[24] Allessie MA, Bonke FL, Schopman FJ. Circus movement in rabbit atrial muscles as a mechanism for tachycardia. III. The leading circle concept: A new model of circus movement in cardiac tissue without the involvement of anatomical obstacles. Circulation Research 1977;41: 9-18.

[25] Panfilov A, Pertsov A. Ventricular fibrillation: evolution of the multiple-wavelet hypothesis. Philosophical Transactions of the Royal Society of London (A) 2001; 359: 1315-1325.

[26] Scherf D. Studies on auricular tachycardia caused by aconitine administration. Proceedings of the Society for Experimental Biology and Medicine 1947;64: 233-239.

[27] Kisch B. The mechanics of flutter and fibrillation. A short review of a century of studies. Cardiologia 1950;17: 244-250

[28] Jervell A, Lange-Nielsen F. Congenital deaf-mutism, functional heart disease with prolongation of the QT interval, and sudden death. American Heart Journal 1957;54: 59-68.

[29] Dessertenne F. La tachycardie ventriculaire a deux foyers opposes variables. Archiv des maladies du coeur et des vaisseaux 1966;59(2): 263–272

[30] Keating MT, Sanguinetti MC. Molecular and cellular mechanisms of cardiac arrhythmias. Cell 2001;104(4): 569-580.

[31] Arvanataki A. Recherches sur la résponse oscillatoire locale de l'axone géant isolé de Sepia. Archiv Internal Physiologie 1939;49: 209-223.

[32] Bozler E. The initiation of impulses in cardiac muscle. American Journal of Physiology 1943;138: 273-282.

[33] Belardinelli L, Shryock JC, Fraser H. Inhibition of the late sodium current as a potential cardioprotective principle: Effects of late sodium current inhibitor ranolazine. Heart 2006;92: iv6-iv14.

[34] Roden DM. Long QT syndrome: Reduced repolarization reserve and the genetic link. Journal of Internal Medicine 2006;259(1): 59-69.

[35] Schmitt FO, Erlanger J. Directional differences in the conduction of the impulse through heart muscle and their possible relation to extrasystolic and fibrillatory contractions. American Journal of Physiology 1928;87: 326-347.

[36] January CT, Riddle JM. Early afterdepolarizations: Mechanism of induction and block. Circulation Research 1989;64: 977-990.

[37] Choi B, Burton F, Salama G. Cytosolic Ca2+ triggers early afterdepolarization and Torsades de Pointes in rabbit hearts with type 2 long QT syndrome. Journal of Physiology 2002;543.2: 615-631.

[38] Volders PGA, Vos MA, Szabo B, Sipido KR, de Groot SHM, Gorgels APM , Wellens HJJ, Lazzara R. Progress in the understanding of cardiac early afterdepolarizations and torsades de pointes: Time to revise current concepts. Cardiovascular Research 2000;46: 376–392.

[39] Pogwizd SM, Schlotthauer K, Li L, Yuan W, Bers DM. Arrhythmogenesis and contractile dysfunction in heart failure: Roles of sodium-calcium exchange, inward rectifier potassium current, and residual β-adrenergic responsiveness, Circulation Research 2001;88: 1159-1167.

[40] Marx SO, Reiken S, Hisamatsu Y, Jayaraman T, Burkhoff D, Rosemblit N, Marks AR. PKA phosphorylation dissociates FKBP12.6 from the calcium release channel (ryanodine receptor): Defective regulation in failing hearts. Cell 2000;101(4): 365-376.

[41] Ai X, Curan JW, Shannon TR, Bers DM, Pogwizd SM. Ca2+/calmodulin-dependent protein kinase modulates cardiac RyR2 phosphorylation and SR Ca2+ leak in heart failure. Circulation Research 2005;97: 1314-1322.

[42] Endo M. Calcium release from the sarcoplasmic reticulum. Physiological Reviews 1977; 57: 71-108.

[43] Fabiato A. Calcium-induced release of calcium from the cardiac sarcoplasmic reticulum. American Journal of Physiology 1983;245: C1–C14.

[44] Fleckenstein A. Specific pharmacology of calcium in myocardium, cardiac pacemakers, and vascular smooth muscle. Annual Reviews Pharmacology Toxicology 1977;17: 149-166

[45] Inui M, Saito A, Fleischer S. Purification of the ryanodine receptor and identity with feet structures of junctional terminal cisternae of sarcoplasmic reticulum from fast skeletal muscle. Journal of Biological Chemistry 1987;262(4): 1740-1747.

[46] Kresge N, Simoni RD, Hill RL. Ion transport in the sarcoplasmic reticulum: The work of David H. MacLennan. Journal of Biological Chemistry 2006;281(25): e20.

[47] Tada M. Katz AM. Phosphorylation of the sarcoplasmic reticulum and sarcolemma. Annual Review of Physiology 1982;44: 401-423.

[48] Tada M, Kirchberger MA, Repke DI, Katz AM. *The stimulation of calcium transport in cardiac sarcoplasmic reticulum by adenosine 3′:5′-monophosphate-dependent protein kinase. Journal of Biological Chemistry* 1974;249: 6174-*6180.*

[49] Van Winkle WB, Pitts BJ, Entman ML. Rapid purification of canine cardiac sarcoplasmic reticulum Ca2+-ATPase. Journal of Biological Chemistry 1978;253(24): 8671-8673.

[50] Pitts BJR. Stoichiometry of sodium-calcium exchange in cardiac sarcolemmal vesicles. Journal of Biological Chemistry 1979;254: 6232-6235.

[51] Reeves JP, Hale CC. The stoichiometry of the cardiac sodium-calcium exchange system. Journal of Biological Chemistry 1984;259: 7733-7739.

[52] Allen DG, Blinks JR. Calcium transients in aequorin-injected frog cardiac muscle. Nature 1978;273: 509-513.

[53] Grynkiewicz G, Poenie M, Tsien RY. A new generation of Ca2+ indicators with greatly improved fluorescence properties. Journal of Biological Chemistry 1985;260(6): 3440-3350.

[54] Neef S, Dybkova N, Sossalla S, Ort KR, Fluschnik N, Neumann K, Seipelt R, Schondube FA, Hasenfuss G, Maier LS. CaMKII-dependent diastolic SR Ca2+ leak and elevated diastolic Ca2+ levels in right atrial myocardium of patients with atrial fibrillation. Circulation Research 2010;106: 1134-1144. Shan J, Xie W, Betzenhauser M, Reiken S, Chen B, Wronska A, Marks AR. Calcium leak through ryanodine receptors leads to atrial fibrillation in three mouse models of catecholaminergic ventricular tachycardia. Circulation Research 2012; doi:10.1161/ CIRCRESAHA.112.273342 .

[55] Wehrens XH, Lehnart SE, Reiken SR, Marks AR. Ca2+/calmodulin-dependent protein kinase II phosphorylation regulates the cardiac ryanodine receptor. Circulation Research 2004;94: e61-e70.

[56] Anderson DC, Betzenhauser MJ, Reiken S, Meli AC, Umanskaya A, Xie W, Shiomi T, Zalk R, Lacampagne A, Marks AR. Ryanodine receptor oxidation causes intracellular calcium leak and muscle weakness in aging. Cell Metabolism 2011;14(2): 196-207.

[57] Ben-David J, Zipes DP. Alpha-adrenoceptor stimulation and blockade modulates cesium-induced early afterdepolarizations and ventricular tachyarrhythmias in dogs. Circulation 1990;82: 225-233.

[58] Kimura S, Cameron JS, Koslovskis PL, Bassett AL, Myerburg RJ. Delayed afterdepolarizations and triggered activity induced in feline Purkinje fibers by alpha-adrenergic stimulation in the presence of elevated calcium levels. Circulation 1984;70(6): 1074-1082.

[59] Molina-Viamonte V, Anyukhovsky EP, Rosen MR. An alpha-1-adrenergic receptor subtype is responsible for delayed afterdepolarizations and triggered activity during simulated ischemia and reperfusion of isolated canine Purkinje fibers. Circulation 1991;84: 1732-1740

[60] Lo LW, Chen YC, Chen YJ, Wongcharoen W, Lin CI, Chen SA. Calmodulin kinase II inhibition prevents arrhythmic activity induced by alpha and beta adrenergic agonists in rabbit pulmonary veins. European Journal of Pharmacology 2007;571(2-3): 197-208.

[61] Wacker MJ, Kosloski LM, Gilbert WJR, Touchberry CD, Moore DS, Kelly JK, Brotto M, Orr JA. Inhibition of thromboxane A2-induced arrhythmias and intracellular calcium changes in cardiac myocytes by blockade of the inositol trisphosphate pathway. Journal of Pharmacology and Experimental Therapeutics 2009;331: 917–924. Xiao J, Liang D, Zhao H, Liu Y, Zhang H, Lu X, Liu Y, Li J, Peng L, Chen YH. 2-Aminoethoxydiphenyl borate, a inositol 1,4,5-triphosphate receptor inhibitor, prevents atrial fibrillation. Experimental Biology Medicine 2010;235: 862–868.

[62] Anderson ME, Braun AP, Wu Y, Lu T, Schulman H, Sung RJ. KN-93, an inhibitor of multifunctional Ca2+/calmodulin-dependent protein kinase, decreases early afterdepolarization. Journal of Pharmacological and Experimental Therapeutics 1998;287: 996-1006.

[63] Anderson ME. The fire from within. The biggest Ca2+ channel erupts and dribbles. Circulation Research 2005;97: 1213-1215.

[64] Shuttleworth TJ. Orai3 – the 'exceptional' Orai? Journal of Physiology 2012;590.2: 241-2

[65] Berg D, Vassalle M. Oscillatory zones and their role in normal and abnormal sheep Purkinje fiber automaticity. Journal of Biomedical Science 2000;7(5): 364-379.

[66] Cerbai E, Mugelli A. I_f in non-pacemaker cells: Role and pharmacological implications. Pharmacological Research 2006;53: 416-423.

[67] Nuss HB, Kaab S, Kass DA, Tomaselli GF, Marban E. Cellular basis of ventricular arrhythmias and abnormal automaticity in heart failure. American Journal of Physiology 1999;277: H80–H91.

[68] Robichaux RP, Dosdall DJ, Osorio J, Garner NW, Li L, Huang J. Periods of highly synchronous, non-reentrant endocardial activation cycles occur during long-duration ventricular fibrillation. Journal of Cardiovascular Electrophysiology 2010;21: 1266–1273.

[69] Li L, Jin Q, Dosdall DJ, Huang J, Pogwizd SM, Ideker RE. Activation becomes highly organized during long-duration ventricular fibrillation in canine hearts. American Journal of Physiology 2010;298(6): H2046-H2053.

[70] Berridge MJ. Inositol trisphosphate and diacylglycerol as second messengers. Biochemical Journal 1984;220(2): 345–360. Streb H, Irvine R F, Berridge M J, Schulz I. Release of Ca2+ from a non-mitochondrial intracellular store in pancreatic acinar cells by inositol-1,4,5-trisphosphate. Nature 1983;306: 67–69.

[71] Szlufcik K, Missiaen L, Parys JB, Callewaert G, De Smedt H. Uncoupled IP3 receptor can function as a Ca2+-leak channel: Cell biological and pathological consequences. Biology of the Cell 2006;98: 1-14.

[72] Zhu X, Jiang M, Peyton MJ, Boulay G, Hurst R, Stefani E, Birnbaumer L. *trp*, a novel mammalian gene family essential for agonist-activated capacitative Ca2+ entry. Cell 1996;85: 661–71.

[73] Sabourin J, Robin E, Raddatz E. A key role of TRPC channels in the regulation of electromechanical activity of the developing heart. Cardiovascular Research 2011;92: 226–236.

[74] Montell C, Rubin GM. Molecular characterization of the Drosophila trp locus: a putative integral membrane protein required for phototransduction. Neuron 1989;2(4): 1313-23.

[75] Birnbaumer L. The TRPC class of ion channels: A critical review of their roles in slow, sustained increases in intracellular Ca2+ concentrations. Annual Review of Pharmacology & Toxicology 2009;49: 395–426.

[76] Montell C, Birnbaumer L, Flockerzi V. The TRP channels, a remarkably functional family. Cell 2002;08(5): 595-598.

[77] Van Wagoner DR. Oxidative stress and inflammation in atrial fibrillation: Role in pathogenesis and potential as a therapeutic target. Journal of Cardiovascular Pharmacology 2008;52: 306-313.

[78] Putney JW. A model for receptor-regulated calcium entry. Cell Calcium 1986;7(1): 1-12.

[79] Putney JW. Origins of the concept of store-operated calcium entry. Frontiers in Biosciences 2011;3: 980-984.

[80] Williams RT, Senior PV, Van Stekelenburg L, Layton JE, Smith PJ, Dziadek MA. Stromal interaction molecule 1 (STIM1), a transmembrane protein with growth suppressor activity, contains an extracellular SAM domain modified by N-linked glycosylation. Biochimica Biophysica Acta 2002;1596(1):131-137.

[81] Liou J, Kim ML, Heo WD, Jones JT, Myers JW, Ferrell JE Jr, Meyer T. STIM is a Ca2+ sensor essential for Ca2+-store-depletion-triggered Ca2+ influx. Current Biology 2005;15(13): 1235–1241.

[82] Luik RM, Wu MM, Buchanan J, Lewis RS. The elementary unit of store-operated Ca2+ entry: Local activation of CRAC channels by STIM1 at ER-plasma membrane junctions. Journal of Cell Biology 2006;174(6): 815-25.

[83] Muthalif MM, Benter IF, Uddin MR, Malik KU. Calcium/calmodulin-dependent protein kinase IIalpha mediates activation of mitogen-activated protein kinase and cytosolic phospholipase A2 in norepinephrine-induced arachidonic acid release in rabbit aortic smooth muscle cells. Journal of Biological Chemistry 1996;271(47): 30149-30157

[84] Lipp P, Laine M, Tovey SC, Burrell KM, Berridge MJ, Li WH, Bootman MD. Functional InsP3 receptors that may modulate excitation-contraction coupling in the heart. Current Biology 2000;10: 939–942. Bootman MD, Higazi DR, Coombes S, Roderick HL. Calcium signaling during excitation-contraction coupling in mammalian atrial myocytes. *Journal of Cell Science* 2006;119(19): 3915–3925. Mackenzie L, Roderick HL, Proven A, Conway SJ, Bootman MD. Inositol-1,4,5- trisphosphate receptors in the heart. Biological Research 2004;37: 553–557.

[85] Mohler PJ, Davis JQ, Bennett V. Ankyrin-B coordinates the Na/K ATPase, Na/Ca exchanger, and InsP(3) receptor in a cardiac T-Tubule/SR microdomain. PLoS Biology 2005;3(12): e423.

[86] Go LO, Moschella MC, Watras J, Handa KK, Fyfe BS, Marks AR. Differential regulation of two types of intracellular calcium release channels during end-stage heart failure. Journal of Clinical Investigation 1995;95: 888–894.

[87] Gorza L, Schiaffino S, Volpe P. Inositol 1,4,5-trisphosphate receptor in heart: evidence for its concentration in Purkinje myocytes of the conduction system. Journal of Cell Biology 1993;121(2): 345-53.

[88] Stuyvers BD, Dun W, Matkovich S, Sorrentino V, Boyden PA, ter Keurs HEDJ. Calcium sparks and waves in canine Purkinje cells: a triple layered system of calcium activation. Circulation Research 2005;97: 35-43.

[89] Ju YK, Chu Y, Chaulet H, Lai D, Gervasio OL, Graham RM, Cannell MB, Allen G. Store-operated calcium influx and expression of TRPC genes in mouse sinoatrial node. Circulation Research 2007;100: 1605–1614.

[90] Demion M, Bois P, Launay P, Guinamard R. TRPM4, a Ca2+-activated nonselective cation channel in mouse sino-atrial node cells. Cardiovascular Research 2007;73: 531–538.

[91] Zima AV, Blatter LA. Inositol-1,4,5-trisphosphate-dependent Ca2+ signaling in cat atrial excitation–contraction coupling and arrhythmias. Journal of Physiology 2004;555: 607–615.

[92] Li X, Zima AV, Sheikh F, Blatter LA, Chen J. Endothelin-1-induced arrhythmogenic Ca2+ signaling is abolished in atrial myocytes of inositol-1,4,5-trisphosphate-receptor type 2–deficient mice. *Circulation Research* 2005;96: 1274-1281.

[93] Hirose M, Takeishi Y, Niizeki T, Shimojo H, Nakada T, Kubota I, Nakayama J, Mende U, Yamada M. Diacylglycerol kinase inhibits Gaq-induced atrial remodeling in transgenic mice. Heart Rhythm 2009;6: 78-84.

[94] Mende U, Kagen A, Cohen A. Transient cardiac expression of constitutively active Gaq leads to hypertrophy and dilated cardiomyopathy by calcineurin-dependent and independent pathways. Proceedings of the National Academy of Sciences (USA) 1998;95: 13893-13898.

[95] Vaidya D, Morley GE, Samie FH, Jalife J. Reentry and fibrillation in the mouse heart. A challenge to the critical mass hypothesis. Circulation Research 1999;85(2): 174-181.

[96] Hirose M, Takeishi Y, Niizeki T, Nakada T, Shimojo H, Kashihara T, Horiuchi-Hirose M, Kubota I, Mende U, Yamada M. Diacylglycerol kinase zeta inhibits ventricular tachyarrhythmias in a mouse model of heart failure – Roles of canonical Transient Receptor Potential (TRPC) channels. Circulation Journal 2011;75: 2333-2342.

[97] Schwarz G, Droogmans G, Nilius B. Multiple effects of SK&F 96365 on ionic currents and intracellular calcium in human endothelial cells. Cell Calcium 1994;15: 45-54. Prakash AS, Pabelick CM, Sieck GC. Store-operated calcium entry in porcine airway smooth muscle. American Journal of Physiology 2004;286: L909-L917.

[98] Lewis RS. The molecular choreography of a store-operated calcium channel. Nature 2007;446: 284-287.

[99] Lewis RS, Cahalan M D. Mitogen-induced oscillations of cytosolic Ca2+ and transmembrane Ca2+ current in human leukemic T cells. Cell Regulation 1989;1: 99–112.

[100] Braun FJ, Aziz O, Putney JW. 2-Aminoethoxydiphenyl borane activates a novel calcium-permeable cation channel. Molecular Pharmacology 2003; 63: 1304–1311.

[101] Peinelt C, Lis A, Beck A, Fleig A, Penner R. 2-APB directly facilitates and indirectly inhibits STIM1-dependent gating of CRAC channels. Journal of Physiology 2008;586: 3061-3073.

[102] DeHaven WI, Smyth JT, Boyles RR, Bird GS, Putney JW. Complex actions of 2-aminoethydiphenyl borate on store-operated calcium entry. Journal of Biological Chemistry 2008;293: 19265–19273.

[103] Wolkowicz PE, Wu HC, Urthaler F, Ku DD. 2-APB induces instability in rat left atrial mechanical activity. Journal of Cardiovascular Pharmacology 2007;49: 325–335.

[104] Wolkowicz PE, Grenett HE, Huang J, Wu HC, Ku DD, Urthaler F. A pharmacological model for calcium overload-induced tachycardia in isolated rat left atria. European Journal of Pharmacology 2007;576: 122–131.

[105] Wolkowicz PE, Huang J, Umeda PK, Sharifov OF, Tabengwa E, Halloran BA, Urthaler F, Grenett HE. Pharmacological evidence for Orai channel activation as a source of cardiac abnormal automaticity. European Journal of Pharmacology 2011;668: 208–216.

[106] Wang P, Umeda PK, Sharifov OF, Halloran BA, Tabengwa E, Grenett HE, Urthaler F, Wolkowicz PE. Evidence that 2-aminoethoxydiphenyl borate provokes fibrillation in perfused rat hearts via voltage-independent calcium channels. European Journal of Pharmacology 2012;681: 60–67.

[107] Nattel S. Driver regions in atrial fibrillation associated with congestive heart failure: where are they and what are they telling us? Journal of Cardiovascular Electrophysiology 2005;16: 1359–1361.

[108] Watanabe H, Takahashi R, Zhang X, Goto Y, Hayashi H, Ando J, Isshiki M, Seto M, Hidaka H, Niki I, Ohno R. An essential role of myosin light-chain kinase in the regulation of agonist- and fluid flow-stimulated Ca2+ influx in endothelial cells. FASEB Journal 1998;12: 341-348. Smyth JT, DeHaven WI, Bird GS, Putney JW. Calcium-store-dependent and -independent reversal of Stim1 localization and function. Journal of Cell Science 2008;121: 762-772.

[109] Shannon TR, Pogwizd SM, Bers DM. Elevated sarcoplasmic reticulum Ca2+ leak in intact ventricular myocytes from rabbits in heart failure. Circulation Research 2003;93: 592-594.

[110] Corda, S., Spurgeon, H.A., Lakatta, E.G., Capogrossi, M.C., Ziegelstein, R.C. Endoplasmic reticulum Ca depletion unmasks a caffeine-induced Ca influx in human aortic endothelial cells. Circulation Research 1995;77: 927-935.

[111] Berenfeld O, Zaitsev AV, Mironov SF, Pertsov AM, Jalife J. Frequency-dependent breakdown of wave propagation into fibrillatory conduction across the pectinate muscle network in the isolated sheep right atrium. Circulation Research 2002;90(11): 1173-1180.

[112] Stiber J, Hawkins A, Zhang ZS, Wang S, Burch J, Graham V, Ward CC, Seth M, Finch E, Malouf N, Williams RS, Eu JP, Rosenberg P. STIM1 signaling controls store-operated calcium entry required for development and contractile function in skeletal muscle. Nature Cell Biology 2008;10: 688-697..

[113] Haïssaguerre M, Shah DC, Jaïs P, Shoda M, Kautzner J, Arentz T, Kalushe D, Kadish A, Griffith M, Gaïta F, Yamane T, Garrigue S, Hocini M, Clémenty J. Role of Purkinje

conducting system in triggering of idiopathic ventricular fibrillation. Lancet 2002;359: 677-678.

[114] Zhang F, Davis MC, McCall KS, Distelhorst CW. Bcl-2 differentially regulates Ca2+ signals according to the strength of T cell receptor activation. Journal of Cell Biology 2006;172: 127-137.

[115] McCarthy BA, Boyle E, Wang XP, Guzowsk D, Paul S, Catera R, Trott J, Yan X, Croce CM, Damle, Yancopoulos S, Messmer BT, Lesser M, Allen SL, Rai KR, Chiorazzi N. Surface expression of Bcl-2 in chronic lymphocytic leukemia and other B-Cell leukemias and lymphomas without a Breakpoint t(14;18). Molecular Medicine 2008;14(9-10): 618-627.

[116] Manero F, Gautier F, Gallenne T, Cauquil N, Gree D, Cartron P, Geneste O, Gree R, Vallette FM, Juin P. The small organic compound HA14-1 prevents Bcl-2 interaction with Bax to sensitize malignant glioma cells to induction of cell death. Cancer Research 2006;66(5): 2757-2764.

[117] Cao X, Rodarte C, Zhang L, Morgan CD, Littlejohn J, Smythe WR. Bcl2/bcl-xl inhibitor engenders apoptosis and increases chemo-sensitivity in mesothelioma. Cancer Biology Therapy 2007;6(2): 246-252.

[118] Palmer A, Jin C, Reed JC, Tsien RY. Bcl-2-mediated alterations in endoplasmic reticulum Ca2+ analyzed with an improved genetically encoded fluorescent sensor. Proceedings of the National Academy of Sciences (USA). 2004;101(50): 17404-17409.

[119] Voss V, Senft C, Lang V, Ronellenfitsch MW, Steinbach JP, Seifert V, Kögel D. The pan-Bcl-2 inhibitor (−)-gossypol triggers autophagic cell death in malignant glioma. Molecular Cancer Research 2010;8(7): 1002–1016.

[120] Huo R, L, Z, Lu C, Xie Y, Wang B, Tu YJ, Hu JT, Xu CQ, Yang BF, Dong DL. Inhibition of 2-aminoethoxydiphenylborate induced rat atrial ectopic activity by antiarrhythmic drugs. Cellular Physiology & Biochemistry 2010;25: 425-432.

Chapter 6

Thrombogenesis in Atrial Fibrillation

Hanan Ahmed GalalAzzam

Additional information is available at the end of the chapter

http://dx.doi.org/10.5772/53613

1. Introduction

Atrial fibrillation is the most common sustained cardiac arrhythmia, which is associated with a high risk of stroke and thromboembolism. Increasing evidence suggests that the thrombogenic tendency in atrial fibrillation is related to several underlying pathophysiological mechanisms. Virchow's triad, a time-honored paradigm that offers mechanistic insights for thrombus initiation and development regardless of origin, does indeed apply to atrial fibrillation thrombogenesis [1,2].

2. Mechanisms of thrombogenesis in atrial fibrillation

More than 150 years ago, Rudolf Virchow proposed a triad of events needed for thrombus formation ie, abnormal changes of the vessel wall, blood flow, and blood constituents [2]. In the 21st century, we now recognize Virchow's triad as: endothelial or endocardial damage or dysfunction (and related structural abnormal changes); abnormal blood stasis; and abnormal haemostasis, platelets, and fibrinolysis (Figure 1). Extensive abnormal changes of these variables are clearly evident in atrial fibrillation. Thus, atrial fibrillation could in fact drive a prothrombotic or hypercoagulable state, by virtue of its fulfillment of Virchow's triad for thrombogenesis [3].

Abnormal changes shown in the vessel wall (eg, atrial tissue changes, endothelial damage and dysfunction), in fl ow (stasis—eg, in the left atrial appendage), and in blood constituents (eg, haemoconcentration, platelets, coagulation cascade activation, infl ammation); all factors contribute to propensity for thrombus formation (thrombogenesis) in atrial fi brillation. vWf=von Willebrand factor.

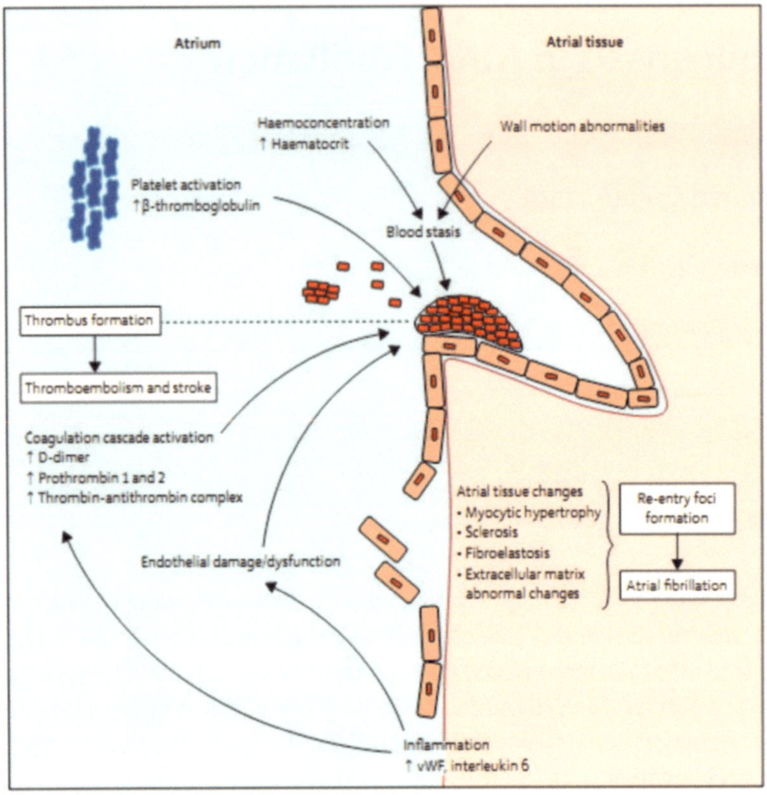

Figure 1. Components of Virchow's triad for thrombogenesis in atrial fibrillation [4](with permission)

2.1. Anatomical and structural considerations:

Attached to each atria is a blind-ended passage known as an appendage. The left atrial appendage (LAA) is long with a narrow inlet, thereby predisposing to blood stasis. Thus, the LAA is the most common site of intra-atrial thrombus formation, not only in atrial fibrillation, but also in patients with sinus rhythm [5,6].

Changes in the dimensions of the left atrium and LAA occur as a consequence of atrial fibrillation, with some correlation to subsequent thromboembolism. Detailed descriptions of endothelial damage in the context of atrial fibrillation are well described and can be visualised by scanning electron microscopy, especially within the appendages. Goldsmith and colleagues [7] have reported more severe endocardial changes in the LAA than in the right-atrial appendages, especially in atrial fibrillation (compared with sinus rhythm) and in mitral stenosis (compared with mitral regurgitation). Similarly, Masawa and co-workers [8] have described a "rough endocardium" with a wrinkled appearance attributable to oedema and fibrinous transformation; small areas of endothelial denudation and thrombotic aggregation have also been noted in patients with atrial fibrillation and cerebral embolism.

Extracellular matrix turnover is a dynamic structure, which continually undergoes a process of structural remodeling [9]. Structural remodelling of the atria could contribute to the hypercoagulable state, by virtue of both enhanced blood stasis and an abnormal endocardium. Structural remodeling of the left atrial appendage to include the pectinate muscles and multiple lobes of the lumen occurs in patients with permanent atrial fibrillation [10]. Morphologic studies have shown larger volumes and luminal surface areas when compared to patients without atrial fibrillation; however, both the absolute and relative surface areas of the pectinate muscles are reduced. In addition, there is significant endocardial thickening with fibrous and elastic tissue (endocardialfibroelastosis) [10].

Several studies have shown that patients with atrial fibrillation have altered amounts of collagen degradation products and impaired matrix degradation, with abnormal plasma concentrations of various matrix metalloproteinases (MMPs), their inhibitors (tissue inhibitor of MMPs [TIMPs]), and various growth factors (eg, transforming growth factor β1) reported [11-13]. These proteins are important in the breakdown of various collagens and hence their regulation is key to ensuring healthy matrix turnover.

Evidence suggests that abnormal changes in the extracellular matrix are not related to the presence of atrial fibrillation in itself, but are probably a consequence of various coexisting comorbidities (eg, hypertension). Nevertheless, MMPs and TIMPs could have a link with the prothrombotic state, as exemplified by a correlation with prothrombin fragments 1 and 2, markers of thrombogenesis [12]. Further studies have identified disruption of other extracellular matrix components, although most have focused on these factors as a cause for the arrhythmia or explanation for remodelling and chamber dilatation [14-17]. One study suggested that some of the changes in MMPs were due to concomitant mitral valve disease [16], whereas another reported changes in the ventricular myocardium, albeit to a lesser extent [17]. Similarly, in patients with ventricular dysfunction (a potent risk factor for atrial fibrillation), various studies have also shown striking atrial structural changes [18,19].

2.2. Abnormal blood stasis

In addition to stasis consequent on the failure of atrial systole, the presence of non-valvular atrial fibrillation seems to promote progressive left atrial (LA) dilatation [20], thus amplifying the potential for stasis. In the presence of mitral stenosis, LA dilatation is increased and leads to further stasis and propensity to thrombosis [21]. The contribution of LA dilatation to thrombogenesis (at least, in non-valvular atrial fibrillation) is indicated by the finding that atrial size corrected for body surface area is an independent risk factor for stroke [22,23].

The contribution of valvular heart disease to thrombogenesis in atrial fibrillation cannot be ignored. In mitral stenosis, up to 75% of patients with cerebral emboli on computed tomography or autopsy are identified to have atrial fibrillation, presumably due to alterations in LA emptying and transmitral flow [24]. By contrast, moderate-to-severe (non-rheumatic) mitral regurgitation seems to reduce the risk of stroke with atrial fibrillation [25]. Defining patients with atrial fibrillation and mitral valve disease who are at the greatest risk of stroke has proved complex. The risk of emboli increases with age and in individuals with a lower cardiac index, but seems to correlate poorly with clinical classification or mitral valve area.

Studies assessing the degree of LA dilatation have also proven inconsistent. However, an initial embolic event is highly predictive for subsequent or recurrent thromboemboli [26].

Abnormal stasis in the LA and LAA can be visualized on TEE with spontaneous echo contrast (SEC) or pulsed-wave doppler during paroxysms of atrial fibrillation [27-30]. In sinus rhythm, aquadriphasic pattern of blood flow can be seen in the LAA, affording minimum blood stasis [31]. This pattern in blood flow is thought to be related to the intimate yet slightly delayed relations between atrial and ventricular passive and active filling. In atrial fibrillation, SEC has been shown to independently predict increased risk of thromboembolism [32].

2.3. Abnormal blood constituents

The main intravascular promoters of thrombogenesis are platelets and the various proteins of the coagulation cascade. In atrial fibrillation, abnormal changes in both these promoters and other blood constituents (eg, inflammatory cytokines, growth factors) are evident, thereby completing Virchow's triad.

2.3.1. Abnormal changes in coagulation

Abnormal haemostasis and coagulation are well described in atrial fibrillation (figure 1,table1). In particular, increased fibrin turnover has been reported in patients with acute onset or chronic atrial fibrillation [33-39]. These changes initially seemed to be unrelated to the cause of atrial fibrillation or structural heart disease [38,39]. However, abnormal concentrations of prothrombotic indices (eg, prothrombin fragments 1 and 2 and thrombin-antithrombin complexes) are more prominent in patients with stroke who have atrial fibrillation than in those who have sinus rhythm [40], as well as in patients with atrial fibrillation and many stroke risk factors (eg, diabetes plus heart failure) compared with either risk factor alone [41-43]. Furthermore, some prothrombotic indices are abnormal in the patients with atrial fibrillation only [44,45] and in those with paroxysmal atrial fibrillation [46]. Notably, some markers have been proposed as suitable candidates to refine various stroke risk stratification schema, many of which are reasonably able to identify patients at low risk or high risk of stroke, but poor at identifying patients at moderate risk [47].

An association between various prothrombotic indices, stasis, and intracardiac thrombus has been described [48,49]. In one study, congestive cardiac failure, a history of recent embolus, and fibrin D-dimer were shown to independently predict the presence of LAA thrombi on TEE, leading the researchers to conclude that D-dimer could be useful in predicting the absence of LAA thrombi [49].

The prothrombotic state also correlates with the degree of LAA dysfunction [50,51]. Furthermore, a relation to TEE indices of stroke risk has been described. For example, SEC that is visible during TEE shows a significant correlation to prothrombin fragments 1 and 2, fibrinopeptide A, and thrombin-antithrombin III complex in non-valvular atrial fibrillation [52,53]. Patients with atrial flutter and impaired LAA function (shown by pulsed-wave doppler) have increased amounts of of D-dimer and â -thromboglobulin[53]. In accordance with clinical data suggesting that mitral regurgitation protects against stroke in atrial fibrillation, a greater degree of mitral regurgitation is associated with reduced coagulation activity as estimated by fibrin D-dimer amounts [54], highlighting the important contribution of stasis.

http://dx.doi.org/10.5772/53613

	Study design	Comment
Gustafsson et al.,[55]	20 AF with stroke; 20 AF without stroke; 20 stroke without AF; 40 healthy controls	↑D-dimer, vWF in NV AF with and without stroke
Kumagai et al., [39]	73 AF; 73 controls	↑D-dimer
Asakura et al.,[56]	83 AF vs healthy controls	↑PF1+2, TATIII
Sohara&Miyahara [57]	13 paroxysmal AF vs healthy controls	NS in D-dimer, TATIII
Lip et al., [38]	87 AF; 158 controls	↑D-dimer, vWF
Lip et al., {58]	51 AF; 26 healthy controls	↑D-dimer
Kahn et al., [36]	75 NV AF with or without previous embolic events; 42 controls with or without previous thrombotic stroke	vWF higher in AF after stroke than controls without stroke and similar to controls after stroke
Heppell et al., [48]	109 AF with or without thrombus in left atrium	↑D-dimer, vWF, TATIII in patients with left atrial thrombus compared with patients without thrombus
Shinohara et al., [51]	45 NV AF	↑D-dimer, TATIII in patients with low LAA velocity vs patients with high LAA velocity
Feinberg (SPAF III) et al., [59]	1531 AF	PF1+2 not associated with thromboembolism
Mondillo et al., [44]	45 AF; 35 healthy controls	↑D-dimer, vWF, s-thrombomodulin
Fukuchi et al., [60]	AF vs without AF	↑vWF in atrial appendage tissue
Conway et al., [[61]	1321 AF	↑vWF in high-risk group for stroke
Kamath et al., [62]	93 AF; 50 healthy controls	↑D-dimer
Vene et al., [63]	113 AF	↑D-dimer in AF with cardiovascular events vs no events
Nakamura et al., [64]	LAA tissue samples of 7 NV AF vs 4 without AF	↑vWF, TF expression
Conway et al., [65]	994 AF	vWF not a significant predictor of stroke and vascular events
Kamath et al., [66]	31 acute onset AF; 93 permanent AF; 31 healthy controls	Haematocrit raised in acute AF; ↑D-dimer in permanent AF, but not in acute AF
Sakurai et al., [67]	28 AFL; 27 controls	↑D-dimer in patients with impaired LAA function
Inoue et al., [42]	246 NV AF; 111 healthy controls	↑D-dimer in NV AF with risk factors, NS in PF1+2
Kumagai et al., [68]	16 AF post mortem	↑vWF mRNA and protein in AF with enlarged atriums
Marin et al., [33]	24 acute onset AF; 24 chronic AF vs 24 coronary artery disease in sinus rhythm; 24 healthy controls	↑D-dimer, vWF, s-thrombomodulin in all AF groups with no significant after cardioversion
Nozawa et al., [69]	509 AF; 111 healthy controls	↑D-dimer, NS in PF1+2
Freestone et al., [70]	59 AF; 40 healthy controls	↑Vwf
Nozawa et al., [71]	509 NV AF	↑D-dimer but not PF1+2 with predictive significance for thromboembolic events
Ohara et al., [43]	591 NV AF; 129 controls	↑D-dimer, PF1+2, platelet factor 4, and â-thromboglobulin in NV AF; D-dimer, prothrombin fragments correlated with accumulation of clinical risk factors for stroke

AF=atrial fibrillation. NV=non-valvular. TATIII=thrombin-antithrombin III complex. AFL=atrial flutter. vWf=von Willebrand factor. LAA=left atrial appendage. TF=tissue factor. NS=non-significant. PF1+2=prothrombin fragments 1 and 2. s-thrombomodulin=soluble thrombomodulin

Table 1. Coagulation abnormal changes in atrial fibrillation [4] (with permission).

2.3.2. Von Willebrand factor (vWf)

Further insight into the hypercoagulable state in atrial fibrillation is provided by studies of vWf, which is a well-established index of endothelial damage and dysfunction. Raised vWf concentrations independently predict presence of LAA thrombus in atrial fibrillation [48]. Furthermore, increased LAA endocardial expression of vWf has been described [60], especially in those with an overloaded appendage, which seems to correlate with the presence of adherent platelet thrombus. Furthermore, increased expression of vWf in the endocardium has been shown to associate with enlarged LA dimensions in mitral valve disease and increased myocyte diameter [68].

Both vWf and tissue factor are overexpressed in the atrial endothelium in patients with atrial fibrillation who have ahistory of cardiogenic thromboembolism—specifically in the endothelial sites containing inflammatory cells and denuded endocardium, which indicate features of persistent myocarditis [64]. Plasma vWf and D-dimer are also positively correlated in patients receiving either aspirin or no antithrombotic treatment, but not in those receiving warfarin [38], further indicating the ability of warfarin to modulate the thrombogenic process.

Furthermore, a positive association between atrial fibrillation and plasma vWf was seen in the Rotterdam study [72]. This relation was most apparent in female patients, which could explain the excess risk of stroke due to atrial fibrillation in women compared with men. Furthermore, plasma vWf amounts were associated with the presence of four independent risk factors for stroke (heart failure, previous stroke, age, and diabetes) and stroke risk stratification schema [61,65]. Follow-up data from this study suggests that vWf concentrations might independently predict subsequent stroke and vascular events [65,73]. However, such applications will probably be hampered by the non-specificity of vWf, concentrations of which are also increased in various other disorders [74,75].

2.3.3. Tissue factor

An understanding of left atrial—left atrial appendage thrombogenesis may have its roots in distinguishing hemostatic and thrombotic clotting. Studies performed by Hoffman and Monroe [76] offer potential mechanistic insight. In a series of wounding experiments, skin punch biopsy tissue was placed on the dorsal skin of C57 black mice. Samples containing the wound specimens were then collected. For comparison, thrombus was provoked in saphenous veins by application of 10% ferric chloride. After complete occlusion, tissue blocks containing the clotted vessels were collected. Histologic evaluation revealed extensive tissue factor staining within saphenous vein thrombi. In distinct contrast, tissue factor staining in hemostatic clots was localized to squamous endothelial cells at the wounds edges—not within the thrombus itself.

The experimental findings suggest that a large volume of blood must flow over an injured surface, such as the left atrial—left atrial appendage endocardium in a person with atrial fibrillation for significant tissue factor, derived from both circulating cells and microparticles [77,78], to accumulate in high concentrations. Further, and of fundamental teleological relevance, hemostasis occurs rapidly, with tissue factor of local origin determining the rate of thrombus development.

The cell-based model of coagulation translates well to left atrial-left atrial appendage thrombogenesis and supports

a primary role for tissue factor-based thrombin generation, with a secondary role being played by platelets. While the results of clinical trials [79,80], and meta-analyses are consistent with this hypothesis, several biological constructs potentially provide a mechanistic platform as well.

The integrated complexity of coagulation in general and platelet-dependent thrombin generation in particular is becoming evident. One of the most interesting and clinically relevant observations over the past decade is the concomitant interdependence and independence of platelet activation and thrombin generation. The former is best considered in the context of primary hemostasis and possibly arterial thrombosis-both highly dependent on platelet

activation, platelet aggregation and thrombin generation (in concentrations sufficient to provoke further platelet activation). In the latter instance, platelet subpopulations with distinct intracellular calcium signaling properties yield procoagulant domains [81]. The down regulation of platelet aIIb/b3, in turn, attenuates proaggregatory potential.

2.3.4. *Platelets*

Many studies indicate a potential role for platelets in the hypercoagulable state (table 2). However, the results of many of these studies have been conflicting, representing the diverse aspects of platelet physiology that have been measured and possibly confounding from interlaboratory assay variability. The available data support the notion that abnormal changes of platelets in atrial fibrillation do exist, but the relation between these measures and increased thrombotic risk remains uncertain, and many of such abnormal changes could simply indicate underlying vascular comorbidities.

Choudhury and colleagues [82] recently showed that patients with atrial fibrillation had far higher amounts of platelet microparticles and soluble P-selectin than healthy controls in sinus rhythm, but no difference was seen between patients with atrial fibrillation and disease-matched controls, implying that the abnormal changes detected were a consequence of the underlying comorbidities rather than atrial fibrillation itself. Increased amounts of β-thromboglobulin, a platelet-specific protein that indicates platelet activation and is released from α-granules during platelet aggregation and subsequent thrombus formation, have been shown in patients with both valvular and non-valvular atrial fibrillation compared with controls in sinus rhythm [51,58,62,83-86]. Substantially higher β-thromboglobulin amounts have been measured in patients with the lowest LAA flow velocities, who had greater left-atrial dimensions [51], suggesting that platelet activation could be enhanced in patients with a greater degree of intra-atrial stasis.

Despite the presence of enhanced platelet activation in atrial fibrillation, any firm clinical evidence indicating that it directly enhances thrombotic risk is lacking. A substudy from the

Stroke Prevention in Atrial Fibrillation III (SPAF-III) trial [59] recorded no association between plasma β -thromboglobulin amounts and subsequent thromboembolic events. By contrast, the population-based Rotterdam study [87] showed that plasma concentrations of soluble P-selectin were predictive of adverse clinical outcomes in elderly patients with atrial fibrillation.

	Patient group	Results
Yamauchi et al., [87]	26 V AF; 73 NV AF; 57 healthy controls	↑ BTG in AF, NS in PF4
Furui et al., [95]	20 AF; 15 healthy controls	BTG increase greater in AF than in controls after treadmill exercise
Gustafsson et al., [55]	20 AF with stroke; 20 AF without stroke; 20 stroke with sinus rhythm; 40 healthy controls	↑BTG, PF4 in NV AF with and without stroke
Sohara et al., [57]	13 paroxysmal AF vs healthy controls	NS in BTG, PF4
Lip et al., [58]	51 AF; 26 healthy controls	↑BTG
Heppell [48]	109 AF with or without thrombus in left atrium	↑BTG, PF4 in patients with left atrial thrombus compared with patients without thrombus
Minamino et al., [86]	25 AF vs healthy controls	↑mP-sel
Shinohara et al., [51]	45 NV AF	↑BTG, PF4 in patients with low LAA velocity vs patients high LAA velocity
Feinberg et al., SPAF III) [59]	1531 AF	BTG not associated with thromboembolism
Minamino et al., [93]	28 AF	↑BTG, mP-sel
Mondillo et al., [44]	45 AF; 35 healthy controls	↑BTG, PF4
Kamath et al., [45]	93 AF; 50 healthy controls	↑BTG, soluble GPV; NS in platelet aggreagation
Conway et al., [61]	1321 AF	sP-sel was independent of risk for stroke
Conway et al., [65]	994 AF	sP-sel not a significant predictor of stroke and vascular events
Atalar et al., [96]	15 paroxysmal AF; 25 chronic AF; 22 healthy controls	Higher BTG, PF4 in chronic AF than in paroxysmal AF and after conversion to sinus rhythm
Nozawa et al., [69]	509 AF; 111 healthy controls	↑BTG, PF4
Sakurai et al., [53]	28 AFL; 27 controls	↑BTG in patients with impaired LAA function
Inoue et al., [42]	246 NV AF; 111 controls	↑BTG, NS in PF4
Nozawa et al., [69]	509 NV AF	BTG, PF4 did not predict thromboembolic events
Choudhury et al., [97]	121 NV AF; 65 healthy controls; 78 disease-matched controls	Similar but raised levels of CD62P, CD63 and sP-sel in AF and disease-matched controls compared with healthy controls
Choudhury et al., [82]	70 NV AF; 46 disease controls; 33 healthy controls	↑PMP and sP-sel in AF and disease controls, but AF not an independent determinant

Atrial fibrillation. V=valvular. NV=non-valvular. AFL=atrial flutter. BTG= β-thromboglobulin. PF4=platelet factor 4. sPsel=soluble P-selectin. mP-sel=matrix P-selectin. GPV=glycoprotein V. LAA=left atrial appendage. NS=non-significant. PMP=platelet microparticles.

Table 2. Studies of platelet function in atrial fibrillation [4] (with permission)

However, Nagao et al., [88] suggests that thromboembolism in atrial fibrillation is probably due to enhancement of various components of the coagulation system due to stasis of blood in the inordinate and irregular atria, rather than to platelet activation perse. The relative role of coagulation versus platelet activation in the pathogenesis of thrombogenesis in patients with atrial fibrillation can roughly be inferred from the results of antithrombotic drug interventions that have been tested in randomized clinical trials [89-91]. These results indicate that inhibition of coagulation remains the mainstay in preventing atrial fibrillation –related thrombogenesis. The lesser but significant role of platelets- best inhibited by a combined antiplatelet drug regimen – is presumably related to the platelet activation seen in this arrhythmia could contribute to thrombogenesis indirectly. For example, increased expression of P-selectin on platelets associated with reduced concentrations of nitric oxide has also been shown to be a risk factor for silent cerebral infarction in patients with atrial fibrillation [92]. Moreover, raised amounts of P-selectin and CD63 have both been associated with the embolic and pre-embolic status of patients with non-rheumatic atrial fibrillation [93]. Or the prominent involvement of platelets in the pathogenesis of atherothrombotic (that is, non-cardiombolic) events [94].

2.3.5. Abnormal changes in fibrinolysis

Few studies have focused on fibrinolytic function in atrial fibrillation. Enhanced fibrinolysis, shown by increased concentrations of tissue-plaminogen activator (t-PA) antigen and t-PA inhibitor (PAI)-1 and reduced amounts of plasmin-antiplasmin complex can be attributable to a pathophysiological response to the prothrombotic state [95,66]. However, the available data are not consistent and conflicting results have also been reported [35]. In the Stroke Prevention in Atrial Fibrillation (SPAF) III study [99], increased concentrations of plasmin-antiplasmin complexes were independently associated with thromboembolic risk factors such as older age (>75 years), recent congestive heart failure, decreased fractional shortening, and recent onset of atrial fibrillation. A significant correlation can be also shown between t-PA amounts and left-atrial diameter in atrial fibrillation [35]. Predictably, anticoagulation leads to some improvement in fibrinolytic markers in rheumatic atrial fibrillation [98].

Increased amounts of t-PA and PAI-1 can indicate the coexistence of confounders, such as hypertension, heart failure, or ischaemic heart disease, all of which can cause endothelial dysfunction, damage, and inflammation. However, studies in patients with atrial fibrillation only confirm that presence of the disorder does modulate these markers. [35,95,99]. Thus, the high amounts of t-PA and PAI-1 in atrial fibrillation could be a consequence of endothelial damage and dysfunction or represent systemic inflammation [100,101]. PAI-1 concentrations are also predictive of successful cardioversion [102], and are independent predictors of the development of atrial fibrillation after cardiopulmonary bypass [103].

It is unclear whether increased amounts of t-PA or PAI-1 in atrial fibrillation are due to endothelial dysfunction, inflammation, fibrinolysis, or vascular disease, or a combination. Nevertheless, abnormal changes in the fibrinolytic system might relate not only to thrombogenesis but also to structural remodelling of the atria, in view of the strong links to extracellular matrix turnover.

2.3.6. Restoration of sinus rhythm

Some evidence suggests that activation of the coagulation system could be adversely affected by cardioversion of atrial fibrillation [104]. Electrical cardioversion has been associated with more prominent activation of the coagulation system than a pharmacological strategy [105]. One study found a positive correlation between the energy delivered for cardioversion to sinus rhythm and plasma D-dimer values on day 7 [105]. Additionally, an extended duration of atrial fibrillation could lead to a more prominent hypercoagulable state (estimated by D-dimer value) after cardioversion[106]. The hypercoagulable state after cardioversion has been seen despite optimum anticoagulation with warfarin [107]. Nevertheless, patients receiving therapeutic low-molecular-weight heparin (LMWH) before cardioversion seem to have reduced hypercoagulability [108].

2.4. What drives the prothrombotic state in atrial fibrillation?

Several mechanisms have been purported to drive then prothrombotic state in atrial fibrillation (figure 2), but recent evidence has focused on the potential role of inflammation and the release of various growth factors.

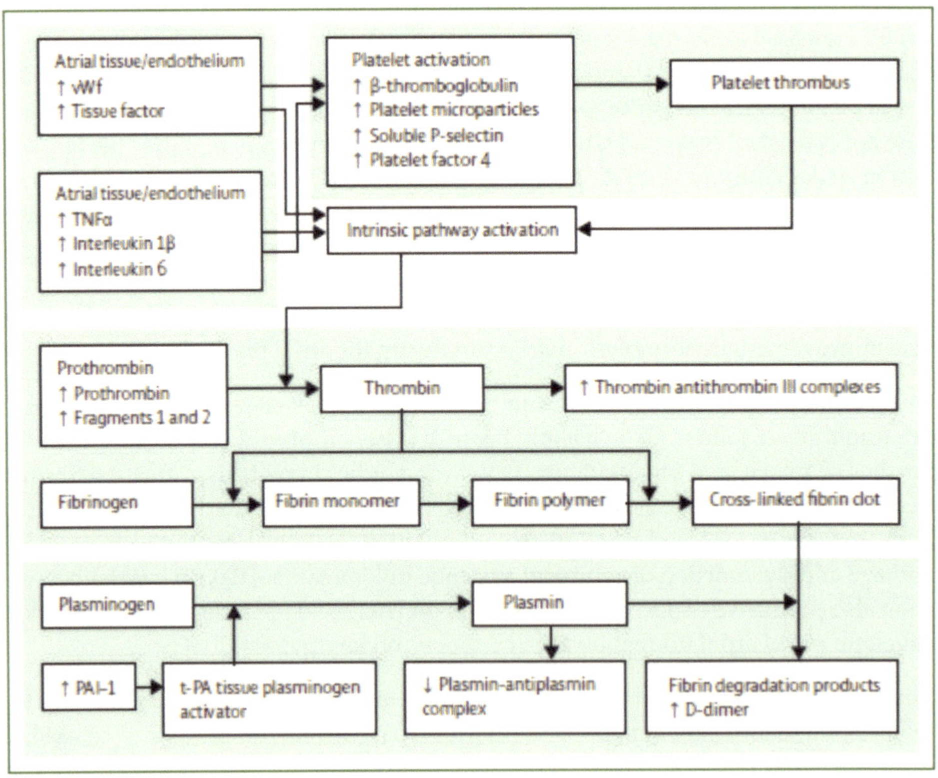

Figure 2. Abnormal changes in coagulation during atrial fibrillation [4] (with permission)

2.4.1. *Inflammation*

In atrial fibrillation, inflammation might not only result in endothelial damage, dysfunction, or activation, but also be linked directly to thrombogenesis. Increasing evidence has supported a link between inflammation and the initiation and perpetuation of atrial fibrillation [109-113]. Furthermore, abnormal changes in systemic inflammation have been related to prothrombotic indices in atrial fibrillation, suggesting that inflammation could drive the prothrombotic state in atrial fibrillation [109].

Although most cases of atrial fibrillation are associated with various comorbidities, many of which could also enhance the baseline inflammatory state, there may be an underlying direct link between atrial fibrillation and inflammation. Interleukin-6 concentrations are abnormal in atrial fibrillation, with some prognostic implications shown in one study [114]. Many studies have also shown that amounts of high-sensitivity C-reactive protein (hs-CRP) are greater in patients with atrial fibrillation than in controls in sinus rhythm, with a stepwise increase in hs-CRP with the transition from patient groups with an increasing burden (sinus rhythm to paroxysmal then persistent) in atrial fibrillation [115]. Raised hs-CRP amounts consistently correlate with cardiovascular risk, although not with future atrial fibrillation [109].More recently, high hc-CRP amounts were shown to be predictive of mortality and vascular death in atrial fibrillation, but not stroke itself [116].

How is inflammation linked to thrombogenesis in atrial fibrillation? Both CRP and interleukin 6 stimulate tissue factor production from monocytes in vitro [117, 118]. Furthermore, interleukin 6 increases platelet production and sensitivity to thrombin [119], stimulates transcription of fibrinogen [120], and is linked to both endothelial activation and damage [121,122]. However, no link seems to exist between hs-CRP and thrombin-antithrombin complexes [123]. Tissue factor and high stroke risk are also independent associates of interleukin 6, whereas fibrinogen and plasma viscosity are independent associates of hs-CRP amounts [124].

2.4.2. *Growth factors*

Another potential driver for thrombogenesis could be growth factors. Various pro-angiogenic factors have been identified; concentrations of some of these factors have been shown to alter in atrial fibrillation [70,125,126]. Vascular endothelial growth factor (VEGF) is largely produced by activated platelets [127], and results in upregulation of tissue factor mRNA production and subsequent expression of this compound on the endothelial membrane [128]. VEGF amounts are substantially increased in both persistent and permanent atrial fibrillation, with a corresponding increase in tissue factor [125]. Additionally, raised serum concentrations of transforming growth factor-β1[126] and angiopoetin 2 (but not angiopoetin 1) [70] are also recorded in atrial fibrillation, showing the depth and complexity of modulation of growth factor amounts.

Although the requirements for enhanced angiogenesis in atrial fibrillation are unknown, in view of the intimate association between VEGF and tissue factor, enhanced growth factors could be a crucial driving force behind the hypercoagulable state. Notably, tissue factor acts as a cofactor to factor VIIa and is widely regarded as the physiological trigger to thrombin formation [129]. But, why are factors such as the angiopoietins involved? Angiopoeitin 1 and 2 are natural co-antagonists and both compete for the same binding site on Tie-2, an endothelial tyrosine kinase receptor. With an excess of angiopoeitin 1, stability of the endothelium is favoured, whereas the converse is true with an excess of angiopoeitin 2 [70]. In these circumstances, the balance could ultimately favour endothelial destabilisation and therefore the action of cytokines such as VEGF.

2.4.3. Extracellular matrix turnover

The relationship between atrial fibrillation and remodeling of the left atrium/arterial appendage is traditionally explained by the absence of contractility and altered flow dynamics. This hypothesis is not entirely fulfilling for several reasons, not the least of which is its inability to substantiate the mechanism of progressive structural change. A contemporary view considers the contribution of coagulation factors and thrombus substrate itself as both initiators and perpetuators of the prothrombotic environment that includes remodeling. Thrombin, a serine protease, beyond its widely recognized role in hemostasis and thrombosis, is directly involved in tissue repair and remodeling through an endothelial mesenchymal transdifferentiation process [130]. Thrombin also exerts an effect on endothelial cell junctions (reviewed in [131], endothelial cell and smooth muscle cell migration and smooth muscle cell proliferation via protease activated receptor (PAR)-1 [132].

Thrombin-induced membrane-type matrix metalloproteinase (MMP)-2 gene transcription and activity [133] may also contribute to structural changes in the atrium/atrial appendage, as may thrombin-augmented fibroblast-mediated collagen gel contraction [134]. Locally generated thrombin has been shown in tissue culture to upregulate tissue factor expression and activity [135].

While thrombin is known to possess a variety of cell regulating capabilities, one must not overlook the contribution

of other coagulation proteases in the remodeling process. Indeed, factor Xa has been shown to promote fibroblast proliferation, migration and differentiation into myofibroblasts through a PAR-2 specific mechanism [136]. Accordingly, the development of oral/direct factor Xa and thrombin inhibitors provides an unprecedented opportunity to investigate fundamental pathological mechanisms in atrial fibrillation.

2.4.4. Nitric oxide

Nitric oxide is synthesized by nitric oxide synthase, which is present in large concentrations in the endothelium. The expression of nitric oxide synthase is regulated by flow-mediated shear stress and is consequently downregulated at sites with low flow velocity [137]. Nitric oxide shows potent antithrombotic effects in arterial endothelium, and nitric oxide released from activated platelets inhibits platelet recruitment to the growing thrombus [138], while also inhibiting expression of PAI-1 [139].

http://dx.doi.org/10.5772/53613

In animal models of atrial fibrillation, the loss of atrial contraction and consequent reduction in shear stress seems to reduce LA expression of nitric oxide synthase with a corresponding decrease in nitric oxide bioavailability and increase in PAI-1 expression [140]. In the LAA, nitric oxide concentrations were also significantly reduced compared with control animals, but this finding did not indicate decreased expression of nitric oxide synthase at this site. Since atrial thrombus is frequently formed in the LAA, this finding still has no adequate explanation.

2.4.5. Renin-Angiotensin-Aldosterone System (RAAS)

The RAAS is now appreciated as key to the pathophysiology of various cardiovascular disease states. The extent of these changes seems to relate predominantly to the reduction in angiotensin-II amounts. Atrial tissue has the capacity to produce and use this hormone with local expression of acetylcholinesterase and angiotensin-II receptors, both of which could be upregulated in atrial fibrillation [141]. RAAS could be mechanistically implicated in initiation and perpetuation of atrial fibrillation [141-143], as well as providing the link to other mechanisms promoting the prothrombotic state in atrial fibrillation.

Angiotensin II has been shown to possess several proinflammatory properties and increases the production of proinflammatory cytokines (eg, interleukin 6 and tumour necrosis factorα [TNFα]), adhesion molecules (eg, vascular-cell adhesion molecule 1), monocyte chemoattractant protein 1, and selectins (eg, P-selectin) [144-146]. Similarly, through release of various chemokines (eg, cytokine-induced neutrophil chemoattractant), angiotensin II can initiate neutrophil recruitment [146]. Expression of angiotensin-II receptors has also been linked with increased atrial cell death and leucocyte infiltration [147]. These data potentially support a complex relation between RAAS, inflammation, and atrial fibrillation.

Additionally, RAAS has been implicated in the activation of various MMPs and thromboxane A2 (a prothrombotic signalling molecule produced by activated platelets). These processes could occur both as a direct effect of angiotensin II and also through induction of interleukin 6 [148]. Furthermore, angiotensin II could accelerate degradation of nitric oxide through production of reactive oxygen species and thereby impair endothelium dependent vasodilatation [149]. Likewise, activation of RAAS increases synthesis of PAI-1, possibly indicating either enhanced endothelial damage or impaired fibrinolysis in atrial fibrillation [150].

3. Conclusion

The mechanisms underlying thrombogenesis in atrial fibrillation are clearly complex and remain only partly understood. Abnormal changes in flow, vessel wall, and blood constituents in atrial fibrillation fulfil Virchow's triad for thrombogenesis, and accord with a prothrombotic or hypercoagulable state in this arrhythmia. That this process is related purely to blood stasis is no longer accepted. Various abnormal changes related both to atrial fibrillation and its comorbidities impart a synergistic effect in maintaining a hypercoagulable state in this condition.

Author details

Hanan Ahmed GalalAzzam

Mansoura university/ Faculty of Medicine, Egypt

References

[1] Lip GYH. Does atrial fi brillation confer a hypercoagulable state? Lancet 1995; 346: 1313–14.

[2] Brotman DJ, Deitcher SR, Lip GY, Martzdorff AC. Virchow's triad revisited. South Med J 2004; 97: 213–14.

[3] Choudhury A, Lip GY. Atrial fibrillation and the hypercoagulable state: from basic science to clinical practice. PathophysiolHaemostThromb 2003–2004; 33: 282–89.

[4] Watson T, Shantsila E, Lip YHG. Mechanisms of thrombogenesis in atrial fibrillation: Virchow's triad revisited. Lancet 2009;373(9658):155-66.

[5] Blackshear JL, Odell JA. Appendage obliteration to reduce stroke incardiac surgical patients with atrial fi brillation.Ann ThoracSurg1996; 61: 755–59.

[6] Pollick C, Taylor D. Assessment of left atrial appendage function bytransesophageal echocardiography. Implications for thedevelopment of thrombus.Circulation 1991; 84: 223–31.

[7] Goldsmith IR, Blann AD, Patel RL, Lip GY. Von Willebrand factor,fibrinogen, and soluble P-selectin levels after mitral valve replacementversus mitral valve repair. Am J Cardiol 2000; 85: 1218–22.

[8] Masawa N, Yoshida Y, Yamada T, Joshita T, Ooneda G. Diagnosis ofcardiac thrombosis in patients with atrial fi brillation in the absenceof macroscopically visible thrombi. Virchows Arch A PatholAnatHistopathol 1993; 422: 67-71..

[9] Dollery CM, McEwan JR, Henney AM. Matrix metalloproteinasesand cardiovascular disease.Circ Res 1995; 77: 863–68.

[10] Shirani J, Alaeddini J. Structural remodeling of the left atrial appendage in patients with chronic non-valvular atrial fibrillation: implications for thrombus formation, systemic embolism, and assessment by transesophageal echocardiography. CardiovascPathol 2000; 9(2):95-101.

[11] Tziakas DN, Chalikias GK, Papanas N, Stakos DA, Chatzikyriakou SV, Maltezos E. Circulating levels of collagen type I degradation marker depend on the type of atrial fi brillation. Europace 2007; 9: 589–96.

[12] Marin F, Roldan V, Climent V, Garcia A, Marco P, Lip GY.Is thrombogenesis in atrial fi brillation related to matrix metalloproteinase-1 and its inhibitor, TIMP-1? Stroke 2003; 34: 1181–86.

[13] Li X, Ma C, Dong J, et al. The fibrosis and atrial fibrillation: is thetransforming growth factor-beta(1) a candidate etiology of atrial fibrillation. Med Hypotheses 2008; 70: 317–19.

[14] Xu J, Cui G, Esmailian F, et al. Atrial extracellular matrix remodeling and the maintenance of atrial fi brillation. Circulation 2004; 109: 363–68.

[15] Nakano Y, Niida S, Dote K, et al. Matrix metalloproteinase-9 contributes to human atrial remodeling during atrial fibrillation. J Am CollCardiol 2004; 43: 818–25.

[16] Anne W, Willems R, Roskams T, et al. Matrix metalloproteinases and atrial remodeling in patients with mitral valve disease and atrial fibrillation.Cardiovasc Res 2005; 67: 655–66.

[17] Mukherjee R, Herron AR, Lowry AS, et al. Selective induction of matrix metalloproteinases and tissue inhibitor of metalloproteinases in atrial and ventricular myocardium in patients with atrial fibrillation. Am J Cardiol 2006; 97: 532–37.

[18] Sanders P, Morton JB, Davidson NC, et al. Electrical remodeling of the atria in congestive heart failure: electrophysiological and electroanatomic mapping in humans. Circulation 2003; 108: 1461–68.

[19] Li D, Fareh S, Leung TK, Nattel S. Promotion of atrial fibrillation by heart failure in dogs: atrial remodeling of a diff erent sort. Circulation 1999; 100: 87–95.

[20] Sanfilippo AJ, Abascal VM, Sheehan M, et al. Atrial enlargement as a consequence of atrial fibrillation. A prospective echocardiographic study.Circulation 1990; 82: 792–97.

[21] Keren G, Etzion T, Sherez J, et al. Atrial fibrillation and atrial enlargement in patients with mitral stenosis. Am Heart J 1987; 114: 1146–55.

[22] The Stroke Prevention in Atrial Fibrillation Investigators. Predictors of thromboembolism in atrial fibrillation: II Echocardiographic features of patients at risk. Ann Intern Med 1992; 116: 6–12.

[23] Di Tullio MR, Sacco RL, Sciacca RR, Homma S. Left atrial size and the risk of ischemic stroke in an ethnically mixed population. Stroke1999; 30: 2019–24.

[24] Salem DN, Stein PD, Al Ahmad A, et al. Antithrombotic therapy in valvular heart disease—native and prosthetic: the seventh ACCP Conference on Antithrombotic and Thrombolytic Therapy. Chest 2004; 126: 457–82S.

[25] Nakagami H, Yamamoto K, Ikeda U, Mitsuhashi T, Goto T, Shimada K. Mitral regurgitation reduces the risk of stroke in patients with nonrheumatic atrial fi brillation. Am Heart J 1998; 136: 528–32.

[26] Chiang CW, Lo SK, Ko YS, Cheng NJ, Lin PJ, Chang CH. Predictors of systemic embolism in patients with mitral stenosis. A prospective study. Ann Intern Med 1998; 128: 885–89.

[27] Pollick C, Taylor D. Assessment of left atrial appendage function by transesophageal echocardiography. Implications for the development of thrombus.Circulation 1991; 84: 223–31.

[28] Asinger RW, Koehler J, Pearce LA, et al. Pathophysiologic correlates of thromboembolism in nonvalvular atrial fi brillation: II Dense spontaneous echocardiographic contrast (The Stroke Prevention in Atrial Fibrillation [SPAF-III] study). J Am SocEchocardiogr 1999; 12: 1088–96.

[29] Handke M, Harloff A, Hetzel A, Olschewski M, Bode C, Geibel A. Left atrial appendage flow velocity as a quantitative surrogate parameter for thromboembolic risk: determinants and relationship to spontaneous echocontrast and thrombus formation—a transesophageal echocardiographic study in 500 patients with cerebral ischemia. J Am SocEchocardiogr 2005; 18: 1366–72.

[30] Obarski TP, Salcedo EE, Castle LW, Stewart WJ. Spontaneous echo contrast in the left atrium during paroxysmal atrial fibrillation.Am Heart J 1990; 120: 988–90.

[31] Jue J, Winslow T, Fazio G, Redberg RF, Foster E, Schiller NB. Pulsed doppler characterization of left atrial appendage flow. J Am SocEchocardiogr 1993; 6: 237–44.

[32] The Stroke Prevention In Atrial Fibrillation Investigators committee on echocardiography. Transesophageal echocardiographic correlates of thromboembolism in high-risk patients with nonvalvular atrial fibrillation. Ann Intern Med 1998; 128: 639–47.

[33] Marin F, Roldan V, Climent VE, et al. Plasma von Willebrand factor, soluble thrombomodulin, and fi brin D-dimer concentrations in acute onset non-rheumatic atrial fi brillation. Heart 2004; 90: 1162–66.

[34] Mahe I, Drouet L, Chassany O, et al. D-dimer: a characteristic of the coagulation state of each patient with chronic atrial fi brillation. Thromb Res 2002; 107: 1–6.

[35] Roldan V, Marin F, Marco P, Martinez JG, Calatayud R, Sogorb F.Hypofibrinolysis in atrial fibrillation. Am Heart J 1998; 136: 956–60.

[36] Kahn SR, Solymoss S, Flegel KM. Nonvalvular atrial fi brillation: evidence for a prothrombotic state. CMAJ 1997; 157: 673–81.

[37] Mitusch R, Siemens HJ, Garbe M, Wagner T, Sheikhzadeh A, Diederich KW. Detection of a hypercoagulable state in nonvalvular atrial fibrillation and the effect of anticoagulant therapy.ThrombHaemost 1996; 75: 219–23.

[38] Lip GY, Lowe GD, Rumley A, Dunn FG. Increased markers of thrombogenesis in chronic atrial fibrillation: effects of warfarin treatment. Br Heart J 1995; 73: 527–33.

[39] Kumagai K, Fukunami M, Ohmori M, Kitabatake A, Kamada T, Hoki N. Increased intracardiovascular clotting in patients with chronic atrial fibrillation. J Am CollCardiol 1990; 16: 377–80.

[40] Turgut N, Akdemir O, Turgut B, et al. Hypercoagulopathy in stroke patients with nonvalvular atrial fibrillation: hematologic and cardiologic investigations. ClinApplThrombHemost 2006; 12: 15–20.

[41] Varughese GI, Patel JV, Tomson J, Lip GY. The prothrombotic risk of diabetes mellitus in atrial fibrillation and heart failure. J ThrombHaemost 2005; 3: 2811–13.

[42] Inoue H, Nozawa T, Okumura K, Jong-Dae L, Shimizu A, Yano K. Prothrombotic activity is increased in patients with nonvalvular atrial fibrillation and risk factors for embolism. Chest 2004; 126: 687–92.

[43] Ohara K, Inoue H, Nozawa T, et al. Accumulation of risk factors enhances the prothrombotic state in atrial fibrillation. Int J Cardiol2008; 126: 316–21.

[44] Mondillo S, Sabatini L, Agricola E, et al. Correlation between left atrial size, prothrombotic state and markers of endothelial dysfunction in patients with lone chronic non-rheumatic atrial fibrillation.Int J Cardiol 2000; 75: 227–32.

[45] Kamath S, Blann AD, Chin BS, Lip GY. A prospective randomized trial of aspirin-clopidogrel combination therapy and dose-adjusted warfarin on indices of thrombogenesis and platelet activation in atrial fibrillation. J Am CollCardiol 2002; 40: 484–90.

[46] Li-Saw-Hee FL, Blann AD, Gurney D, Lip GY. Plasma von Willebrand factor, fibrinogen and soluble P-selectin levels in paroxysmal, persistent and permanent atrial fi brillation. Effects of cardioversion and return of left atrial function.Eur Heart J 2001; 22: 1741–47.

[47] Roldan V, Marin F, Garcia-Herola A, Lip GY. Correlation of plasma von Willebrand factor levels, an index of endothelial damage/ dysfunction, with two point-based stroke risk stratification scores in atrial fibrillation. Thromb Res 2005; 116: 321–25.

[48] Heppell RM, Berkin KE, McLenachan JM, Davies JA. Haemostatic and haemodynamic abnormalities associated with left atrial thrombosis in non-rheumatic atrial fi brillation. Heart 1997; 77: 407–11.

[49] Habara S, Dote K, Kato M, et al. Prediction of left atrial appendage thrombi in nonvalvular atrial fi brillation. Eur Heart J 2007; 28: 2217–22.

[50] Igarashi Y, Kashimura K, Makiyama Y, Sato T, Ojima K, Aizawa Y. Left atrial appendage dysfunction in chronic nonvalvular atrial fibrillation is significantly associated with an elevated level of brain natriuretic peptide and a prothrombotic state. JpnCirc J 2001;65: 788–92.

[51] Shinohara H, Fukuda N, Soeki T, et al. Relationship between flow dynamics in the left atrium and hemostatic abnormalities in patients with nonvalvular atrial fibrillation. Jpn Heart J 1998;39: 721–30.

[52] Tsai LM, Chen JH, Tsao CJ. Relation of left atrial spontaneous echo contrast with prethrombotic state in atrial fi brillation associated with systemic hypertension, idiopathic dilated cardiomyopathy, or no identifiable cause (lone). Am J Cardiol 1998; 81: 1249–52.

[53] Sakurai K, Hirai T, Nakagawa K, et al. Left atrial appendage function and abnormal hypercoagulability in patients with atrial fl utter. Chest 2003; 124: 1670–74.

[54] Lip GY, Rumley A, Dunn FG, Lowe GD. Thrombogenesis in mitral regurgitation and aortic stenosis. Angiology 1996; 47: 1117–25.

[55] Gustafsson C, Blomback M, Britton M, Hamsten A, Svensson J. Coagulation factors and the increased risk of stroke in nonvalvularatrial fibrillation. Stroke 1990; 21: 47–51.

[56] Asakura H, Hifumi S, Jokaji H, et al. Prothrombin fragment F1 + 2 and thrombin-antithrombin III complex are useful markers of the hypercoagulable state in atrial fibrillation. Blood CoagulFibrinolysis 1992; 3: 469–73.

[57] Sohara H, Miyahara K. E ▪ ect of atrial fibrillation on the fibrino-coagulation system-study in patients with paroxysmal atrial fibrillation. JpnCirc J 1994; 58: 821–26.

[58] Lip GY, Lip PL, Zarifis J, et al. Fibrin D-dimer and beta-thromboglobulin as markers of thrombogenesis and platelet activation in atrial fibrillation. E ▪ ects of introducing ultra-low-dose warfarin and aspirin. Circulation 1996; 94: 425–31.

[59] Feinberg WM, Pearce LA, Hart RG, et al. Markers of thrombin and platelet activity in patients with atrial fibrillation: correlation with stroke among 1531 participants in the stroke prevention in atrial fibrillation III study. Stroke 1999; 30: 2547–53.

[60] Fukuchi M, Watanabe J, Kumagai K, et al. Increased von Willebrandfactor in the endocardium as a local predisposing factor for thrombogenesis in overloaded human atrial appendage. J Am CollCardiol 2001; 37: 1436–42.

[61] Conway DS, Pearce LA, Chin BS, Hart RG, Lip GY. Plasma von Willebran factor and soluble P-selectin as indices of endothelial damage and platelet activation in 1321 patients with nonvalvular atrial fibrillation: relationship to stroke risk factors. Circulation 2002; 106: 1962–67.

[62] Kamath S, Blann AD, Chin BS, et al. A study of platelet activation in atrial fibrillation and the e ▪ ects of antithrombotic therapy. Eur Heart J 2002; 23: 1788–95.

[63] Vene N, Mavri A, Kosmelj K, Stegnar M. High D-dimer levels predict cardiovascular events in patients with chronic atrial fibrillation during oral anticoagulant therapy. ThrombHaemost2003; 90: 1163–72.

[64] Nakamura Y, Nakamura K, Fukushima-Kusano K, et al. Tissue factor expression in atrial endothelia associated with nonvalvularatrial fibrillation: possible involvement in intracardiacthrombogenesis. Thromb Res 2003; 111: 137–42.

[65] Conway DS, Pearce LA, Chin BS, Hart RG, Lip GY. Prognostic value of plasma von Willebrand factor and soluble P-selectin as indices of endothelial damage and platelet activation in 994 patients with nonvalvular atrial fi brillation.Circulation 2003; 107: 3141–45.

[66] Kamath S, Blann AD, Chin BS, Lip GY. Platelet activation, haemorheology and thrombogenesis in acute atrial fibrillation: a comparison with permanent atrial fibrillation. Heart 2003; 89: 1093–95.

[67] Sakurai K, Hirai T, Nakagawa K, et al. Prolonged activation of hemostatic markers following conversion of atrial flutter to sinus rhythm. Circ J 2004; 68: 1041–44

[68] Kumagai K, Fukuchi M, Ohta J, et al. Expression of the vonWillebrand factor in atrial endocardium is increased in atrial fibrillation depending on the extent of structural remodeling. Circ J 2004; 68: 321–27.

[69] Nozawa T, Inoue H, Iwasa A, et al. E ▪ ects of anticoagulation intensity on hemostatic markers in patients with non-valvular atrial fibrillation. Circ J 2004; 68: 29–34.

[70] Freestone B, Chong AY, Lim HS, Blann A, Lip GYH. Angiogenicfactors in atrial fibrillation: a possible role in thrombogenesis? Ann Med 2005; 37: 365–72.

[71] Nozawa T, Inoue H, Hirai T, et al. D-dimer level influences thromboembolic events in patients with atrial fibrillation. Int J Cardiol 2006; 109: 59–65.

[72] Conway DS, Heeringa J, Van Der Kuip DA, et al. Atrial fibrillation and the prothrombotic state in the elderly: the Rotterdam Study. Stroke 2003; 34: 413–17.

[73] Lip GY, Lane D, Van Walraven C, Hart RG. Additive role of plasma von Willebrand factor levels to clinical factors for risk stratification of patients with atrial fi brillation. Stroke 2006; 37: 2294–300.

[74] Varughese GI, Patel JV, Tomson J, Lip GY. Effects of blood pressure on the prothrombotic risk in 1235 patients with non-valvular atrial fibrillation. Heart 2007; 93: 495–99.

[75] Lip GY, Pearce LA, Chin BS, Conway DS, Hart RG. Effects of congestive heart failure on plasma von Willebrand factor and soluble P-selectin concentrations in patients with non-valvar atrial fibrillation. Heart 2005; 91: 759–63.

[76] Hoffman M, Whinna HC, Monroe DM. Circulating tissue factor accumulates in thrombi, but not in hemostatic plugs. J ThrombHaemost 2006; 4:2092–2093.

[77] Lechner D, Weltermann A. Circulating tissue factorexposingmicroparticles. Thromb Res 2008; 122:S47–S54.

[78] George FD. Microparticles in vascular diseases.Thromb Res 2008; 122:S55–S59.

[79] Connolly S, Pogue J, Hart R et al., Clopidogrel plus aspirin versus oral anticoagulation for atrial fibrillation in the Atrial fibrillation Clopidogrel Trial with Irbesartan

for prevention of Vascular Events (ACTIVE W): a randomised controlled trial. Lancet 2006; 367:1903–1912.

[80] Healey JS, Hart RG, Pogue J et al., Risks and benefits of oral anticoagulation compared with clopidogrel plus aspirin in patients with atrial fibrillation according to stroke risk: the atrial fibrillation clopidogrel trial with irbesartan for prevention of vascular events (ACTIVE-W). Stroke 2008; 39:1482–1486.

[81] MunnixIC, Kuijpers MJ, Auger J et al., Segregation of platelet aggregatory and procoagulantmicrodomains in thrombus formation: regulation by transient integrin activation. ArteriosclerThrombVascBiol 2007; 27:2484–2490.

[82] Choudhury A, Chung I, Blann AD, Lip GY. Elevated platelet microparticle levels in nonvalvular atrial fi brillation: relationship to P-selectin and antithrombotic therapy. Chest 2007; 131: 809–15

[83] Kaplan KL, Nossel HL, Drillings M, Lesznik G. Radioimmunoassay of platelet factor 4 and beta-thromboglobulin: development and application to studies of platelet release in relation to fibrinopeptideA generation. Br J Haematol 1978; 39: 129–46.

[84] Kunishima S, Hattori M, Kobayashi S, et al. Activation and destruction of platelets in patients with rheumatic heart disease. Eur Heart J 1994; 15: 335–38.

[85] Minamino T, Kitakaze M, Asanuma H, et al. Plasma adenosine levels and platelet activation in patients with atrial fi brillation. Am J Cardiol 1999; 83: 194–98.

[86] Yamauchi K, Furui H, Taniguchi N, Sotobata I. Plasma beta-thromboglobulin and platelet factor 4 concentrations in patients with atrial fibrillation. Jpn Heart J 1986; 27: 481–87.

[87] Heeringa J, Conway DS, van der Kuip DA, et al. A longitudinal population-based study of prothrombotic factors in elderly subjects with atrial fibrillation: the Rotterdam Study 1990–1999. J ThrombHaemost 2006; 4: 1944–49.

[88] Nagao, T.; Hamamoto, M.; Kanda, A.; Tsuganesawa, T.; Ueda, M.; Kobayashi, K.; Miyazaki, T.&Terashi, A. (1995). Platelet activation is not involved in acceleration of the coagulation system in acute cardioembolic stroke with nonvalvular atrial fibrillation. Stroke, Vol.26:pp.1365-8.

[89] Hart, RG.; Pearce, LA.& Aguilar, MI. Meta-analysis: antithrombotic therapy to prevent stroke in patients who have nonvalvular atrial fibrillation. Ann internal Med 2007; 146:857-67.

[90] Lip, GY. & Lim, BS. Atrial fibrillation and stroke prevention. Lancet Neurol 2007; 6: 981-93.

[91] Connolly, SJ., Pogue, J., Hart, RG., Hart, RG., Hohnloser, SH., Pfeffer, M., Chrolavicius, S. & Yusuf, S. Effect of clopidogrel added to aspirin in patients with atrial fibrillation. ACTIVE Investigatiors, N Engl J Med 2009; 360: 2066-78.

[92] Minamino T, Kitakaze M, Sanada S, et al. Increased expression of P-selectin on platelets is a risk factor for silent cerebral infarction in patients with atrial fi brillation: role of nitric oxide. Circulation 1998;98: 1721–27.

[93] Pongratz G, Brandt-Pohlmann M, Henneke KH, et al. Platelet activation in embolic and preembolic status of patients with nonrheumatic atrial fi brillation. Chest 1997; 111: 929–33.

[94] Lip, GYH.; Huber, K.; Andreotti, F.; Arnesen, H.; Airaksinen KJ; Cuisset, T.; Kirchhof, P.& Marin, F. Management of antithrombotic therapy in atrial fibrillation patients presenting with acute coronary syndrome and/or undergoing percutaneous coronary intervention/stenting. ThrombHaemost 2009; 102:1-15.

[95] Furui H, Taniguchi N, Yamauchi K, Sotobata I, Saito H, Inagaki H. Effects of treadmill exercise on platelet function, blood coagulability and fibrinolytic activity in patients with atrial fibrillation. Jpn Heart J 1987; 28: 177–84.

[96] Atalar E, Haznedaroglu IC, Acil T, et al. Patients with paroxysmal atrial fibrillation but not paroxysmal supraventricular tachycardia display evidence of platelet activation during arrhythmia. Platelets 2003; 14: 407–11.

[97] Choudhury A, Chung I, Blann AD, Lip GY. Platelet surface CD62P and CD63, mean platelet volume, and soluble/platelet P-selectin as indexes of platelet function in atrial fibrillation: a comparison of "healthy control subjects" and "disease control subjects" in sinus rhythm. J Am CollCardiol 2007; 49: 1957–64.

[98] Feinberg WM, Macy E, Cornell ES, et al. Plasmin–a2-antiplasmin complex in patients with atrial fibrillation. ThrombHaemost 1999; 82: 100–03.

[99] Marın F, Roldan V, Marco P, et al. Improvement of fibrinolytical function in chronic rheumatic atrial fibrillation after anticoagulation. Rev EspCardiol 1999; 52: 25–30.

[100] Chung MK, Martin DO, Sprecher D, et al. C-reactive protein elevation in patients with atrial arrhythmias. Inflammatory mechanisms and persistence of atrial fi brillation. Circulation 2001; 104: 2886–91.

[101] Dernellis J, Panaretou M. C-reactive protein and paroxysmal atrial fibrillation: evidence of the implication of an inflammatory process in paroxysmal atrial fi brillation. ActaCardiol 2001; 56: 375–80.

[102] Tveit A, Seljeflot I, Grundvold I, Abdelnoor M, Smith P, Arnesen H. Levels of PAI-1 and outcome after electrical cardioversion for atrial fibrillation. Thromb Res 2008; 121: 447–53.

[103] Pretorius M, Donahue BS, Yu C, Greelish JP, Roden DM, Brown NJ. Plasminogen activator inhibitor-1 as a predictor of postoperative atrial fibrillation after cardiopulmonary bypass.Circulation 2007; 116: I1–7.

[104] Oltrona L, Broccolino M, Merlini PA, Spinola A, Pezzano A, Mannucci PM. Activation of the hemostatic mechanism afterpharmacological cardioversion of acute nonvalvular atrial Fibrillation.Circulation 1997; 95: 2003–06.

[105] Giansante C, Fiotti N, Miccio M, Altamura N, Salvi R, Guarnieri G. Coagulation indicators in patients with paroxysmal atrialfibrillation: effects of electric and pharmacologic cardioversion.Am Heart J 2000; 140: 423–29.

[106] Hatzinikolaou-Kotsakou E, Kartasis Z, Tziakas D, et al. Clotting state after cardioversion of atrial fibrillation: a haemostasis index could detect the relationship with the arrhythmia duration. Thromb J 2005; 3: 2.

[107] Jacob K, Talwar S, Copplestone A, Gilbert TJ, Haywood GA. Activation of coagulation occurs after electrical cardioversion in patients with chronic atrial fibrillation despite optimal anticoagulation with warfarin. Int J Cardiol 2004; 95: 83–88.

[108] Zeuthen EL, Lassen JF, Husted SE. Haemostatic activity in patients with atrial fibrillation treated with low-molecular-weight heparin before and after electrical cardioversion. J Thromb Thrombolysis 2004; 17: 185–89.

[109] Boos CJ, Anderson RA, Lip GY. Is atrial fibrillation an inflamatory disorder? Eur Heart J 2006; 27: 136–49.

[110] Hernandez Madrid A, Moro C. Atrial fibrillation and C-reactive protein: searching for local inflammation. J Am CollCardiol 2007; 49: 1649–50.

[111] Engelmann MD, Svendsen JH. Inflammation in the genesis and perpetuation of atrial fibrillation.Eur Heart J 2005; 26: 2083–92.

[112] Gedikli O, Dogan A, Altuntas I, et al. Inflammatory markers according to types of atrial fibrillation. Int J Cardiol 2007; 120: 193–97.

[113] Bruins P, teVelthuis H, Yazdanbakhsh AP, et al. Activation of the complement system during and after cardiopulmonary bypass surgery: postsurgery activation involves C-reactive protein and is associated with postoperative arrhythmia. Circulation 1997; 96: 3542–48.

[114] Conway DS, Buggins P, Hughes E, Lip GY. Prognostic significance of raised plasma levels of interleukin-6 and C-reactive protein in atrial fibrillation. Am Heart J 2004; 148: 462–66.

[115] Chung MK, Martin DO, Sprecher D, et al. C-reactive protein elevation in patients with atrial arrhythmias: inflammatory mechanisms and persistence of atrial fibrillation. Circulation 2001; 104: 2886–91.

[116] Lip GY, Patel JV, Hughes E, Hart RG. High-sensitivity C-reactive protein and soluble CD40 ligand as indices of inflammation and platelet activation in 880 patients with nonvalvular atrial fibrillation: relationship to stroke risk factors, stroke risk stratification schema, and prognosis. Stroke 2007; 38: 1229–37.

[117] Cermak J, Key NS, Bach RR, Balla J, Jacob HS, Vercellotti GM. C-reactive protein induces human peripheral blood monocytes to synthesize tissue factor. Blood 1993; 82: 513–20.

[118] Neumann FJ, Ott I, Marx N, et al. Effect of human recombinant interleukin-6 and interleukin-8 on monocyte procoagulant activity. ArteriosclerThrombVascBiol 1997; 17: 3399–405.

[119] Burstein SA. Cytokines, platelet production and hemostasis.Platelets 1997; 8: 93–104.

[120] Amrani DL. Regulation of fibrinogen biosynthesis: glucocorticoid and interleukin-6 control. Blood Coagul Fibrinolysis 1990; 1: 443–46.

[121] Burstein SA, Peng J, Friese P, et al. Cytokine-induced alteration of platelet and hemostatic function. Stem Cells 1996; 14: 154–62.

[122] Yudkin JS, Stehouwer CD, Emeis JJ, Coppack SW. C-reactive protein in healthy subjects: associations with obesity, insulin resistance and endothelial dysfunction: a potential role for cytokines originating from adipose tissue? ArteriosclerThrombVascBiol 1999; 19: 972–78.

[123] Acevedo M, Corbalan R, Braun S, Pereira J, Navarrete C, Gonzalez I. C-reactive protein and atrial fibrillation: "evidence for the presence of inflammation in the perpetuation of the arrhythmia". Int J Cardiol 2006; 108: 326–31.

[124] Conway DS, Buggins P, Hughes E, Lip GY. Relationship of interleukin-6 and C-reactive protein to the prothrombotic state in chronic atrial fibrillation. J Am CollCardiol 2004; 43: 2075–82.

[125] Chung NA, Belgore F, Li-Saw-Hee FL, Conway DS, Blann AD, Lip GY. Is the hypercoagulable state in atrial fibrillation mediated by vascular endothelial growth factor? Stroke 2002; 33: 2187–91.

[126] Seko Y, Nishimura H, Takanashi N, Ashida T, Nagai R. Serum levels of vascular endothelial growth factor and transforming growth factor-β1 in patients with atrial fibrillation undergoing defibrillation therapy. Jpn Heart J 2000; 41: 27–32.

[127] Webb NJ, Bottomley MJ, Watson CJ, Brenchley PE. Vascular endothelial growth factor (VEGF) is released from platelets during blood clotting: implications for measurement of circulating VEGF levels in clinical disease. Clin Sci (Lond) 1998; 94: 395–404.

[128] Armesilla AL, Lorenzo E, Gomez del Arco P, Martinez-Martinez S, Alfranca A, Redondo JM. Vascular endothelial growth factoractivates nuclear factor of activated T cells in human endothelialcells: a role for tissue factor gene expression. Mol Cell Biol 1999;19: 2032–43

[129] Morrissey JH. Tissue factor: an enzyme cofactor and true receptor. ThrombHaemost 2001; 86: 66–74.

[130] Archiniegas E, Neves CY, Candelle D, Cardier JE.Thrombin and its protease-activated receptor-1 (PAR1) participate in the endothelial–mesenchymaltransdifferentiation process. DNA Cell Biol 2004; 23:815–825.

[131] Vandenbroucke E, Mehta D, Minshall R, Malik AB. Regulation of endothelial junctional permeability. Ann N Y AcadSci 2008; 1123:134–145.

[132] Gluck N, Schwob O, Krimsky M, Yedgar S. Activation of cytosolic phospholipase A2 and fatty acid transacylase is essential but not sufficient for thrombin-induced smooth muscle cell proliferation. Am J Physiol Cell Physiol 2008; 294:C1597–C1603.

[133] Dahi S, Lee JG, Lovett DH, Sarkar R. Differential transcriptional activation of matrix metalloproteinase-2 and membrane type-1 matrix metalloproteinase by experimental deep venous thrombosis and thrombin. J VascSurg 2005; 42:539–545.

[134] Fang Q, Mao L, Kobayashi T et al., PKCdelta mediates thrombin-augmented fibroblast-mediated collagen gel contraction. BiochemBiophys Res Commun 2008; 369:1199–1203.

[135] BelAiba RS, Djordjevic T, Bonello S et al., The serum- and glucocorticoid-inducible kinase Sgk-1 is involved in pulmonary vascular remodeling: role in redox-sensitive regulation of tissue factor by thrombin. Circ Res 2006; 98:828–836.

[136] Borensztajn K, Stiekema J, Nijmeijer S, Reitsma PH, Peppelenbosch MP, Spek CA. Factor Xa stimulates proinflammatory and profibrotic responses in fibroblasts via protease-activated receptor-2 activation. Am J Pathol 2008; 172:309–320.

[137] Davis ME, Cai H, Drummond GR, Harrison DG. Shear stress regulates endothelial nitric oxide synthase expression through c-Srcby divergent signaling pathways. Circ Res 2001; 89: 1073–80.

[138] Freedman JE, Loscalzo J, Barnard MR, Alpert C, Keaney JF, Michelson AD. Nitric oxide released from activated platelets inhibits platelet recruitment. J Clin Invest 1997; 100: 350–56.

[139] Swiatkowska M, Cierniewska-Cieslak A, Pawlowska Z, Cierniewski CS. Dual regulatory effects of nitric oxide on plasminogen activator inhibitor type 1 expression in endothelial cells. Eur J Biochem 2000; 267: 1001–07.

[140] Cai H, Li Z, Goette A, et al. Downregulation of endocardial nitric oxide synthase expression and nitric oxide production in atrial fibrillation: potential mechanisms for atrial thrombosis and stroke. Circulation 2002; 106: 2854–58.

[141] Goette A, Staack T, Rocken C, et al. Increased expression of extracellular signalregulated kinase and angiotensin-converting enzyme in human atria during atrial fibrillation. J Am CollCardiol 2000; 35: 1669–77.

[142] Choudhury A, Varughese GI, Lip GY. Targeting the renin-angiotensinaldosterone-system in atrial fi brillation: a shift from electrical to structural therapy? Expert OpinPharmacother 2005; 6: 2193–207.

[143] Healey JS, Baranchuk A, Crystal E, et al. Prevention of atrial fibrillation with angiotensin-converting enzyme inhibitors and angiotensin receptor blockers: a meta-analysis. J Am CollCardiol 2005; 45: 1832–39.

[144] Das UN. Is angiotensin-II an endogenous pro-inflammatorymolecule? Med SciMonit 2005; 11: 155–62.

[145] Tamarat R, Silvestre JS, Durie M, Levy BI.Angiotensin II angiogeniceffect in vivo involves vascular endothelial growth factorand inflammation-related pathways. Lab Invest 2002; 82: 747–56.

[146] Suzuki Y, Ruiz-Ortega M, Lorenzo O, Ruperez M, Esteban V, Egido J. Infl ammation and angiotensin II. Int J Biochem Cell Biol 2003; 35: 881–900.

[147] Cardin S, Li D, Thorin-Trescases N, Leung TK, Thorin E, Nattel S. Evolution of the atrial fi brillation substrate in experimental congestive heart failure: angiotensin-dependent and –independent pathways. Cardiovasc Res 2003; 60: 315–25.

[148] Takagishi T, Murahashi N, Azagami S, Morimatsu M, Sasaguri Y. Effect of angiotensin II and thromboxane A2 on the production of matrix metalloproteinase by human aortic smooth muscle cells. BiochemMolBiolInt 1995; 35: 265–73.

[149] Griendling KK, Alexander RW. Oxidative stress and cardiovascular disease.Circulation 1997; 96: 3264–65.

[150] Dzau VJ, Bernstein K, Celermajer D, et al; working group on tissue angiotensin-converting enzyme, International Society of Cardiovascular Pharmacotherapy. The relevance of tissue angiotensin-converting enzyme: manifestations in mechanistic and endpoint data. Am J Cardiol 2001; 88: 1–20L.

Section 3

Signal Analysis

Chapter 7

Applications of Signal Analysis to Atrial Fibrillation

José Joaquín Rieta and Raúl Alcaraz

Additional information is available at the end of the chapter

http://dx.doi.org/10.5772/54199

1. Introduction

Currently, atrial fibrillation (AF) guidelines are intended to assist physicians in clinical decision making by describing a range of generally acceptable approaches for the diagnosis and management of AF. However, these guidelines provide no recommendations that takes into account other aspects of the arrhythmia related with its computational analysis. For example, the proper application of spectral analysis, how to quantify different AF patterns in terms of organization, or how to deal with ventricular contamination before AF analysis are some aspects that could provide an improved scenario to the physician in the search of useful clinical information [1].

Both in surface and invasive recordings of AF the presence of ventricular activity has to be considered as a contaminant signal which has to be removed. In this respect, the proper analysis and characterization of AF from ECG recordings requires the extraction or cancellation of the signal components associated to ventricular activity, that is, the QRS complex and the T wave. Unfortunately, a number of facts hinder this operation [2]. Firstly, the atrial activity presents in the ECG much lower amplitude, in some cases well under the noise level, than its ventricular counterpart. Additionally, both phenomena possess spectral distributions notably overlapped, rendering linear filtering solutions unsuccessful. Within this context, several methods have been proposed to deal with this problem during last years. They go from a simple average beat subtraction [3], to the most advanced adaptive methods based on multidimensional signal processing [4] that will be detailed Section § 2.

From a clinical point of view, the estimation of the dominant atrial frequency (DAF), i.e., the repetition rate of the fibrillatory waves, is an important goal in the analysis of ECG recordings in AF. By comparing endocardial electrograms with ECGs, it has been established that the ECG-based AF frequency estimate can be used as an index of the atrial cycle length [5].

AF recordings with low DAF are more likely to terminate spontaneously and to respond better to antiarrhythmic drugs or cardioversion, whereas high DAF is more often associated with persistence to therapy [6]. The likelihood of successful pharmacological cardioversion is higher when the DAF is below 6 Hz [7]. Moreover, the risk of early AF recurrence is higher for patients with higher DAF [8] and, therefore, the DAF may be taken into consideration when selecting candidates for cardioversion. Section § 3 will provide to the reader basic concepts and recent advances in DAF estimation, as well as more elaborated techniques like time-frequency analysis or spectral modeling.

On the other hand, organization deals with strategies to quantify the repetitiveness of the AF signal pattern, thus providing very useful clinical information on the arrhythmia state. This relevant concept will be addressed in Section § 4, where the most important methods will be described [9, 10]. AF organization has demonstrated its clinical usefulness because indices of organization have been related to the electrophysiological mechanisms sustaining AF, or may be useful in the evaluation of strategies for AF treatment, such as catheter ablation or electrical cardioversion [11].

2. Atrial activity extraction

This section describes the most widely used methods to separate atrial from ventricular activities, both on surface and invasive recordings, grouped by they core way of operation. Mathematical notation or equations have been avoided in the interest of readability. Anyway, the reader could find detailed explanations in the corresponding references. Firstly, the methods based on the generation of an average beat, able to represent approximately each individual beat, are detailed. Within these methods, the main idea is to subtract the average beat from every single beat. Next, other group of methods take profit of physiological observations such as atrial and ventricular activities being uncoupled and originated from independent electrical sources. This fact allows the application of signal separation methods to dissociate atrial from ventricular activities, that will be addressed later.

2.1. Average Beat Subtraction methods

The average beat subtraction (ABS) based method was firstly presented by Slocum et al. [3] and still remains as the most widely used on the surface ECG [12, 13]. The ABS methodology takes advantage of the lack of a fixed relationship between atrial and ventricular activities and the consistent morphology of the QRST complexes [3]. In this method, fiducial points from ventricular complexes are detected and aligned [14]. Next, an average beat is generated where the window length is determined by the minimum or mean R–R interval. The window was aligned such that 30% of it preceded the fiducial point and 70% followed it [15]. A template of average beats was constructed and subtracted from the original signal, resulting in the atrial activity with subtracted ventricular activity.

The use of an adaptive template in conjunction with the correct alignment of every QRS complex, both in time and space, has proven to be very effective through the spatiotemporal QRST cancellation [16]. Since ABS is performed in individual leads, it becomes sensitive to alterations in the electrical axis, which are manifested as large QRS-related residuals. However, the effect of such alterations can be suppressed by using the spatiotemporal QRST cancellation in which the average beats of adjacent leads are mathematically combined with

http://dx.doi.org/10.5772/54199

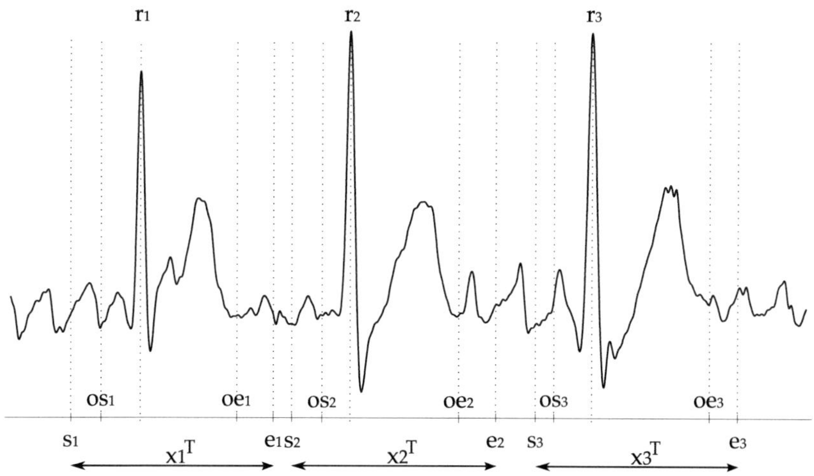

Figure 1. Relevant time instants used by the ASVC algorithm. The points s_i and e_i are the start and end points of the i-th QRST complex which is represented by $\mathbf{x}_i$, respectively. The points os_i and oe_i define the zones, at the beginning and the end of the i-th QRST complex, that will be processed to avoid sudden transitions after ventricular cancellation [13].

the average beat of the analyzed lead in order to optimize cancellation [16]. Other authors have proposed the idea of processing separately the QRS complex and the T wave [17]. This is because the depolarization waveform changes notably as a function of the heart rate, whereas the repolarization waveform remains almost unchanged.

Finally, the most recently ABS method is based on adaptive singular value cancellation (ASVC) of the ventricular activity [13]. Given that the ECG signal presents a high degree of temporal redundancy which could be exploited for ventricular activity cancellation, the ASVC method detected all the R waves making use of the Pan and Tompkins technique [14]. Next, the starting and ending points of each QRS complex were detected and the complexes were aligned using their R peak timing. Figure 1 depicts the fiducial points and relevant time instants described herein. Once all the beats were temporally aligned, their eigenvector sequence was obtained by singular value decomposition (SVD). In this way, the highest variance provided the eigenvector considered as the representative ventricular activity [13]. Thereby, this activity was used as the primary cancellation template. Next the template was adapted to each QRST width and height and was temporally aligned with each R peak in the ECG. Finally, the customized template for each beat was subtracted from every QRST complex and the atrial activity estimation inside the complex was obtained. This SVD–based method provided a more accurate ventricular activity representation adapted to each individual beat and, as a consequence, a higher quality AA extraction in a wide variety of AF recordings [13].

As an illustration on how the ABS-based methods can behave, Figure 2 plots the comparison between the simple ABS method introduced in [3] and the ASVC method presented in [13]. As can be observed, ventricular residua use to be present in the extracted AA, specially for the simple ABS method in (c). In fact, this is the main reason justifying the permanent optimization of atrial activity extraction methods during last years.

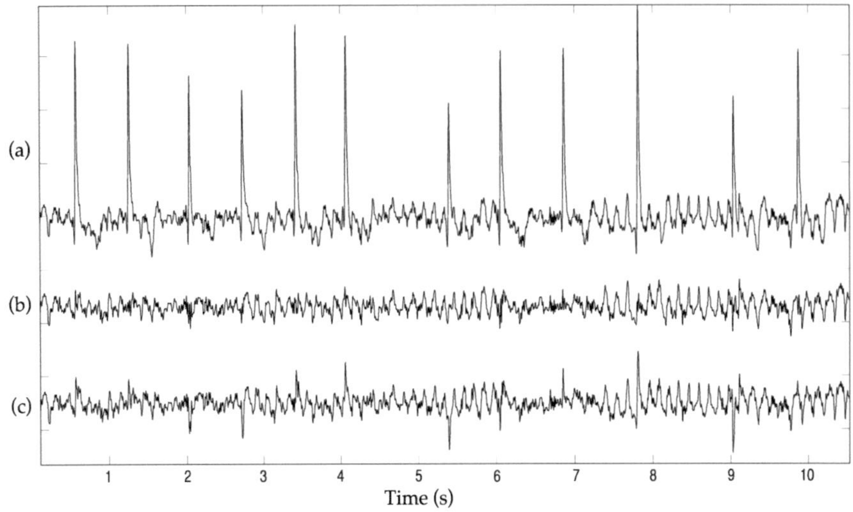

Figure 2. Example of a real ECG segment in AF with irregular QRST shape and the illustration on how the ABS-based method are able to cancel out ventricular activity. (a) ECG ready for ventricular activity cancellation. (b) Atrial activity signal provided by ASVC [13]. (c) Atrial activity signal provided by ABS [3].

2.2. Signal separation methods

Other recently proposed alternative consist of applying signal separation algorithms, which are able to use the multi-lead information provided by the ECG to obtain a unified atrial activity. They can be based on principal component analysis (PCA) [18] or blind source separation (BSS) [4]. These methodologies have been compared in a joint study proving their coincident results in the estimation of AF spectra on the surface ECG [19]. One common drawback to the ABS-based methods is that they are mainly thought to be applied over single lead ECGs. In other words, the application of ABS cancellation techniques to different ECG leads would involve the obtention of an equal number of different atrial activities as well. Consequently, they do not make use of the information included in every lead in an unified way. On the contrary, BSS techniques perform a multi-lead statistical analysis by exploiting the spatial diversity that multiple spatially-separated electrodes may introduce [4, 20].

The blind source separation consists in recovering a set of source signals from the observation of linear mixtures of the sources [21]. The term *blind* emphasizes that nothing is known about the source signals or the mixing structure, the only hypothesis being the source mutual independence [22]. To achieve the source separation, a linear transformation is sought such that the components of the output signal vector become statistically independent, thus representing an estimate of the sources except for (perhaps) scaling and permutation, which are considered as admissible indeterminacies [22]. Some authors have proposed the use of PCA to solve the mixing model between atrial and ventricular activity in AF [23]. However, it is important to remark that the success of PCA relies heavily on the orthogonality of the sources. But, in general, there is no reason why bioelectrical sources of the heart should be spatially orthogonal to one another in the ECG. This orthogonality condition can only be forced through appropriate electrode placement, as previously emphasized in the context of the fetal ECG extraction problem [24] and the cancellation of artifacts in the electroencephalogram [25].

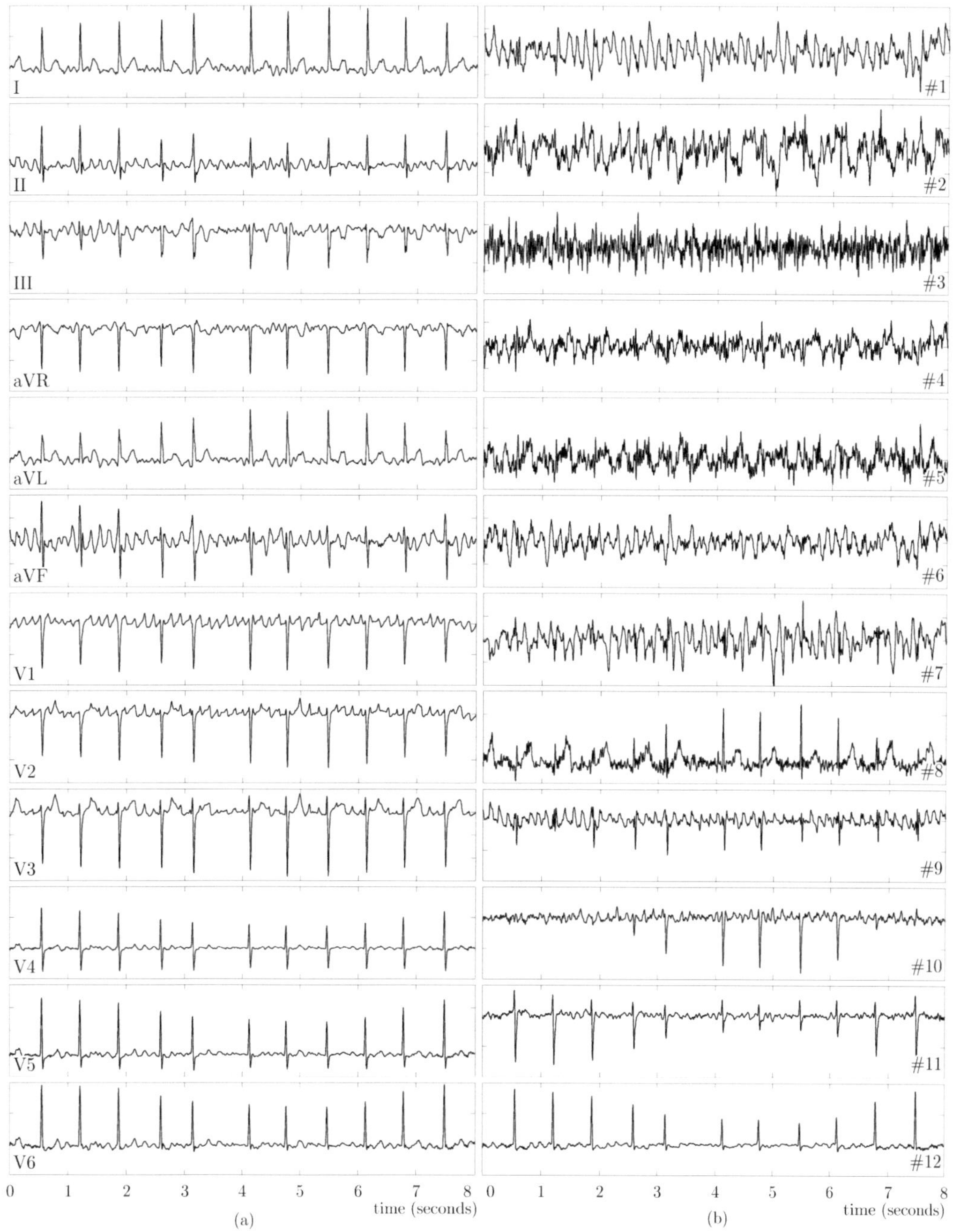

Figure 3. Input and result of the BSS separation process applied to an ECG of atrial fibrillation. (a) 12-lead ECG segment from a patient in AF. The multi-lead information will be used by BSS to yield a unified atrial activity. (b) Estimated sources obtained via BSS and reordered from lower to higher kurtosis value. The unified atrial activity is contained in source #1 [4].

When BSS is applied to an ECG in AF, a set of different sources can be observed as illustrated in Figure 3. Consequently a crucial step in BSS-based atrial activity extraction is to identify the sources(s) which contains atrial activity. The first algorithm proposed for this purpose made use of a kurtosis-based reordering of the components, relying on the assumption that sub-Gaussian sources are associated with atrial activity, approximately Gaussian ones with various types of noise and artifacts, whereas super-Gaussian sources are associated with ventricular activity [4]. Since information on kurtosis alone is insufficient for accurate identification of the atrial component, kurtosis reordering was combined with power spectral analysis of the sub-Gaussian components to detect when a dominant spectral peak, reflecting atrial rate, was present or not. It is commonly accepted that atrial rate is reflected by a peak whose frequency is confined to the interval 3–9 Hz [4]. In this respect Figure 4 shows the power spectral density associated to the separated sources with lower kurtosis in Figure 3. As can be appreciated, source #1 is the one representing the typical spectrum of an atrial activity.

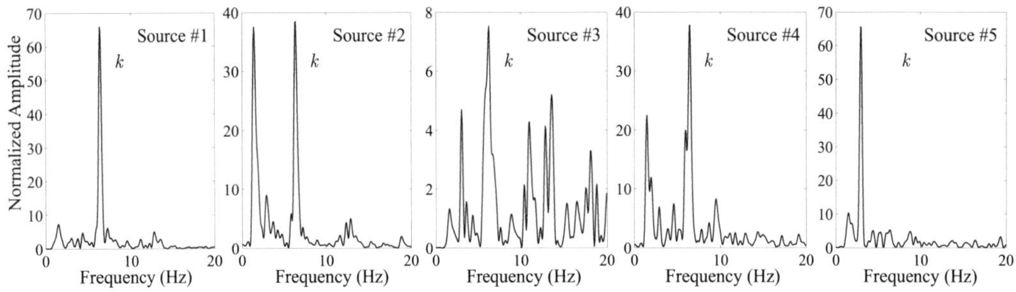

Figure 4. Power spectral densities from several BSS-estimated sources of Fig. 3. After kurtosis-based reordering only five sources have subgaussian kurtosis, and the one with lowest kurtosis (source #1) presents a power spectral density typically associated with the atrial activity in AF episodes [4].

Another approach to atrial component identification was later presented in [20], where kurtosis reordering and spectral analysis are supplemented with another technique with which ventricular components are excluded from further processing and only components with possible atrial activity are retained. Since the kurtosis of the ventricular components is usually very high, they can be excluded with a simple threshold test. It was found that a threshold of about 1.5 retained components with atrial activity, but excluded components with QRS complexes. The block diagram of this technique is represented in Figure 5.

The nonventricular components, i.e., atrial activity, noise, and artifacts, with kurtosis close to zero, are separated using second-order blind identification (SOBI). This technique aims at separating a mixture of uncorrelated sources with different spectral content through second-order statistical analysis which also takes into consideration the source temporal information [20].

2.3. Specific methods for invasive recordings

In the same way as with surface ECG recordings, other relevant point of view to understand the pathophysiological mechanisms of AF is the analysis and interpretation of atrial electrograms (AEG), which are recordings obtained on the atrial surface. More precise and successful therapies can be developed through this analysis, like guided radio-frequency ablation [26], analysis of antiarrhythmic drug effects [27] or performance improvement of

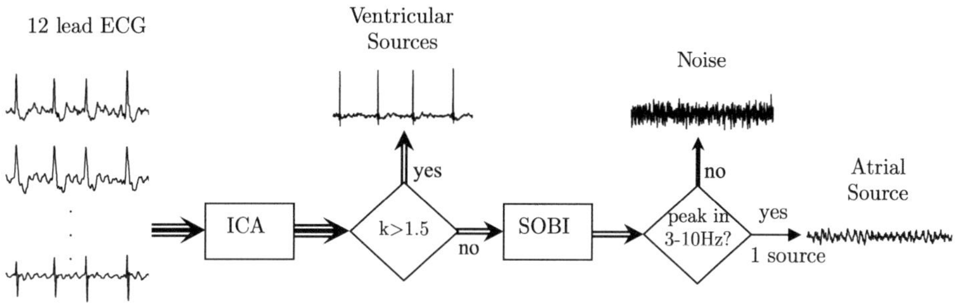

Figure 5. Block diagram of the BSS method, implemented by independent component analysis (ICA), and SOBI for atrial activity extraction in multi-lead ECGs of AF. It can be observed that components whose kurtosis exceed 1.5 are excluded from the SOBI stage [20].

atrial implantable cardioverter-defibrillators [28]. Within this context, ABS (or a similar methodology) has been applied to the AEG in order to discriminate sinus rhythm from AF [15], to measure AF organization [9] and synchronization [29] and to monitor the effects of ablation procedures and antiarrhythmic drugs [30].

However, ABS tends to distort the resulting atrial signal when the AEG under analysis corresponds to a well organized AF, as Figure 6 shows. Observe in Fig. 6.a that the atrial rhythm is well organized and uncoupled with the ventricular rhythm. The AEG shows ventricular depolarization contamination and the remaining three signals are the resultant atrial activity after applying ventricular reduction with the corresponding algorithm. Observe how ABS can modify the atrial waveform within the atrial segments. In contrast, Fig. 6.b shows a disorganized AF episode. In this case, thanks to the irregularity of the atrial signal, ABS performs better, preserving the atrial waveform and reducing ventricular peaks.

Because of the aforementioned problems with ABS, alternative methods have been introduced in the literature [31]. Firstly, adaptive ventricular cancellation (AVC) can be considered. This method is based on an adaptive filter that operates on the reference channel to produce an estimate of the interference, which is then subtracted from the main channel [32]. In this case the main channel was the recorded AEG containing both atrial and ventricular components. On the other hand, the reference channel was lead II from the standard surface ECG. The motivation to select this lead was based on the large ventricular amplitude that can be observed on it, and the precise time alignment existing between the QRS complex of lead II and the AEG [12, 33]. The resulting atrial activity provided by the AVC method can be observed in Figure 6 for two different types of AF recordings.

The last approach introduced to deal with AA extraction from the AEG has been based also in BSS through the use of independent component analysis (ICA) [31]. This is because in the context of AF patients, atrial and ventricular activities can be considered as decoupled electrical processes that appear mixed at the electrode output [4]. Therefore, it should be possible to dissociate atrial from ventricular activity in one AEG lead by using the proper reference signal which, in this case, has been the surface standard lead II by the same reasons as with AVC. In this case, the dimension is 2×2 where the observations are composed of the AEG and lead II, and the sources are the atrial and ventricular components to be dissociated. The FastICA algorithm was preferred to perform the ICA process due to its fast convergence and robust performance, previously demonstrated in a variety of different applications [34].

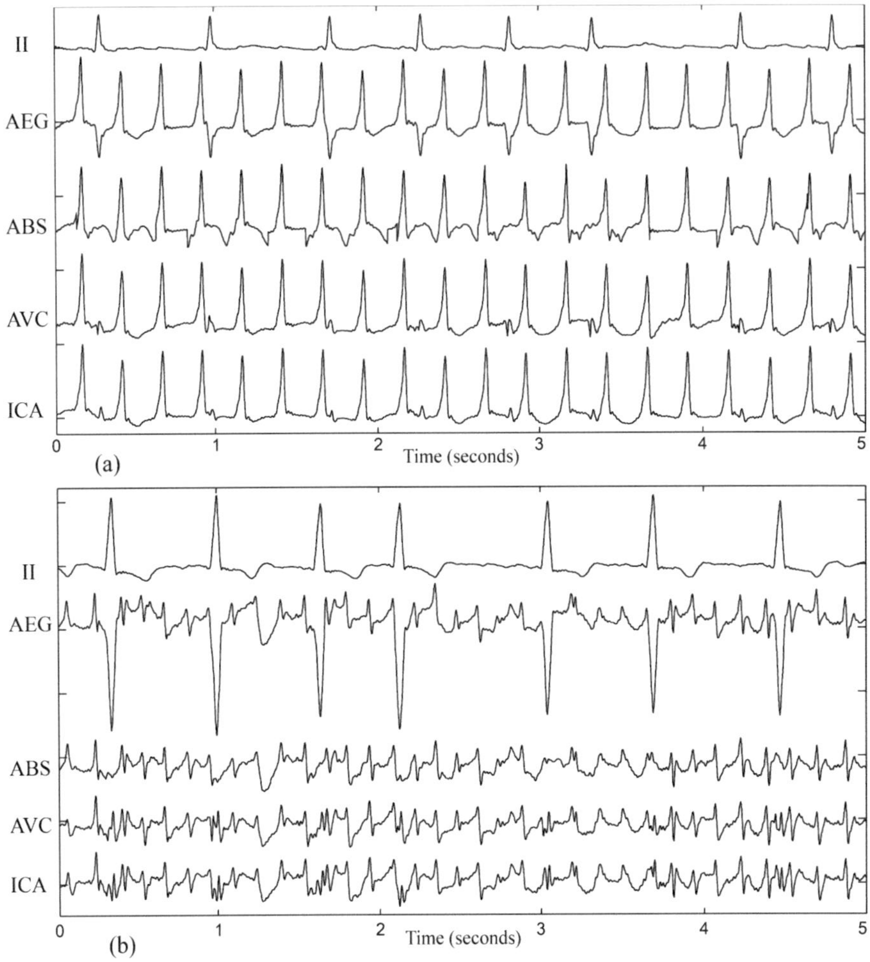

Figure 6. (a) From top to bottom, Lead II of an organized AF ECG shown for reference, the corresponding epicardial atrial electrogram (AEG), result of ventricular reduction with average beat subtraction (ABS), adaptive ventricular cancellation (AVC) and independent component analysis (ICA). (b) This panel plots the same information as panel (a) for a disorganized AF ECG. Note how ABS does not distort the resulting signal in this latter case [31].

The results provided by ICA in separating the atrial activity from ventricular contamination in AEGs are considered as better than those provided by ABS or AVC regarding how the atrial waveforms are preserved and the amount of ventricular residue removed [31], see Figure 6.

3. Frequency analysis of AF

When an atrial activity signal is available after QRST cancellation, the power spectral analysis door can be opened for the purpose of locating the dominant atrial frequency. This will be the first aspect to be addressed in this section. However, it is well known that the fibrillatory waves present time-dependent properties that may be blurred through a basic spectral analysis. As a consequence, when more detailed information and robust spectral estimation are needed, time-frequency analysis may be the way to go. In this respect, concepts like the spectral profile or the spectral modeling have proven to be efficient techniques that will be detailed by the end of this section.

3.1. Power spectral analysis

The computation of power spectral analysis on the atrial activity signal is the most common approach to determine the DAF [7]. Basically, the technique consist of locating the largest spectral peak within the power spectrum. The spectrum is usually defined as the discrete Fourier transform of the autocorrelation function of the signal. In this case, the signal is the atrial activity which is divided into shorter, overlapping segments, where each segment is subjected to proper windowing, e.g., using commonly the Welch's method [35]. Finally, the desired power spectrum is obtained by averaging the power spectra of the respective segments.

Primarily there exist two ways to compute the power spectral density of a discrete signal. First, estimate its autocorrelation function and then take its Fourier transform. Second, compute the Fourier transform of the signal and, next, square its magnitude to obtain the periodogram. Normally, the second way is the most commonly applied because of the great computational efficiency of the fast Fourier transform algorithm [36].

Depending on prior information about the signal, spectral estimation can be divided into two categories: nonparametric and parametric approaches. Nonparametric approaches explicitly estimate the autocorrelation function or the power spectral density of the process without any prior information. On the other hand, parametric approaches assume that the underlying random process has a certain structure, for example, an autoregressive (AR) model, which can be described using a small number of parameters and estimate the parameters of the model [37]. A widely used nonparametric estimation approach is the periodogram, which is based on the fast Fourier transform (FFT). A common parametric technique is maximum entropy spectral estimation, which involves fitting the observed signal to an AR model [36].

The raw periodogram is not a statistically stable spectral estimate since there is not much averaging on its computation. In fact, the periodogram is computed from a finite-length observed sequence that is sharply truncated. This sharp truncation effectively spreads the original signal spectrum into other frequencies, which is called spectral leakage [37]. The spectral leakage problem can be reduced by multiplying the finite sequence by a windowing function before the FFT computation, which reduces the sequence values gradually rather than abruptly. In order to reduce the periodogram variance, averaging can be applied. This modified algorithm is called Welch's method, which is the most widely used in nonparametric spectral estimation [35]. In order to increase the number of segments being averaged in a finite-length sequence, the sequence can be segmented with overlap; for example, 50% overlap can duplicate the number of segments of the same length [35]. Segment length can be considered as the most important parameter in AF spectral analysis since it determines the estimation accuracy of the DAF by restricting spectral resolution. It is advisable that the segment length is chosen to be at least a few seconds so as to produce an acceptable variance of the power spectrum [1, 2].

With respect to the surface ECG lead selection for AF power spectral analysis, this lead use to be V1. This is because lead V1 contains the fibrillatory waves with largest amplitude and, therefore, the associated DAF peak will be the largest in this lead [12]. As an example of

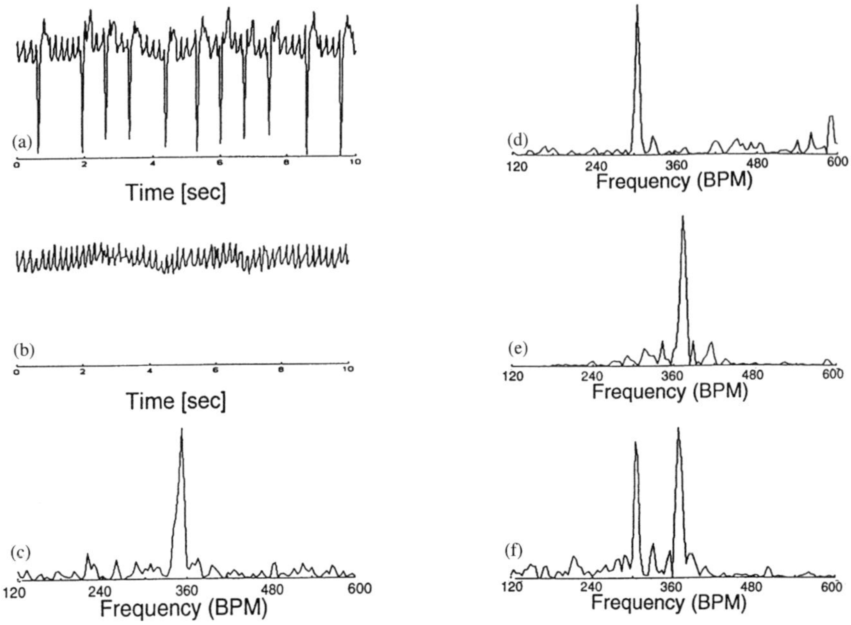

Figure 7. Example of AF power spectral analysis. (a) Surface ECG lead V1 from a patient in AF ready to be analyzed. (b) Atrial activity extracted from lead V1. (c) Atrial activity power spectral density. (d) and (e) Right and left atrium invasive recording PSDs of a different patient in which a notable frequency contrast between both atria was observed. (f) Surface lead V1 PSD of the patient in (d) and (e) proving how power spectral analysis can be useful in the study of AF [7].

power spectral analysis of AF, Figure 7 plots several situations related to this analysis. Firstly, the left panel shows the traditional procedure for AF spectral analysis, where the original ECG in AF is presented in Fig. 7.a. Next, the extracted atrial activity after QRST cancellation can be observed in Fig. 7.b. Finally, the power spectrum associated to that activity is shown in Fig. 7.c. In this example, the atrial activity signal was downsampled to 100Hz and processed with a Hamming window [38]. Next, a 1024-point FFT was applied and the PSD was displayed by computing the squared magnitude of each sample frequency. Remark that the frequency axis use to be traditionally expressed in Hz but, in some studies, clinicians prefer to express the fibrillatory frequencies in beats per minute (BPM). Furthermore, the right panel of Fig. 7 shows how AF power spectral analysis of the surface ECG is able to show the difference in the right and left atrial frequency. Hence, Fig. 7.d shows the right atrium invasive recording PSD, whereas Fig. 7.e plots the left atrium PSD. Finally, Fig. 7.f shows the PSD associated to the analysis of surface lead V1 from the same patient [1].

3.2. Time-frequency analysis

As demonstrated previously, power spectral analysis reflects the average signal behavior during the analyzed time interval, the robust location of the DAF being the main goal with clinical interest. However, this analysis may not be able to characterize temporal variations in the DAF. From an electrophysiological point of view, there are solid reasons to believe that the atrial fibrillatory waves have time-dependent properties, since they reflect complex patterns of electrical activation wavefronts. Therefore, it is advisable to employ time-frequency analysis in order to track variations in AF frequency when more detailed

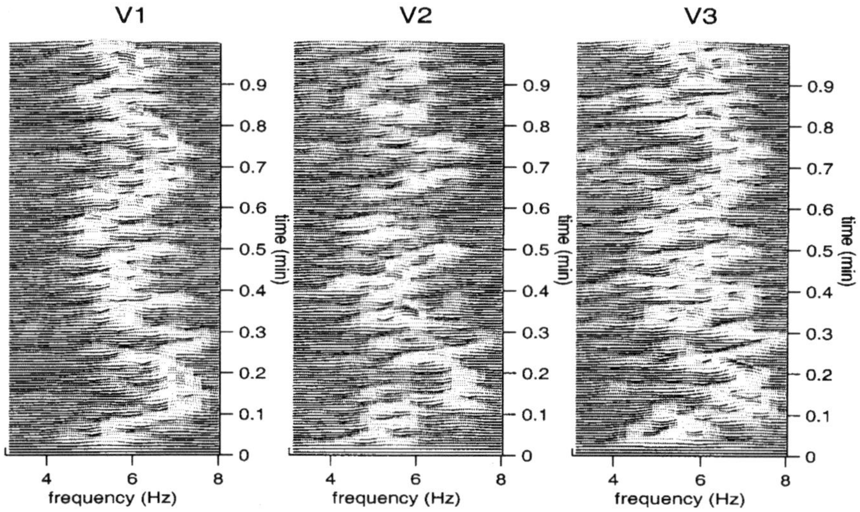

Figure 8. Spectrogram of a one minute atrial activity signal computed with a 128 point FFT using a 2.5 seconds window length. Surface leads V1 to V3 are shown for comparison [39].

information is needed [39]. The DAF is known to be influenced by autonomic modulation and its variations over time have been studied in terms of the effects of parasympathetic and sympathetic stimulation as well as with respect to circadian rhythm. It has been shown that AF frequency decreases during the night and increases in the morning [40].

The simplest way to apply time-frequency analysis to AF recordings consists of dividing the continuous-time atrial signal into short, consecutive and overlapping segments. Next, each of the segments will be subjected to spectral analysis. The resulting series of spectra reflects the time-varying nature of the signal [36, 39]. The most common approach to time-frequency analysis is the nonparametric, i.e., Fourier-based spectral analysis applied to each AF segment. This operation is known as the short-time Fourier transform (STFT) [41]. In this approach, the definition of the Fourier transform is modified so that a sliding time window defines each time segment to be analyzed. As a result, a two-dimensional function will be obtained in which the resolution in time and frequency will always have to be a trade-off compromise between both domains [37]. In the same way as with the periodogram, the spectrogram of a signal can be obtained by computing the squared magnitude of the STFT [41], thus making it possible to get a PSD representation of the signal in the time-frequency domain. An example on how an AF spectrogram looks like is shown in Figure 8, where three surface ECG leads are shown for comparison. As can be appreciated, the DAF trend presents great similarities but, also, some differences between leads. However, remark that the spectrogram frequency resolution cannot be better because of the time window length selected.

Because of the conflicting requirements between time and frequency resolution needed to be satisfied by the STFT, other techniques for time-frequency analysis have been proposed [42]. Basically, while the STFT depends linearly on the signal, these new techniques depend quadratically, thus providing much better resolution. One of the most successfully applied time-frequency distribution to AF recordings is the cross Wigner-Ville distribution (XWVD). Its selection was considered primarily because of its excellent noise performance for signals

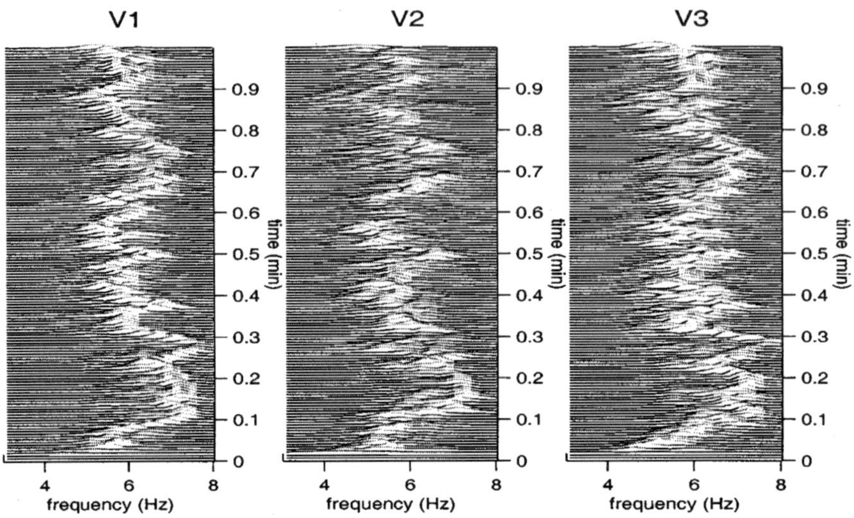

Figure 9. Cross Wigner-Ville distribution of the same atrial activity signal presented in Fig. 8. As shown, frequency resolution has been improved notably [39].

that are long compared to the window length [43], but also because it reflected precisely the variations in the DAF [39]. In order to illustrate how the XWVD is able to improve time-frequency analysis in AF, Figure 9 shows the same analyzed lead as in Fig. 8 but, this time, computed via the XWVD. As can be observed, frequency resolution has been improved notably, thus allowing to follow subtle changes in the DAF that would remain masked under STFT analysis [39].

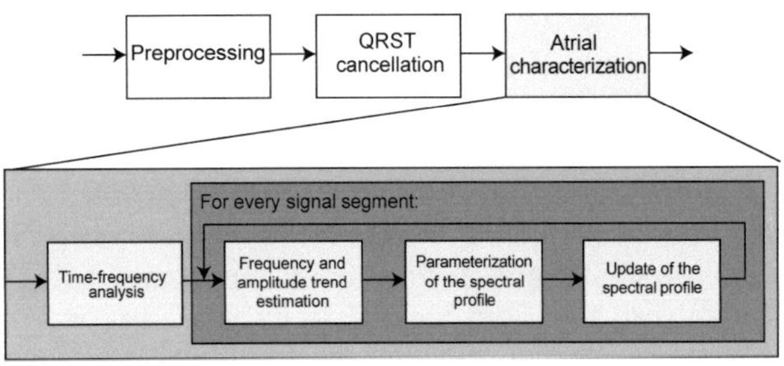

Figure 10. Block diagram of the spectral profile method for time-frequency analysis of atrial signals. Each new time slice, the time-frequency distribution is aligned to the spectral profile in order to find estimates of the frequency and amplitude. The spectral profile is then parameterized and updated [44].

3.3. The spectral profile

The aforementioned spectral analysis techniques had the limitation of only considering the fundamental spectral peak of the atrial activity, but its harmonics have not been put under consideration. However, harmonics could improve DAF estimation and, furthermore, their pattern may be of clinical interest [45]. To alleviate this problem the spectral profile has been proposed [44], its block diagram being depicted in Figure 10. Its main idea is to obtain a time-frequency distribution of successive short segments from the atrial signal. Next, the distribution is decomposed into a spectral profile and a number of parameters

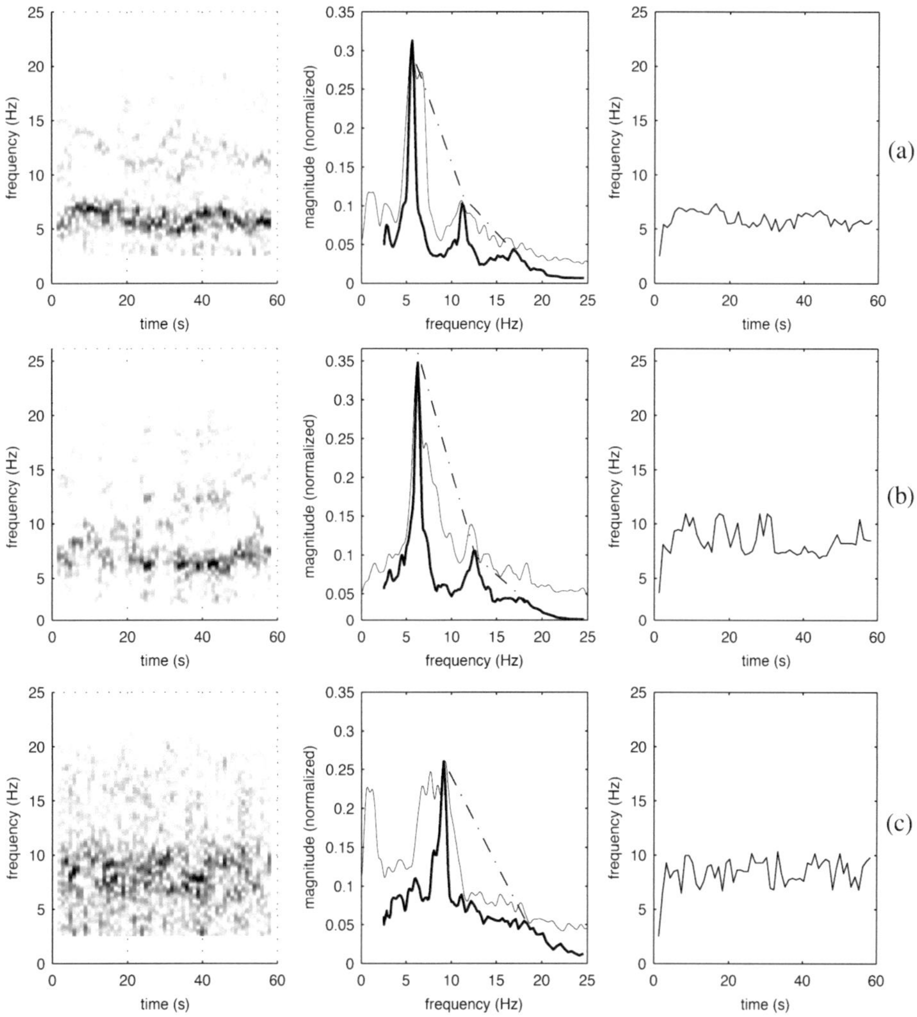

Figure 11. Illustration of the spectral profile technique for three one-minute recordings of atrial fibrillation. The left panel shows the logarithmic time-frequency distribution of the atrial signals. The middle panel shows the spectral profile in solid thick line, the conventional magnitude power spectrum in solid thin line and the fitted spectral line model in dashed line. Finally, the DAF trend is shown in the right panel.(a) Spectral profile for a rather organized AF. (b) Similar to (a) but with notably larger DAF variations. (c) A noisy case with a very high DAF together with a large trend variation [44].

able to describe variations in the DAF as well as in the fibrillatory waves morphology are extracted. Hence, each spectrum is modeled as a frequency-shifted and amplitude-scaled version of the spectral profile. The transformation to the frequency domain is performed by using a nonuniform discrete-time Fourier transform with a logarithmic frequency scale. This particular scale allows for two spectra to be matched by shifting, even though they have different fundamental frequencies and related harmonics [44].

The spectral profile is dynamically updated from previous spectra, which are matched to each new spectrum using weighted least squares estimation. The frequency shift needed to achieve optimal matching then yields a measure on instantaneous fibrillatory rate and

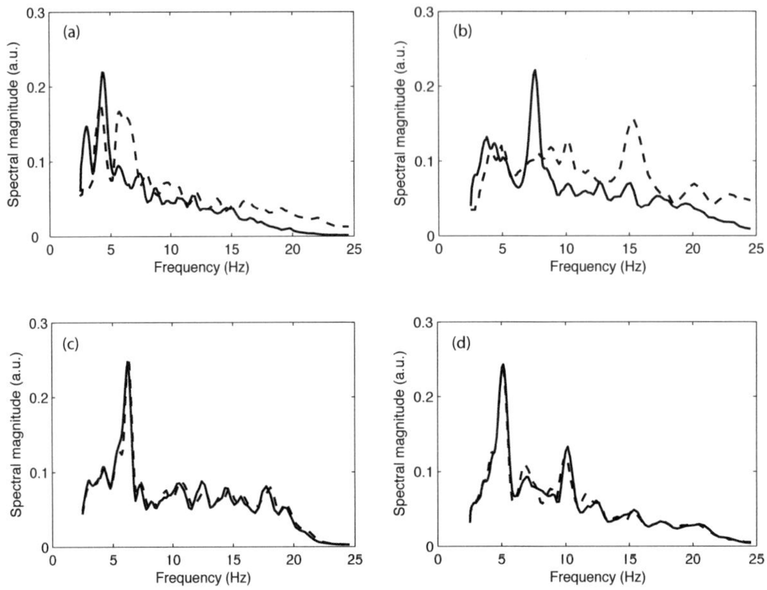

Figure 12. Spectral profile of different atrial signals (dashed line) and the corrected spectral profile obtained by spectral modeling applying the exclusion criteria (solid line). (a) and (b) atrial activity signals with a considerable amount of QRS residua. (c) and (d) atrial activities without noise contamination [46].

is trended as a function of time. An important feature of this approach is that, due to the alignment procedure, the peaks of the spectral profile become more prominent than the corresponding peaks of the conventional power spectrum. As a result, the spectral profile lends itself much better to analysis of the harmonics whose amplitudes reflect the shape of the fibrillatory waveforms and are related with AF organization [44].

Three different examples of the spectral profile technique are shown in Figure 11. Firstly, Fig. 11.a shows the results of a rather organized case of atrial fibrillation, with a DAF of about 6 Hz and a variation within 5–7 Hz. The high degree of organization in the signal is reflected in the presence of two harmonics in the spectral profile (thick solid line in the middle panel). Comparing the spectral profile to the magnitude spectrum (thin solid line), it is evident that the fundamental peak of the former spectrum is narrower and that its harmonics are much more easily discerned. Such a behavior is, of course, expected since the spectral profile represents an average of spectra from successive signal intervals where each individual spectrum, prior to averaging, has been shifted such that the fundamental is optimally aligned to the fundamental frequency of the spectral profile [44]. The example in Fig. 11.b has a DAF of about 7 Hz with a relatively large variation and one harmonic. Finally, Fig. 11.c presents a much more disorganized atrial activity, with a DAF around 8.5 Hz and lack of harmonic behavior. As can be appreciated in the three examples, the spectral profile notably improves DAF and harmonics estimation, specially in the presence of noisy signals.

3.4. Improved spectral estimation

A drawback of the spectral profile-based method is its lack of control of what goes into the spectral profile: a spectrum reflecting large QRS residuals is just as influential as a spectrum reflecting clear atrial activity. Although the spectral profile has a slow adaptation

http://dx.doi.org/10.5772/54199

rate, making it less sensitive to single noisy segments, a short sequence of bad segments causes the spectral profile to lose its structure, and thus, the frequency estimates become incorrect. Furthermore, once the spectral profile has lost its structure, the recovery time until the frequency estimates are valid again becomes unacceptably long, even if the segments have an harmonic structure.

Unfortunately, there are clinical situations in which sequences of noisy segments are common, e.g., during stress testing and ambulatory monitoring and, accordingly, the spectral profile is bound to become corrupt. Therefore, an improved spectral profile method has been proposed able to test the spectrum of each data segment before entering the spectral profile update [46]. A model defined by a superimposition of Gaussian functions, which represent the peaks of the fundamental and harmonics of the AF spectrum, has been proposed (see Fig. 12). These parameters are used to decide whether a new spectrum should be included in the spectral profile or not. The parameters are descriptors of the spectrum and designed so as to verify if a spectrum exhibits the typical harmonic pattern of AF, i.e., a fundamental component and, possibly, few harmonics [46].

Finally, a recently presented approach to improve AF spectral estimation is to use a hidden Markov model (HMM) to enhance noise robustness when tracking the DAF. With a HMM, short-time frequency estimates that differ significantly from the frequency trend can be detected and excluded or replaced by estimates based on adjacent frequencies [47]. A Markov model consists of a finite number of states with predefined state transition probabilities [48]. Based on the observed state sequence, the Viterbi algorithm retrieves the optimal sequence by exploiting the state transition matrix, incorporating knowledge of AF characteristics, and the observation matrix, incorporating knowledge of the frequency estimation method and signal-to-noise ratio [47].

4. Arrhythmia organization

During last years several methods to estimate the degree of AF organization have been presented. Primarily, organization estimation was introduced making use of invasive recordings, in which the atrial signal is of notably higher amplitude. However, in recent years, new methods have emerged in the estimation of organization from surface recordings, thus been able to provide clinical useful information through very cheap procedures. The next subsections will describe some of the most recent and extended methods to estimate atrial fibrillation organization.

4.1. Invasive organization methods

The observation that some degree of organization is present during AF has motivated many investigators to develop algorithms quantifying this degree of organization. Nevertheless, the term *organization* is ambiguous, because of the lack of a standard and common definition within the context of AF. As a consequence, several methods have been proposed to quantify different aspects of AF organization, which are related to different electrophysiological properties or AF mechanisms [49]. According to the number of endocardial recording places involved in the analysis, single-site measurements [50, 51] provide information on the local electrical activity of specific atrial areas, while multi-site algorithms [52–54] introduce the concept of spatial coordination between different regions.

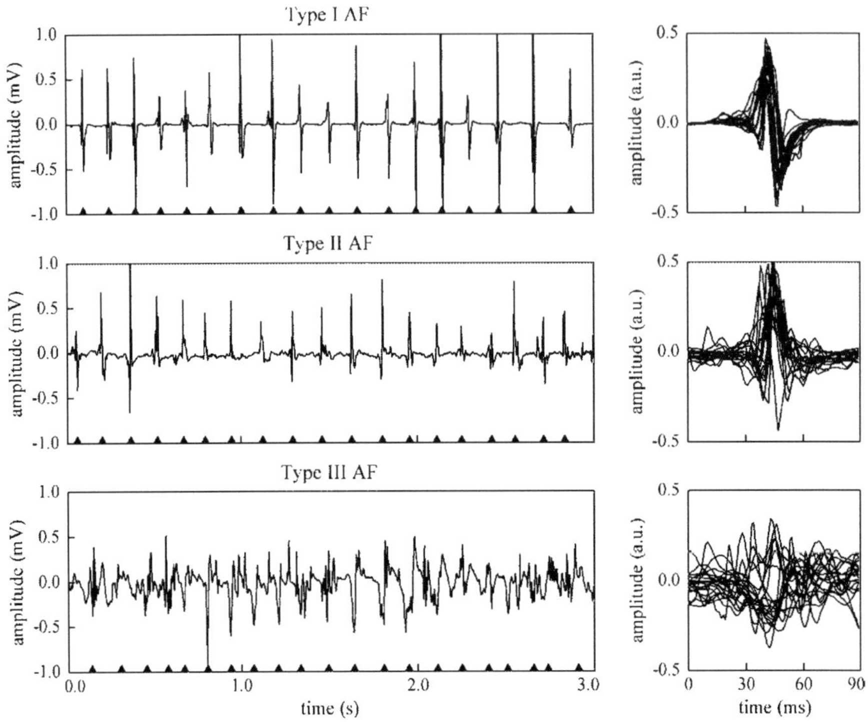

Figure 13. Analysis of the local activation waves for AF episodes with different complexity class. From top to bottom, bipolar electrograms of type I, type II, and type III AF following Wells classification. Filled triangles indicate the time of local activation waves detection. On the right panels, superposition of the normalized activation times obtained from the signals of the left panels [9].

Regarding single-site measurements, Wells et al. [55] published one of the earliest studies examining relative differences in atrial fibrillation electrograms. From right atrial bipolar electrograms after open-heart surgery, Wells classified atrial fibrillation recordings into four categories based on the discreteness of the electrograms and the stability of the baseline. However, the greatest weakness of this method is its subjectivity because it requires manual interpretation and over-reading of the epicardial recordings. Nonetheless, later works have implemented automated methods based on these criteria [56]. In this case, the method was based on comparing diverse features of the parameters describing the dynamic, morphological and spectral properties of intraatrial bipolar electrograms during AF. Next, by making use of that parameters an algorithm was designed for automated AF classification.

On the other hand, organization has also been used in the frequency domain. Given that the AF waveform can be effectively analyzed in the frequency domain, as described in Section § 3, some authors have hypothesized that analysis of the spectra of short segments of an interatrial electrogram during AF would show a correlation of the variance of the signal and the amplitude of harmonic peaks with defibrillation efficacy [51]. Furthermore, the same authors hypothesized that the spatiotemporal organization of AF would vary over time and tried to determine the optimal sampling window to optimize defibrillation predictability.

Nonlinear analysis has also been used to evaluate single-site AF electrograms. In this respect one of the first works specifically applied to atrial fibrillation electrograms was introduced by

Hoekstra et al. [57]. They analyzed epicardial mapping data obtained from atrial fibrillation patients undergoing surgical correction of an accessory pathway. The nonlinear applied techniques were correlation dimension and correlation entropy on the epicardial signals. It was found that these measures discriminated between the various types of electrograms as defined by Wells, thus suggesting that nonlinear dynamics plays a relevant role in atrial fibrillation and can also be used to quantify AF organization.

Finally, one interesting work quantifying AF organization from single-site measurements was introduced by Faes et al. [9] and relied on wave morphology similarity. The algorithm quantified the regularity of an atrial electrogram by measuring the extent of repetitiveness over time of its consecutive activation waves. Since the analysis was focused on the shape of the waveforms occurring in correspondence to the local activations of the atrial tissue, the morphology of the atrial activations was the element by which the algorithm differentiated among various degrees of AF organization. As an example, Figure 13 plots the local activation waves associated to three different AF episodes with different complexity. As can be seen, the method is able to generate a pattern which, later, can be quantified following the organization criteria. The same team introduced an automatic organization estimation method based on features extraction, selection and classification of the AF patterns [58].

With respect to multi-site measurements, this viewpoint would imply that activity at one site should be judged in relation to the activity at another site. Furthermore, when distances between the recording sites are known, and especially when more than two sites are used to compute the organization, spatial organization concepts are also incorporated into these measures [11]. One interesting comparison of methods for estimating AF synchronization between two atrial sites was published by Sih et al. [53]. In this study, after filtering and scaling short segments (300 ms) of atrial fibrillation, the electrograms were passed through two parallel linear adaptive filters, as shown in Figure 14. One way of interpreting an adaptive filter is that it attempts to predict one electrogram through linear filtering of a second electrogram. If the two electrograms are linearly related, then the prediction process would theoretically be perfect. However, if there are non-linearities between the electrograms, the adaptive filter would yield a prediction error. This algorithm defines organization according to the prediction errors from the parallel adaptive filters. The algorithm was theoretically extensible to account for non-linear relationships between electrograms by simply altering the nature of the adaptive filters. This group used the algorithm to quantify organization differences between acute and chronic models of atrial fibrillation [59].

Other works have quantified AF organization between two different atrial sites making use of nonlinear techniques. In this way, Censi et al. [60] quantified the duration of stable recurrence patterns through the use of recurrent plots as well as a measure of entropy in the recurrence plots. The authors suggested that there may exist nonlinear relationships between electrograms from the right versus the left atrium that would otherwise be missed by algorithms relying on linear analyses.

Finally, cardiac mapping tools have brought a wealth of information to cardiac electrophysiology, where the concept of a combined spatial and temporal organization is most easily realized. Within this context, the concept of coupling between several endocardial signal has been introduced. In this respect a two-dimensional analysis by evaluating the simultaneous presence of morphological similarity in two endocardial signals, in order

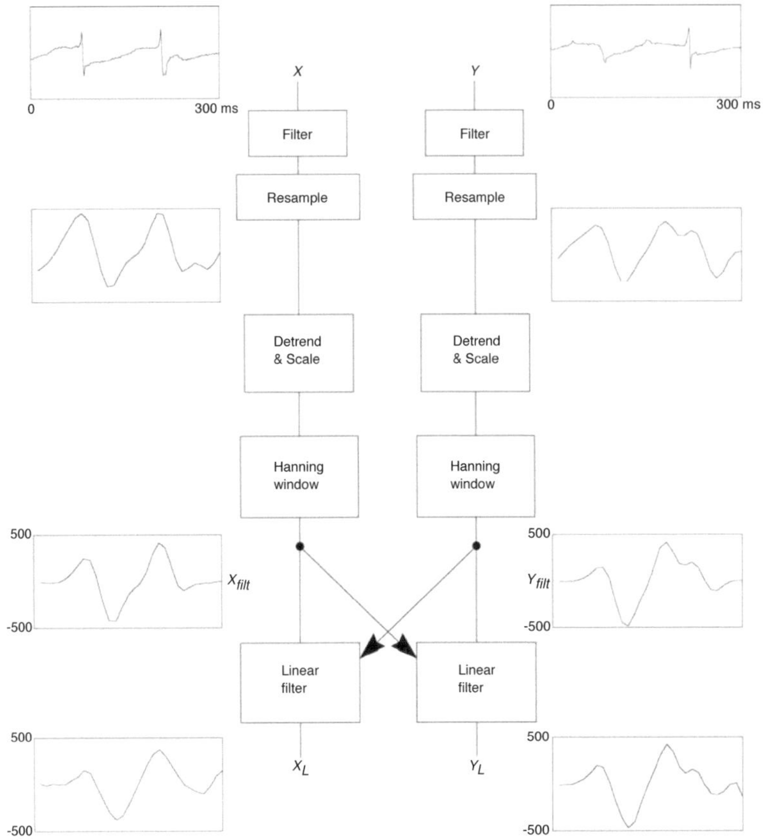

Figure 14. Example of a multi-site AF organization method based on the application of adaptive filtering to the electrograms under study. If there are nonlinearities between the two electrograms, the adaptive filters would yield a concrete prediction error, thus allowing to quantify the degree of synchronization between the electrograms [53].

to quantify their degree of coupling has been introduced [49]. The method considers the atrial activation times on every recording place and estimates the cross-probability of finding similar local activation waves between the considered recordings places, as shown in Figure 15. On the other hand, Mainardi et al. [54] introduced a comparative study for the analysis among atrial electrical activities in different sites during AF. They characterized the properties of pairs between atrial signals making use of a linear parameter obtained from the cross-correlation function and by a nonlinear association estimator. Furthermore, they also studied synchronization through the application of an index based on the corrected cross-conditional entropy [61]. The most recent advances in the study of propagation patterns in AF have been introduced by Richter and co-workers. They investigated propagation patterns in intracardiac signals using a approach based on partial directed coherence, which evaluated directional coupling between multiple signals in the frequency domain [62]. Furthermore, the same team recently presented an improvement in propagation pattern analysis based on sparse modeling through the use of the partial directed coherence function derived from fitting a multivariate autoregresive model to the observed signal [63].

http://dx.doi.org/10.5772/54199

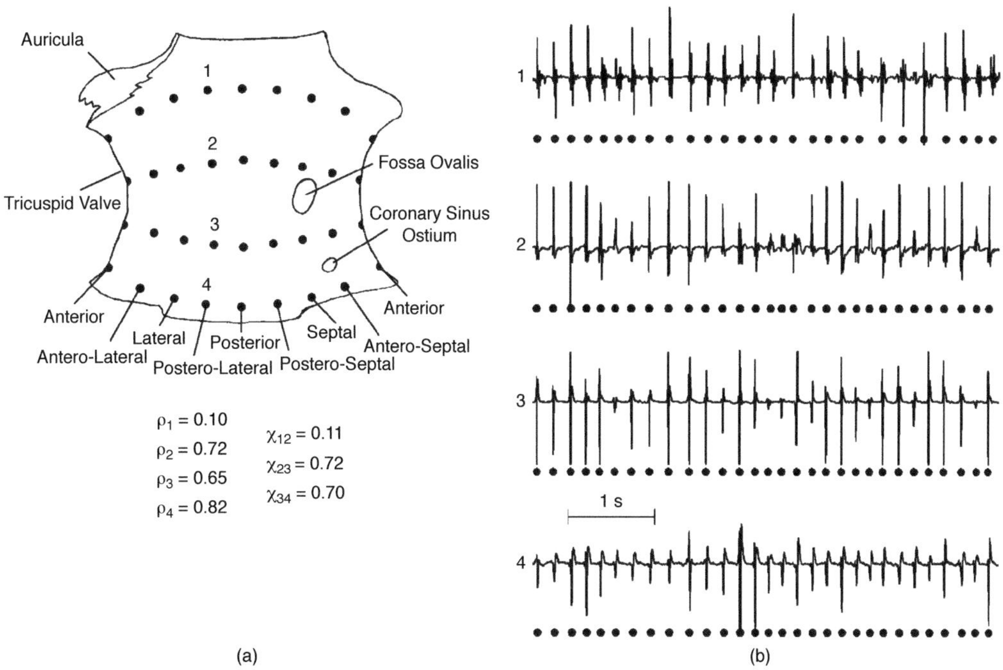

Figure 15. Example of regularity and coupling indices obtained for endocardial signals recorded by a multipolar basket catheter in the human right atrium during AF. (a) Schematic representation of the internal surface of the right atrium with the position of the sites of bipolar signal acquisition. (b) Endocardial recordings taken during AF, from the four electrodes placed in the postero-lateral wall along with the detected activation times (circles). The regularity index (ρ) associated with the four signals and the coupling (χ) between pairs of signals recorded on adjacent sites are indicated [49].

4.2. Surface organization methods

From a clinical point of view, the assessment of AF organization from the standard surface ECG would be very interesting, because it can be easily and cheaply obtained and could avoid the risks associated to invasive procedures [12]. However, only few indirect non-invasive AF organization estimates from this recording have been proposed in the literature. Firstly, the DAF, which has been described in Section § 3. Its inverse has been directly related to atrial refractoriness [64] and, hence, to atrial cycle length [5]. Moreover, it has been suggested that the DAF is directly related to the number of simultaneous wavelets [65]. On the other hand, the second way to get a non-invasive estimate of AF organization has been based on a nonlinear regularity index, such as sample entropy [66]. This index has been proposed to estimate the amount of repetitive patterns existing in the fibrillatory waves from the fundamental waveform of the atrial activity signal, which have been named as main atrial wave (MAW) in the literature. Through the application of sample entropy to the MAW, it has been possible to predict a number of AF-reated events. For example, the onset of paroxysmal AF, its spontaneous termination, its time course from the beginning up to the end of the episode or the outcome of electrical cardioversion in persistent AF [10].

Obviously, the drawback of non-invasive organization estimation is the lack of strict accuracy in the process, given that both sample entropy and DAF are only able to assess fibrillatory waves regularity indirectly. However they have been recently validated by comparison with

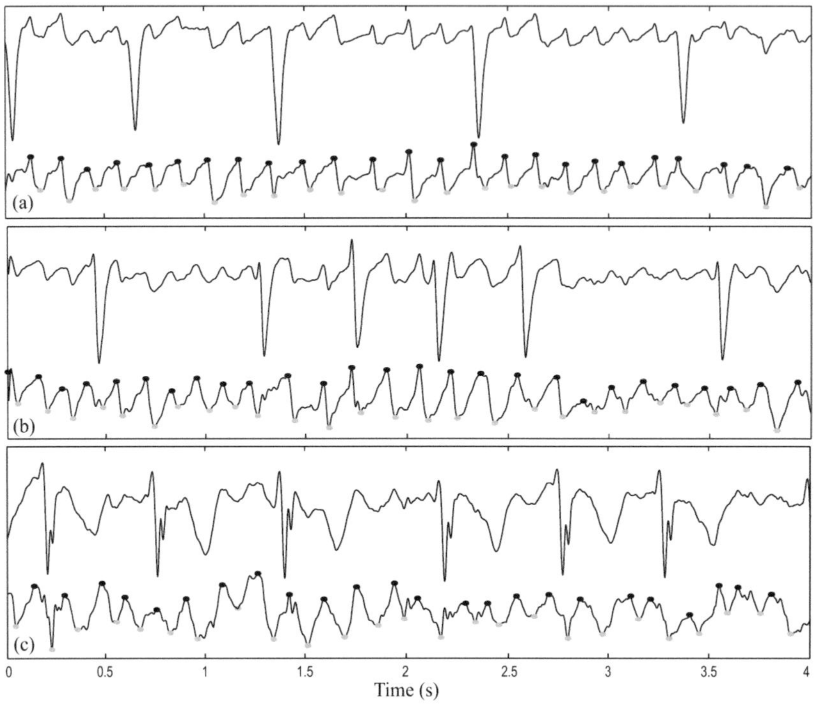

Figure 16. Delineation of the fibrillatory waves for typical 4 second segments corresponding to (a) type I, (b) type II and (c) type III AF episodes, respectively. For each segment, the ECG and atrial activity, after QRST cancellation, are displayed. The upper black circles mark the maximum associated to each activation, whereas lower gray circles indicate their boundaries [70].

invasive recordings [67]. On the other hand, an additional disadvantage of these estimators is that the proper DAF identification in the AA spectral content, computed via the fast Fourier transform, depends significantly on the analyzed segment length, because it determines the spectral resolution [68]. It is advisable that segment length is chosen to be, at least, several seconds for an appropriate DAF identification and to produce an acceptable variance of the frequency estimate [69]. On the other hand, although AF organization could be successfully estimated by analyzing a segment as short as 1 second with sample entropy, the proper MAW obtention depends on an adequate DAF computation [10]. Thereby, it could be considered that the two aforesaid estimators can only yield an average AF organization assessment, thus blurring the possible information carried by each single activation.

One solution to the aforementioned limitations has been recently proposed which is able to quantify directly and in short-time AF organization from the surface ECG. The method quantifies every single fibrillatory wave regularity by measuring how repetitive its morphology is along onward atrial activations [70]. Basically, the atrial activity was delineated through mathematical morphology operators [71]. A combination of erosion and dilation operations was applied to the atrial activity with two structuring elements. The first one was adapted to the fibrillatory waves by an even triangular shape with duration proportional to the DAF. The second was designed as a rectangular shape of length larger to the DAF to suppress the drift between atrial cycles [70]. Finally, the resulting impulsive signal was used to extract atrial activations by peak detection [70]. An example of the potential applications offered by this method, able to work from the surface ECG, is shown

http://dx.doi.org/10.5772/54199

in Figure 16 where several recordings and the corresponding delineation result have been plotted. As can be observed, the method is able to provide precise and automatic fibrillatory waves delineation, making it possible to quantify non-invasively AF organization in short time.

5. Conclusions

The recent advances in signal analysis and processing have provided powerful solutions for the improved knowledge of atrial fibrillation. In this respect, intensive research has been carried out to separate atrial activity from ventricular activity in the ECG and invasive recordings. Furthermore, the proper extraction of an atrial signal has opened the possibilities of developing advanced analysis techniques to gain as much information as possible on the fibrillatory waves. Within this context, relevant information, like the atrial fibrillatory frequency or arrhythmia organization, have been reliably assessed from surface and invasive recordings using digital signal processing methods.

Acknowledgements

This work was supported by projects TEC2010–20633 from the Spanish Ministry of Science and Innovation and PPII11–0194–8121 from Junta de Comunidades de Castilla-La Mancha.

Author details

José Joaquín Rieta[1,*] and Raúl Alcaraz[2]

* Address all correspondence to: jjrieta@upv.es

[1]Biomedical Synergy, Electronic Engineering Department, Universidad Politécnica de Valencia, Gandia, Spain
[2]Innovation in Bioengineering Research Group, University of Castilla-La Mancha, Cuenca, Spain

References

[1] Andreas Bollmann, Daniela Husser, Luca Mainardi, Federico Lombardi, Philip Langley, Alan Murray, José Joaquín Rieta, José Millet, S. Bertil Olsson, Martin Stridh, and Leif Sörnmo. Analysis of surface electrocardiograms in atrial fibrillation: Techniques, research, and clinical applications. *Europace*, 8(11):911–926, Nov 2006.

[2] Leif Sörnmo, Martin Stridh, Daniela Husser, Andreas Bollmann, and S Bertil Olsson. Analysis of atrial fibrillation: from electrocardiogram signal processing to clinical management. *Philos Transact A Math Phys Eng Sci*, 367(1887):235–53, Jan 2009.

[3] J Slocum, E Byrom, L McCarthy, A Sahakian, and S Swiryn. Computer detection of atrioventricular dissociation from surface electrocardiograms during wide qrs complex tachycardias. *Circulation*, 72(5):1028–1036, 1985.

[4] José Joaquín Rieta, Francisco Castells, César Sánchez, Vicente Zarzoso, and José Millet. Atrial activity extraction for atrial fibrillation analysis using blind source separation. *IEEE Trans Biomed Eng*, 51(7):1176–1186, Jul 2004.

[5] M. Holm, S. Pehrson, M. Ingemansson, L. Sörnmo, R. Johansson, L. Sandhall, M. Sunemark, B. Smideberg, C. Olsson, and S. B. Olsson. Non-invasive assessment of the atrial cycle length during atrial fibrillation in man: Introducing, validating and illustrating a new ECG method. *Cardiovasc Res*, 38(1):69–81, Apr 1998.

[6] Shinichi Niwano, Takeshi Sasaki, Sayaka Kurokawa, Michiro Kiryu, Hidehira Fukaya, Yuko Hatakeyama, Hiroe Niwano, Akira Fujiki, and Tohru Izumi. Predicting the efficacy of antiarrhythmic agents for interrupting persistent atrial fibrillation according to spectral analysis of the fibrillation waves on the surface ecg. *Circ J*, 73(7):1210–8, Jul 2009.

[7] A. Bollmann, N. K. Kanuru, K. K. McTeague, P. F. Walter, D. B. DeLurgio, and J. J. Langberg. Frequency analysis of human atrial fibrillation using the surface electrocardiogram and its response to ibutilide. *Am J Cardiol*, 81(12):1439–1445, Jun 1998.

[8] J J Langberg, J C Burnette, and K K McTeague. Spectral analysis of the electrocardiogram predicts recurrence of atrial fibrillation after cardioversion. *J Electrocardiol*, 31 Suppl:80–4, 1998.

[9] Luca Faes, Giandomenico Nollo, Renzo Antolini, Fiorenzo Gaita, and Flavia Ravelli. A method for quantifying atrial fibrillation organization based on wave-morphology similarity. *IEEE Trans Biomed Eng*, 49(12 Pt 2):1504–1513, Dec 2002.

[10] Raul Alcaraz and Jose Joaquin Rieta. A review on sample entropy applications for the non-invasive analysis of atrial fibrillation electrocardiograms. *Biomed Signal Process Control*, 5:1–14, 2010.

[11] HJ Sih. Measures of organization during atrial fibrillation. *Annali dell'Istituto superiore di sanità*, 37(3):361–9, 01 2001.

[12] Simona Petrutiu, Jason Ng, Grace M Nijm, Haitham Al-Angari, Steven Swiryn, and Alan V Sahakian. Atrial fibrillation and waveform characterization. A time domain perspective in the surface ECG. *IEEE Eng Med Biol Mag*, 25(6):24–30, 2006.

[13] Raúl Alcaraz and José Joaquín Rieta. Adaptive singular value cancellation of ventricular activity in single-lead atrial fibrillation electrocardiograms. *Physiol Meas*, 29(12):1351–1369, Oct 2008.

[14] J. Pan and W. J. Tompkins. A real-time QRS detection algorithm. *IEEE Trans Biomed Eng*, 32(3):230–236, Mar 1985.

[15] S. Shkurovich, A. V. Sahakian, and S. Swiryn. Detection of atrial activity from high-voltage leads of implantable ventricular defibrillators using a cancellation technique. *IEEE Trans Biomed Eng*, 45(2):229–234, Feb 1998.

[16] M. Stridh and L. Sörnmo. Spatiotemporal QRST cancellation techniques for analysis of atrial fibrillation. *IEEE Trans Biomed Eng*, 48(1):105–111, Jan 2001.

[17] Mathieu Lemay, Jean-Marc Vesin, Adriaan van Oosterom, Vincent Jacquemet, and Lukas Kappenberger. Cancellation of ventricular activity in the ECG: Evaluation of novel and existing methods. *IEEE Trans Biomed Eng*, 54(3):542–546, Mar 2007.

[18] D. Raine, P. Langley, A. Murray, S. S. Furniss, and J. P. Bourke. Surface atrial frequency analysis in patients with atrial fibrillation: Assessing the effects of linear left atrial ablation. *Journal of Cardiovascular Electrophysiology*, 16(8):838–844, 2005.

[19] Philip Langley, José Joaquín Rieta, Martin Stridh, José Millet, Leif Sörnmo, and Alan Murray. Comparison of atrial signal extraction algorithms in 12-lead ECGs with atrial fibrillation. *IEEE Trans Biomed Eng*, 53(2):343–346, Feb 2006.

[20] F Castells, J J Rieta, J Millet, and V Zarzoso. Spatiotemporal blind source separation approach to atrial activity estimation in atrial tachyarrhythmias. *IEEE Transactions on Biomedical Engineering*, 52(2):258–267, 2005.

[21] P. Comon. Independent component analysis, a new concept? *Signal Processing*, 36(3):287–314, 1994.

[22] J. F. Cardoso. Blind signal separation: Statistical principles. *Proceedings of the IEEE*, 86(10):2009–2025, 1998.

[23] P. Langley, J. P. Bourke, and A. Murray. Frequency analysis of atrial fibrillation. In *Conf Proc IEEE Comput Cardiol*, volume 27, pages 65–68, Los Alamitos, CA, 2000. IEEE.

[24] V. Zarzoso and A. K. Nandi. Noninvasive fetal electrocardiogram extraction: blind separation versus adaptive noise cancellation. *IEEE Trans. Biomed. Eng*, 48(1):12–18, 2001.

[25] T. P. Jung, S. Makeig, C. Humphries, T. W. Lee, M. J. McKeown, V. Iragui, and T. J. Sejnowski. Removing electroencephalographic artifacts by blind source separation. *Psychophysiology*, 37(2):163–178, 2000.

[26] K Nademanee, J McKenzie, E Kosar, M Schwab, B Sunsaneewitayakul, T Vasavakul, C Khunnawat, and T Ngarmukos. A new approach for catheter ablation of atrial fibrillation: mapping of the electrophysiologic substrate. *J Am Coll Cardiol*, 43(11):2054–2056, 2004.

[27] Z Shan, PH Van Der Voort, Y Blaauw, M Duytschaever, and MA Allessie. Fractionation of electrograms and linking of activation during pharmacologic cardioversion of persistent atrial fibrillation in the goat. *J. Cardiovasc. Electrophysiol.*, 15(5):572–580, 2004.

[28] DJ Dosdall and RE Ideker. Intracardiac atrial defibrillation. *Heart Rhythm*, 4(3):S51–56, 2007.

[29] M. Mase, L. Faes, R. Antolini, M. Scaglione, and F. Ravelli. Quantification of synchronization during atrial fibrillation by shannon entropy: validation in patients and computer model of atrial arrhythmias. *Physiological Measurement*, 26(6):911–923, Dec 2005.

[30] RP Houben and MA Allessie. Processing of intracardiac electrograms in atrial fibrillation. diagnosis of electropathological substrate of af. *IEEE Engineering in Medicine and Biology Magazine*, 25(6):40–51, 2006.

[31] Jose Joaquin Rieta and Fernando Hornero. Comparative study of methods for ventricular activity cancellation in atrial electrograms of atrial fibrillation. *Physiol Meas*, 28(8):925–936, 2007.

[32] B. Widrow, J. R. Glover, J. M. McCool, and et al. Adaptive noise cancelling: Principles and applications. *Proceedings of the IEEE*, 63(12):1692–1716, 1975.

[33] J. Malmivuo and R. Plonsey. *Bioelectromagnetism: Principles and Applications of Bioelectric and Biomagnetic Fields*. Oxford University Press, 1995.

[34] A. Hyvarinen, J. Karhunen, and E. Oja. *Independent Component Analysis*. John Wiley & Sons, Inc., 2001.

[35] P. D. Welch. Use of Fast Fourier Transform for estimation of power spectra: A method based on time averaging over short modified periodograms. *IEEE Trans. Audio and Electroacustics*, 15(2):70–73, 1967.

[36] Dimitris G Manolakis, Vinay K Ingle, and Stephen M Kogon. *Statistical and adaptive signal processing: spectral estimation, signal modeling, adaptive filtering, and array processing*. Artech House, Boston, 2005.

[37] Mohamed Najim. *Modeling, estimation and optimal filtering in signal processing*. Digital signal and image processing series. J. Wiley & Sons, London, 2008.

[38] R. W Hamming. *Digital filters*. Prentice-Hall signal processing series. Prentice-Hall, Englewood Cliffs, N.J., 1977.

[39] M. Stridh, L. Sörnmo, C. J. Meurling, and S. B. Olsson. Characterization of atrial fibrillation using the surface ECG: Time-dependent spectral properties. *IEEE Trans Biomed Eng*, 48(1):19–27, Jan 2001.

[40] Frida Sandberg, Andreas Bollmann, Daniela Husser, Martin Stridh, and Leif Sörnmo. Circadian variation in dominant atrial fibrillation frequency in persistent atrial fibrillation. *Physiol Meas*, 31(4):531–42, Apr 2010.

[41] Antonia Papandreou-Suppappola. *Applications in time-frequency signal processing*. CRC Press, Boca Raton, 2003.

[42] Leon Cohen. *Time-frequency analysis*. Prentice Hall PTR, Englewood Cliffs, N.J, 1995.

[43] B. Boashash. Estimating and interpreting the instantaneous frequency of a signal. ii. algorithms and applications. *Proceedings of the IEEE*, 80(4):540 –568, apr 1992.

[44] Martin Stridh, Leif Sörnmo, Carl J Meurling, and S. Bertil Olsson. Sequential characterization of atrial tachyarrhythmias based on ECG time-frequency analysis. *IEEE Trans Biomed Eng*, 51(1):100–114, Jan 2004.

[45] T H Everett, 4th, J R Moorman, L C Kok, J G Akar, and D E Haines. Assessment of global atrial fibrillation organization to optimize timing of atrial defibrillation. *Circulation*, 103(23):2857–61, Jun 2001.

[46] Valentina D A Corino, Luca T Mainardi, Martin Stridh, and Leif Sörnmo. Improved time–frequency analysis of atrial fibrillation signals using spectral modeling. *IEEE Trans Biomed Eng*, 55(12):2723–30, Dec 2008.

[47] Frida Sandberg, Martin Stridh, and Leif Sörnmo. Frequency tracking of atrial fibrillation using hidden markov models. *IEEE Trans Biomed Eng*, 55(2 Pt 1):502–11, Feb 2008.

[48] Benjamin Schuster-Böckler and Alex Bateman. An introduction to hidden markov models. *Curr Protoc Bioinformatics*, Appendix 3:Appendix 3A, Jun 2007.

[49] L Faes and F Ravelli. A morphology-based approach to the evaluation of atrial fibrillation organization. *Engineering in Medicine and Biology Magazine, IEEE*, 26(4):59–67, 2007.

[50] V Barbaro, P Bartolini, G Calcagnini, F Censi, S Morelli, and A Michelucci. Mapping the organization of atrial fibrillation with basket catheters. part i: Validation of a real-time algorithm. *Pacing and clinical electrophysiology : PACE*, 24(7):1082–8, 07 2001.

[51] T H Everett, 4th, L C Kok, R H Vaughn, J R Moorman, and D E Haines. Frequency domain algorithm for quantifying atrial fibrillation organization to increase defibrillation efficacy. *IEEE Trans Biomed Eng*, 48(9):969–78, Sep 2001.

[52] GW Botteron and JM Smith. A technique for measurement of the extent of spatial organization of atrial activation during atrial fibrillation in the intact human heart. *IEEE transactions on bio-medical engineering*, 42(6):579–86, 06 1995.

[53] H. J. Sih, D. P. Zipes, E. J. Berbari, and J. E. Olgin. A high-temporal resolution algorithm for quantifying organization during atrial fibrillation. *IEEE Trans Biomed Eng*, 46(4):440–450, Apr 1999.

[54] Luca T Mainardi, Valentina D A Corino, Leonida Lombardi, Claudio Tondo, Massimo Mantica, Federico Lombardi, and Sergio Cerutti. Linear and nonlinear coupling between atrial signals. Three methods for the analysis of the relationships among atrial electrical activities in different sites. *IEEE Eng Med Biol Mag*, 25(6):63–70, 2006.

[55] J.L. Wells, R.B. Karp, N.T. Kouchoukos, WA MacLean, TN James, and AL Waldo. Characterization of atrial fibrillation in man: studies following open heart surgery. *Pacing and Clinical Electrophysiology (PACE)*, 1(4):426–438, 1978.

[56] V Barbaro, P Bartolini, G Calcagnini, S Morelli, A Michelucci, and G Gensini. Automated classification of human atrial fibrillation from intraatrial electrograms. *Pacing and clinical electrophysiology : PACE*, 23(2):192–202, 02 2000.

[57] B P Hoekstra, C G Diks, M A Allessie, and J DeGoede. Nonlinear analysis of epicardial atrial electrograms of electrically induced atrial fibrillation in man. *J Cardiovasc Electrophysiol*, 6(6):419–40, Jun 1995.

[58] G Nollo, M Marconcini, L Faes, F Bovolo, F Ravelli, and L Bruzzone. An automatic system for the analysis and classification of human atrial fibrillation patterns from intracardiac electrograms. *IEEE Transactions on Biomedical Engineering*, 55(9):2275, 2008.

[59] H. J. Sih, D. P. Zipes, E. J. Berbari, D. E. Adams, and J. E. Olgin. Differences in organization between acute and chronic atrial fibrillation in dogs. *J Am Coll Cardiol*, 36(3):924–931, Sep 2000.

[60] F Censi, V Barbaro, P Bartolini, G Calcagnini, A Michelucci, G F Gensini, and S Cerutti. Recurrent patterns of atrial depolarization during atrial fibrillation assessed by recurrence plot quantification. *Ann Biomed Eng*, 28(1):61–70, Jan 2000.

[61] L T Mainardi, A Porta, G Calcagnini, P Bartolini, A Michelucci, and S Cerutti. Linear and non-linear analysis of atrial signals and local activation period series during atrial-fibrillation episodes. *Med Biol Eng Comput*, 39(2):249–54, Mar 2001.

[62] U Richter, L Faes, A Cristoforetti, M Masè, F Ravelli, M Stridh, and L Sornmo. A novel approach to propagation pattern analysis in intracardiac atrial fibrillation signals. *Annals of biomedical engineering*, 08 2010.

[63] U Richter, L Faes, F Ravelli, and L Sornmo. Propagation pattern analysis during atrial fibrillation based on sparse modeling. *IEEE transactions on bio-medical engineering*, 59(5):1319–28, 05 2012.

[64] A. Capucci, M. Biffi, G. Boriani, F. Ravelli, G. Nollo, P. Sabbatani, C. Orsi, and B. Magnani. Dynamic electrophysiological behavior of human atria during paroxysmal atrial fibrillation. *Circulation*, 92(5):1193–1202, Sep 1995.

[65] A. Bollmann, K. Sonne, H. D. Esperer, I. Toepffer, J. J. Langberg, and H. U. Klein. Non-invasive assessment of fibrillatory activity in patients with paroxysmal and persistent atrial fibrillation using the holter ECG. *Cardiovasc Res*, 44(1):60–66, Oct 1999.

[66] J. S. Richman and J. R. Moorman. Physiological time-series analysis using approximate entropy and sample entropy. *Am J Physiol Heart Circ Physiol*, 278(6):H2039–H2049, Jun 2000.

[67] Raúl Alcaraz, Fernando Hornero, and José J Rieta. Assessment of non-invasive time and frequency atrial fibrillation organization markers with unipolar atrial electrograms. *Physiol Meas*, 32(1):99–114, Jan 2011.

[68] Jason Ng and Jeffrey J Goldberger. Understanding and interpreting dominant frequency analysis of AF electrograms. *J Cardiovasc Electrophysiol*, 18(6):680–5, Jun 2007.

[69] Jason Ng, Alan H Kadish, and Jeffrey J Goldberger. Technical considerations for dominant frequency analysis. *J Cardiovasc Electrophysiol*, 18(7):757–64, Jul 2007.

[70] Raúl Alcaraz, Fernando Hornero, Arturo Martínez, and José J Rieta. Short-time regularity assessment of fibrillatory waves from the surface ecg in atrial fibrillation. *Physiol Meas*, 33(6):969–84, Jun 2012.

[71] P Maragos. Morphological filters–part I: Their set-theoretic analysis and relations to linear shift-invariant filters. *IEEE Transactions on Acoustics, Speech and Signal Processing*, 35(8):1153 – 1169, 1987.

Chapter 8

The Contribution of Nonlinear Methods in the Understanding of Atrial Fibrillation

Raúl Alcaraz and José Joaquín Rieta

Additional information is available at the end of the chapter

http://dx.doi.org/10.5772/53407

1. Introduction

Analysis of cardiac time series by nonlinear metrics has recently gained great interest, because the latter observations suggest that the mechanisms involved in cardiovascular regulation likely interact with each other in a nonlinear way [1]. Furthermore, chaotic behavior can be appreciated in the diseased heart with atrial fibrillation (AF) at cellular level and atrial electrophysiological remodeling during this arrhythmia is a far-from-linear process [2]. Hence, the purpose of this chapter is to review the use of nonlinear methods in the analysis of AF, highlighting the clinically useful revealed information that can improve the understanding of this arrhythmia mechanisms and the existing treatments.

Considering that the atrial activity (AA) can be viewed as uncoupled to the ventricular activity (VA) during AF [3], the applications of nonlinear metrics to AA and VA are addressed separately. Regarding the AA study, different measures of irregularity, chaos and complexity of time series have provided a successful assessment of the fibrillatory (f) wave regularity from both single-lead invasive and surface recordings. This evaluation of temporal organization of AF has been directly associated with the number of active reentries wandering throughout the atrial tissue [4], which maintain and can perpetuate the arrhythmia [5, 6]. In agreement with this relation, nonlinear metrics have shown powerful prognostic information in the prediction of AF organization-dependent events, including spontaneous termination of paroxysmal AF, successful electrical cardioversion (ECV) of persistent AF patients, atrial remodeling time course during the arrhythmia or infusion effects of different drugs. In addition, these nonlinear analysis methods have also been applied to every signal collected by basked catheters, thus providing an estimation of spatial organization of AF by comparing different atrial sites. On the other hand, the application of nonlinear coupling approaches to intraatrial electrograms (EGMs) recorded simultaneously from different atrial places has reveal differences in the spatio-temporal organization of AF consistent with clinical studies [7]. Thus, differences between paroxysmal and persistent AF episodes and among patients with different organization degree, classified by following Wells' criteria [8], have been statistically detected. Moreover, patients successfully cardioverted making use of anti-arrhythmic drugs or ECV have been appropriately identified. Finally, with regard to the VA analysis, ventricular response has been widely characterized by quantifying nonlinear dynamics in interval series between successive R peaks, i.e., RR-interval series [9]. In this respect, multiple measures of fractal fluctuations, irregularity and geometric structure of time series have shown ability to evaluate the cardiovascular autonomic regulation before, during and after AF onset and characterize the main electrophysiological characteristics of the atrioventricular (AV) node.

2. Preprocessing of cardiac recordings

Prior to the application of nonlinear indices to surface ECG recordings and intraatrial EGMs, they requires at least the basic preprocessing described in the following subsections.

2.1. Surface ECG recording

The surface ECG recording provides a widely used and non-invasive way to study AF. Some advantages of using the ECG include the ability to record data for a long period of time and the minimal costs and risks involved for the patient, in comparison with invasive procedures [10]. However, because of ECG represents the heart's electrical activity recorded on the thorax's surface, the signal is corrupted by different types of noise, which are picked up by the volume conductor constituting the human body. Thereby, in order to improve later analysis, these recordings need to be preprocessed. Filtering operations have been typically applied to the ECG for the reduction of noise sources, like baseline wandering, high frequency noise and powerline interference [11]. Thus, baseline wander is often removed making use of high-pass filtering (0.5 Hz cut-off frequency), high frequency noise with a low-pass filtering (70 Hz cut-off frequency) and powerline interference with an adaptive notch filtering.

Additionally, the f wave analysis from surface ECG recordings is complicated by the simultaneous presence of VA, which is of much higher amplitude. Thereby, the dissociation of atrial and ventricular components is mandatory [12]. Nowadays, several methods to extract the AA signal from surface ECG recordings exist. The most powerful techniques are those that exploit the spatial diversity of the multilead ECG, such as the method that solves the blind source separation problem [3] or the spatiotemporal QRST cancellation strategy [13]. However, the performance of these techniques is seriously reduced when recordings are obtained from Holter systems for paroxysmal AF analysis. The reason is that, generally, Holter systems use no more than two or three leads, which are not enough to exploit the ECG spatial information. For single-lead applications, the most widely used alternative to extract the AA is the averaged beat subtraction (ABS). This method relies on the assumption that the average beat can represent, approximately, each individual beat [12]. Recently, a variety of extensions for this method have been proposed [12, 14].

2.2. Intraatrial EGM

Nowadays, a variety of intraatrial recording modalities exists, such as bipolar and unipolar recordings from endocardial and epicardial electrodes, optical mapping and noncontact mapping [15]. Although recordings from each one of these modalities have their own characteristics, unipolar recordings are generally characterized by a substantial far-field contamination, such as VA, whereas bipolar recordings contains local atrial activations of the place in which the electrodes are located. Nonetheless, these recordings are also affected by ventricular interference, especially in recording sites closer to the ventricles, even if its effect is less evident than on unipolar EGMs and surface ECG recordings. Thereby, for the VA cancellation both from unipolar and bipolar recordings, an averaged ventricular interference complex, as in ABS, is usually computed and subtracted from each atrial signal [16, 17]. Only remark that the ventricular activations are habitually detected from a surface ECG recording simultaneously acquired for more accuracy.

On the other hand, given that atrial dynamics can be analyzed both from simple EGMs and local atrial period (LAP) series, i.e., the sequence of temporal distances between two consecutive local atrial activations, the appropriate identification of these points is a important task in this context. For this purpose, EGMs are habitually high-pass filtering (40–250 Hz) to remove baseline shifts and high-frequency noise [18]. The filtered signal is then rectified, introducing low-frequency components related to the amplitude of the high-frequency oscillations of the original signal. The modulus of the filtered signal is further low-pass filtered (cut-off at 20 Hz) to extract a waveform proportional to the amplitude of the components of occurring at 40–250 Hz. The atrial activations are then detected by threshold crossing and their occurrence time can be identified by different methods, including the local maximum peak, maximum slope of the atrial depolarization or their barycenter [19].

3. Nonlinear time series analysis

3.1. Fractal fluctuations quantification

The dynamics of a time series can be explored through its correlation properties, or in other words, the time ordering of the series. Fractal analysis is an appropriate method to characterize complex time series by focusing on the time-evolutionary properties on the data series and on their correlation properties. In this context, the *detrended fluctuation analysis* (DFA) method was developed specifically to distinguish between intrinsic fluctuations generated by complex systems and those caused by external or environmental stimuli acting on the system [20]. The DFA method can quantify the temporal organization of the fluctuations in a given non-stationary time series by a single scaling exponent α, a self-similarity parameter that represents the long-range power-law correlation properties of the signal. The scaling exponent α is obtained by computing the root-mean-square fluctuation $F(n)$ of integrated and detrended time series at different observation windows of size n and plotting $F(n)$ against n on a log-log scale. Fractal signals are characterized by a power law relation between the average magnitudes of the fluctuations $F(n)$ and the number of points n, $F(n) \sim n^{\alpha}$. The slope of the regression line relating $\log(F(n))$ to $\log(n)$ determines the scaling exponent α.

3.2. Chaos degree quantification

The principle of chaos analysis is to transform the properties of a time series into the topological properties of a geometrical object (attractor) constructed out of a time series, which is embedded in a *state/phase space*. The concept of phase space reconstruction is central to the analysis of nonlinear dynamics. A valid phase space is any vector space in which the state of the dynamical system can be unequivocally defined at any point [21]. The most used way of reconstructing the full dynamics of the system from scalar time measurements is based on the embedding theorem [21], which justifies the transformation of a time series into a m-dimensional multivariate time series. This is done by associating to each m successive samples distant a certain number τ of samples, a point in the phase space.

Several methods and algorithms are currently available to characterize a reconstructed phase space. Thus, two features widely used to emphasize the geometrical properties of the attractor are the *correlation dimension* (CD) and the *correlation entropy* (CorEn). The CD is a measure of the dimensionality of the attractor, i.e., of the organization of points in the phase space. Although there are several algorithms for its estimation, the CD can be computed by first calculating the correlation sum of the time series, which is defined as the number of points in the phase space that are closer than a certain threshold r [21]. Then, the CD is defined as the slope of the line fitting the log-log plot of the correlation sum as a function of the threshold. On the other hand, the CorEn is a measure of how fast the distance between two initially nearby states in phase space grows in time. This can be envisaged by taking a point in the reconstructed phase space, which corresponds to a segment in the time series. Another point in phase space located closely to the first one refers to a different segment in the time series. Thus, the CorEn is a measure of how fast these time segments loose their resemblance when both the segments are lengthened.

Lyapunov exponents (LEs) are also found habitually in the literature to enhance the dynamics of trajectories in the phase space. Precisely, these exponents quantify the exponential divergence or convergence of initially close phase space trajectories. LEs quantify also the amount of instability or predictability of the process. An m-dimensional dynamical system has m exponents but in most applications it is sufficient to compute only the largest LE (LLE), which can be computed as follows. First, a starting point is selected in the reconstructed phase space and all the points which are closer to this point than a predetermined distance, ϵ, are found. Then the average value of the distances between the trajectory of the initial point and the trajectories of the neighboring points are calculated as the system evolves. The slope of the line obtained by plotting the logarithms of these average values versus time gives the LLE. To remove the dependence of calculated values on the starting point, the procedure is repeated for different starting points and the LLE is taking as the average.

3.3. Information content quantification

Symbolic time series analysis involves the transformation of the original time series into a series of discrete symbols that are processed to extract useful information about the state of the system generating the process [20]. The first step of symbolic time series analysis is, hence, the transformation of the time series into a symbolic/binary sequence using a context-dependent symbolization procedure. After symbolization, the next step is the construction of words from the symbol series by collecting groups of symbols together in temporal order. This process typically involves definition of a finite word-length template that can be moved along the symbol series one step at a time, each step revealing a new sequence.

Quantitative measures of word sequence frequencies include statistics of words (word frequency or transition probabilities between words) and information theoretic based on entropy measures. Thus, a complexity measures widely used is the proposed by Lempel and Ziv [20], which will be referred to as *Lempel-Ziv complexity* (LZC). This metric provides a measure of complexity related to the number of distinct substrings and the rate of their occurrence along a given sequence, larger values of LZC corresponding to more complex series. Another metric habitually used is the *Shannon entropy* (ShEn) [21]. This index gives a number that characterize the probability that different words occur. Thus, counting the relative frequency of each word, the ShEn is estimated as the sum of the relative frequencies weighted by the logarithm of the inverse of the relative frequencies (i.e. when the frequency is low, the weight is high, and vice versa). For a very regular binary sequence, only a few distinct words occur. Hence, ShEn would be small because the probability for these patterns is high and only little information is contained in the whole sequence. For a random binary sequence, all possible words occur with the same probability and the ShEn is maximal.

3.4. Irregularity quantification

Approximate entropy (ApEn) provides a measure of the degree of irregularity or randomness within a series of data. ApEn assigns a non-negative number to a sequence or time series, with larger values corresponding to greater process randomness or serial irregularity, and smaller values corresponding to more instances of recognizable features or patterns in the data [21]. ApEn measures the logarithmic likelihood that runs of patterns that are close (within a tolerance window r) for length m continuous observations remain close (within the same tolerance r) on next incremental comparison. The input variables m and r must be fixed to calculate ApEn. The method can be applied to relatively short time series, but the amounts of data points has an influence on the value of ApEn. This is due to the fact that the algorithm counts each sequence as matching itself to avoid the occurrence of $\ln(0)$ in the calculations. The *sample entropy* (SampEn) algorithm excludes self-matches in the analysis and is less dependent of the length of data series [22].

On the other hand, the *multiscale entropy* (MSE) has been developed as a more robust measure of regularity of physiological time series which typically exhibit structure over multiple time scales [23]. For its computation, the sample mean inside each non-overlapping window of the original time series is calculated, thus constituting this set of sample means a new time series. Repeating the process N times with a set of window lengths starting from 1 to a certain length N, this will give a set of N time series of sample means. The MSE is obtained by computing any entropy measure (SampEn is suggested) for each time series, and displaying it as a function of the number of data points N inside the window (i.e. of the scale).

Another index that can be used to quantity the regularity of a time series is the *conditional entropy* (CE) [24]. This index computed for a time series measures the amount of information carried by its most recent sample which is not explained by the knowledge of a predetermined conditioning vector containing information about the past of the observed multivariate process. The CE computation can be expressed as the difference between the ShEn calculated for the time series divided both in L and $L-1$ sample-length patterns. Thus, this index measures the amount of information obtained when the pattern length is augmented from $L-1$ to L. If a process is periodic (i.e. perfectly predictable) and has been observed for a sufficient time, it will be possible to predict the next samples. Therefore, there will be no increase of information by increasing the pattern length and CE will go to zero after a certain L. Nonetheless, this algorithm requires a corrective term to estimate accurately the CE. The correction is thought to counteract the bias toward a reduction of the CE which occurs increasing the size of the conditioning vectors and depends strongly on the length of the time series [24].

It is interesting to remark that a slightly modified version of the CE, such as *Cross-CE* (CCE), is able to assess the coupling degree between two time series [24]. Synchronization occurs when interactive dynamics between two signals are repetitive. In this line, this index computes the amount of information included in the most recent sample of a times series when the past L-sample-length pattern of the other series is given. Given that CCE suffers from the same limitation as CE, it has to be corrected in the same way.

Finally, other measure proposed to estimate coupling between time series is the *causal entropy* (CauEn) [25]. This index is an asymmetric, time-adaptive, event-based measure of the regularity of the phase- or time-lag with which point i fires after point j. It is calculated from two components: a non-parametric time-adaptive estimate of the probability density of spike time lag between two points i and j such that i follows j (and, independently, the distribution of j following i), and a cost function estimate of the spread and stability of the distribution. Although a variety of alternatives exists to compute this metric, CauEn can be easily estimated by choosing an event-normalized histogram as the time-adaptive density estimator and the ShEn as the cost function [25].

3.5. Geometric structure quantification

A *Recurrence plot* (RP) is a visual representation of all the possible distances between the points constituting the phase space of a time series [21]. Whenever the distance between two points is below a certain threshold, there is a recurrence in the dynamics: i.e. the dynamical system visited multiple times a certain area of the phase space. From this transformation, well suited for the study of short non-stationary signals, many geometric features can be extracted. In this sense, there are four main elements characterizing a RP: isolated points (reflecting stochasticity in the signal), diagonal lines (index of determinism) and horizontal/vertical lines (reflecting local stationarity in the signal). The combination of these elements creates large-scale and small-scale patterns from which is possible to compute several features, mainly based on the count of number of points within each element.

On the other hand, the *Poincaré plots* (PPs) are a particular case of phase space representation created selecting $m = 2$ and $\tau = 1$; that corresponds to displaying a generic sample n of the time series as a function of the sample $n - 1$ [21]. This is also known as a return map or a Lorenz plot. The main limitation of this technique is that assumes that a low dimensional representation of a dynamical attractor is enough to detect relevant features of the dynamics. Despite its simplicity, this transformation has been successfully employed also with high dimensional systems. The benefit is that, given the low dimensionality, it is possible to easily design and visualize several types of geometric features. These features are based on an ellipse fitted to the PP. These features can be seen as measures of nonlinear autocorrelation. If successive values in the time series are not linearly correlated, there will be a deviation from a line that is often properly modeled using an ellipse. The different features involve the centroid of the ellipse, the length of the two axes of the ellipse, the standard deviation in the direction of the identity line (called SD2) and the standard deviation in the direction orthogonal to the identity line (called SD1).

http://dx.doi.org/10.5772/53407

4. Atrial activity analysis

Although the mechanisms of AF still are unclear, several studies have demonstrated that this arrhythmia is associated with the propagation, throughout the atrial tissue, of multiple activation wavelets, resulting in complex ever-changing patterns of electrical activity [5]. As a consequence, the morphology of the registered f waves during AF changes constantly both in time and space showing different levels of organization, according to a definition of organization as repetitive wave morphologies in the AF signals [19]. Given that various morphologies reflect different activation patterns such as slow conduction, wave collision, and conduction blocks [26], AF organization analysis plays an important role to understand the mechanisms responsible for its induction and maintenance. In addition, the analysis of the degree of complexity characterizing the shape of the activation waves could provide useful information to improve AF treatment, which still is unsatisfactory, and contribute to take the appropriate decisions on its management [27].

Since a rigorous definition of organization does not exist, a variety of nonlinear indices have been applied to the AA signal extracted from both surface ECG recordings and intraatrial EGMs to quantify AF pattern dynamic and morphology. In the next subsections, the state of the art related to the AF organization estimation by using nonlinear methods is summarized.

4.1. Surface organization assessment

From a clinical point of view, the assessment of AF organization from the standard surface ECG is very interesting, because it can be easily and cheaply obtained [10]. Previous works have shown that structural changes into surface f waves reflect the intraatrial activity organization variation [28, 29]. Thus, it has been observed that ECGs acquired during intraatrial organized rhythms present f waves with well-defined and repetitive morphology and ECGs recorded during highly disorganized AA with fragmented activations contain surface f waves with very dissimilar morphologies [30]. Taking advantage of this finding, several nonlinear indices have been applied to single-lead ECG recordings to estimate the amount of repetitive patterns existing in their extracted AA signal. Leads V1 and II have been most often selected for this purpose, because the atrial signal is larger in these recordings [10].

The first proposed method to estimate non-invasively temporal organization of AF is based on the application of SampEn to the fundamental waveform of the AA signal, which have been named as main atrial wave (MAW) in the literature [4]. Note that SampEn computation directly from the AA has also been investigated, but an unsuccessful AF organization assessment has been reported by several authors [4]. The presence of ventricular residua and other nuisance signals together with the SampEn sensitivity to noise have been considered the main reasons for this poor result [4]. In contrast, the MAW-SampEn strategy has provided ability to reliably reflect the intraatrial fibrillatory activity dynamics [29] and has been validated by predicting successfully a variety of AF organization-dependent events. In this respect, the method has shown a high diagnostic accuracy in the paroxysmal AF termination prediction, presenting more regular f waves for terminating than non-terminating episodes [4]. This result is in agreement with the decrease in the number of reentries prior to sinus rhythm (SR) restoration observed in previous invasive studies, where AF termination was achieved by using different therapies [6]. In a similar way, according with the invasive observation that self-sustained AF is associated with more circulating wavelets that non-sustained AF [6], the method has noticed higher organization levels for paroxysmal than persistent AF episodes [31].

On the other hand, the MAW-SampEn method has also presented a high discriminant ability in the prediction of ECV result before the procedure is attempted. According with previous invasive findings [32], SampEn reported higher AF organization levels in those patients who maintained SR during the first month post-cardioversion [4]. In addition, analyzing SampEn after each needed electrical shock to restore SR, a relative entropy decrease was observed for the patients who finally reverted to SR, but the largest variation took place after the first attempt, thus indicating that this shock plays the most important role in the procedure [33]. Finally, remark that the method has also been used to assess the organization evolution along onward episodes of paroxysmal AF and within an specific episode. In the first case, the achieved results, in close agreement with previous findings obtained from invasive recordings [34], proved several relevant aspects of arial remodeling [35]. Thus, a progressive disorganization increase along onward episodes of AF was observed for 63% of the analyzed patients, whereas a stable AF organization degree was appreciated in the remaining 37%. Moreover, a positive correlation between episode duration and SampEn and a remarkable influence of the fibrillation-free interval, preceding each episode, on the corresponding level of AF organization at the onset of the subsequent AF episode were noticed. With respect to the application of the method to track organization variations within each specific episode [4], a decrease in the first minutes after AF onset and an increase within the last minute before spontaneous AF termination were revealed, in coherence with previous works [6].

It is interesting note that f waves regularity has also been assessed through the application of SampEn to the wavelet domain of the AA signal [4]. In this case, the proposed approach reached a slightly lower discriminant ability than the MAW-SampEn method both for paroxysmal AF termination and ECV outcome predictions. Nonetheless, both methodologies showed to provide complementary information, their combination allowing to improve the identification of AF organization time course [4]. A similar result has been recently observed when the variability of the wavelet coefficients computed from the AA signal has been quantified by the central tendency measure [36]. This nonlinear metric is the percentage of points which falls within a certain radius from the centre of the PP of the first difference of the original time series [21] and, in view of the provided results, can be considered as a successful non-invasive estimator of temporal organization of AF.

In addition to SampEn, other nonlinear indices have also been applied to the AA signal time domain. Thus, Kao et al [37] computed the CD, LLE and LZC from the AA signal extracted for the lead V1 in order to distinguish between atrial flutter and AF episodes. According to the expected AF disorganization levels, results showed that during AF, nonlinear parameters concentrated on higher values, which were lower at typical flutter and middle in atypical flutter. In addition, the combination of these parameters by using a neural network classification allowed the differentiation of these arrhythmias with a high diagnostic accuracy around 95%. On the other hand, Sun and Wang [38] have investigated the spontaneous termination of paroxysmal AF by quantifying the RP structure of the AA signal. More precisely, eleven features were extracted from the RP including, among others, the point recurrence rate, the patterns along the main diagonal, the patterns along the 135° diagonal and square-like patterns. Thereafter, a sequential forward search algorithm was utilized to select the feature subset which could predict the AF termination more effectively. Finally, a multilayer perceptron neural network was applied to predict the AF termination with an accuracy higher than 95%.

4.2. Intraatrial organization assessment

As an alternative to the use of surface recordings, AF organization can be quantified from single-lead atrial EGMs by analysis of the whole signal aimed to infer measures related to the dynamical complexity of the signal itself. As for surface ECG recordings, the presence of undisturbed portions of the signal or the repetitiveness over time of similar patterns, are indicative of high regularity, or low dynamical complexity, related to the temporal organization of the arrhythmia. Within this context, Wells et al [8] distinguished three types of AF. In type I AF, the EGMs showed discrete complexes of variable morphology separated by a clear isoelectric baseline. Type II AF EGMs were characterized by discrete atrial beat-to-beat complexes of variable morphology but, in contrast to type I AF, the baseline showed continuous perturbations of varying degrees. During type III AF, highly fragmented atrial EGMs could be observed with no discrete complexes or isoelectric intervals. An analysis looking at these characteristics in AF EGMs has a peculiar electrophysiological relevance, as it may reflect the propagation patterns underlying the maintenance of AF [6]. Indeed, the Wells' approach has been used in several clinical and experimental studies to identify organization patterns in paroxysmal and chronic AF and to support the ablative treatment of AF [39]. In addition, many authors have proposed to quantify automatically single-lead EGMs organization by using analysis of fractal fluctuations and entropy measures.

In this line, the study of Hoekstra et al [40] was the first exhaustive nonlinear analysis of AF in man. The authors estimated the CD and the CorEn of unipolar epicardial EGMs. Both indices were exploited to discriminate among EGMs during induced AF, revealing the presence of nonlinear dynamics in type I AF. In contrast, type II and type III AF did not appear to exhibit features of low-dimensional chaos. Both previous indices were also used to investigate the anti-fibrillatory properties of the class Ic agent cibenzoline in instrumented conscious goats in which sustained AF had been electrically induced [41]. Results showed that during drug administration the nonlinear parameters were not significantly different from control. Nonetheless, scaling regions in the correlation sum were observed after infusion of cibenzoline suggesting that the drug introduced low-dimensional features in the dynamics of AF, whereas SR recorded shortly after cardioversion was very regular. Hence, authors concluded that nonlinear analysis revealed that cibenzoline does not significantly alter the dynamics of sustained AF during pharmacological conversion other than a slowing down of the atrial activation and a somewhat increasing global organization of the atrial activation pattern.

More recently, Mainardi et al [24] have developed a regularity index based on the corrected CE for single-site atrial EGMs and LAP series, which has provided ability to discriminate among different atrial rhythms and, particularly within different AF complexity classes according to Wells' criteria [24, 42]. In a similar way, the index has been able to capture subtle changes due to isoproterenol infusion both during SR and AF [43]. On the other hand, ShEn has been tested as a measure of EGMs complexity for distinguishing complex fractionated atrial electrograms (CFAE) from non-CFAE signals [44]. Given that CFAE have been identified as targets for AF ablation, the development of robust automatic algorithms to objectively classify these signals is clinically relevant. An index of fractional intervals (FI) has been traditionally used and validated as a semiautomatic algorithm to identify CFAE [45]. This measure takes the average interval between deflections of an EGM signal during AF. In contrast, ShEn computation requires each EGM amplitude sample to be classified into bins of defined amplitude ranges. After quantifying EGMs with a bin with of 0.125 their with a bin width of 0.125 times their standard deviation, ShEn provided comparable results to the index of FI in distinguishing CFAE from non-CFAE without requiring user input for threshold levels. Hence, authors claimed that ShEn can be a useful tool in the study of AF pathophysiology as well as help in the classification of CFAE, although its use for EGM-guided approaches in AF ablation requires further validation.

It is interesting note that approaches of nonlinear analysis have also been applied to each one of the bipolar signals collected by basked catheters, thus providing estimates of spatial organization of AF. In this respect, Pitschner et al [46] calculated the CD of the depolarization wavefronts on signals measured during paroxysmal AF and found that the area anterior to the tricuspid valve showed the most pronounced chaotic activity. Later, Berkowitsch et al [47] proposed a combination of symbolic dynamics and adaptive power estimation to compute the normalized algorithmic complexity of single-site bipolar EGMs. The algorithm produces a measure of the "redundancies" in patterns of the AF EGM so that the complexity is inversely related to the number of redundancies found in the analyzed signal. The method was used to show heterogeneous complexity among different atrial regions and complexity changes after drug administration [48]. In a similar way, Cervigón et al [49] analyzed the regularity differences in EGMs captured both from right (RA) and left (LA) atria after propofol administration. Global regularity from each atrium was estimated by applying both MSE and ShEn to each registered single EGM and averaging all the recordings acquired from each atrium. Results revealed differences between the MSE profiles in basal and propofol states and that EGMs at basal condition were sightly less irregular in RA than in LA. In addition, an irregularity decrease in EGMs was noticed, through the MSE, for RA during the proposal infusion. Note that this behavior was observed for all time scales, although MSE decreased on small scales and gradually increases indicating the reduction of complexity on the larger scales. The application of ShEn showed the same upward trend in the LA during propofol infusion, and downward trend in the RA in the anaesthesic state.

In a similar way, both MSE and ShEn have also been used to assess regional organization differences between paroxysmal and persistent AF episodes [50]. In this case, both for paroxysmal and persistent AF patients, no significant differences were found in an intra-atrial analysis (i.e. between the EGMs within the same atrium) in any atria. However, in an inter-atrial analysis, entropy values were higher at the LA than at the RA; i.e. the atrial activations were generally more organized at the RA than at the LA. However, compared with persistent AF, results from the analysis of paroxysmal AF demonstrated larger differences between the atrial chambers. Therefore, a regional gradient from the LA to RA in the organization degree of the atrial electrical activity was found in paroxysmal AF patients, whereas no gradient was found in persistent AF patients.

4.3. Intraatrial synchronization assessment

Spatio-temporal organization of AF has been investigated from mutual analysis of pairs of EGMs simultaneously collected during different atrial rhythms. In this case, measuring organization implies judging the electrical activity at one site in relation to the activity of another. Measures derived in such a way emphasize the concepts of relative temporal behavior and spatial coordination between electrical activations occurring at different sizes. With respect to approaches developed for single-site EGMs, the introduction of algorithms involving two (or more) signals provide complementary information. For instance, synchronization measures have been exploited to investigate the preferential directions of waveforms propagation during arrhythmias, or to reflect the spatial dispersion of electrophysiological parameters such as conduction velocity and refractory period.

To capture and quantify nonlinear interactions among EGMs, some entropy measures have been adapted to the analysis of endocardial signals. Indeed, the studies of Censi et al [51] and Mainardi et al [24] estimated the degree of nonlinear coupling between pairs of bipolar EGMs acquired by decapolar catheters by performing specific multivariate embedding procedures. In particular, Censi et al [51] assessed the organization of the LAP series during AF by means of two indices, namely independence of complexity and independence of predictability. These indices were computed on the basis of a multivariate embedding procedure for the estimation of CD and CorEn. Significant degrees of nonlinear coupling were found in segments belonging to types I and II, while type III EGMs turned out to be only weakly coupled. On the other hand, Mainardi et al [24] estimated spatio-temporal organization in the atria by means of a synchronization index assessing the coupling level between EGMs by means of the corrected CCE. Although this index is sensitive to various signal coupling mechanisms (linear or not), it provides superior performance when compared to linear indices derived from the cross-correlation function, as evidenced in many applications [24]. Thus, it was found to be the best discriminator between organized (sinus rhythm and AF I, classified according to Wells' criteria) and non-organized (AF II and AF III) rhythms [24], showing sensitivity and positive predictability higher than 95%. The index also provided ability to capture subtle changes in atrial dynamics, thus improving the understand the effect of the sympathetic nervous system activity during SR and AF in patients suffering from paroxysmal and persistent AF [43]. In a similar way, the synchronization index showed to be able to underline the effect of the adrenergic stimulation, highlighting variations related to the distance between recording sites [7]. These variations were not detected with the same level of detail by any other linear and nonlinear parameter. Finally, a reduction in the synchronization among EGMs was evidenced by using this index during isoproterenol infusion in both SR and paroxysmal AF episodes [52].

Coupling between atrial EGMs can also be assessed by quantifying the temporal synchronism between activation times in two sites. In this context, researches have focused their attention to either the LAP series or the activation time sequences. Thus, Censi et al [53] exploited RPs to show that a certain degree of organization during AF can be detected as spatio-temporal recurrent patterns of the coupling between the atrial depolarization periods at two atrial sites. They demonstrated a deterministic mechanism underlying the apparently random activation processes during AF. Other approach for the same purpose was proposed by Masé et al [54] who characterized the synchronization between two atrial signals through a measure of the properties of the time delay distribution by the ShEn. Specifically, the values of the propagation delay were quantized into severals bins and the entropy of their distribution was estimated. After introducing a corrective term to reduce the systematic underestimation of ShEn due to the approximation of the probabilities with the corresponding sample frequency, the index was validated with a computer model of atrial arrhythmias. It was shown to discriminate among different AF types and to elicit spatial heterogeneities in the synchronization between different atrial sites. Moreover, a comparison of the real data with simulation results linked the different shapes of the time delay distribution, and thus the proposed index, to different underlying electrophysiological propagation patterns.

Finally, CauEn has been recently used to monitor coupling between temporal variations from two atrial EGMs for paroxysmal and persistent AF episodes [50]. Results showed differences between both atrial chambers with a higher disorganization in the LA than RA in paroxysmal AF patients and a more homogenous behavior along the atria in persistent AF patients. These findings were in strong agreement with the hypothesis that high-frequency periodic sources located in the LA drive AF [55]. Nonetheless, the result may also support the multiple wavelet hypothesis, which have a random movement throughout the atria [5].

5. Ventricular activity analysis

Ventricular response during AF has been widely characterized making use of the heart rate variability (HRV) analysis. Although how the autonomic nervous system exactly modulates the heart rate remains an open question, HRV can be used to quantify several aspects of the autonomic heart rate modulation [56]. Standard time and frequency domain methods of HRV are well described by the Task Force of the European Society of Cardiology and the North American Society of Pacing and Electrophysiology [57], but they fail to show the dynamic properties of the fluctuations. Therefore, nonlinear methods have been typically applied to the HRV for assessing its variability, scaling and correlation properties, thus providing complementary information to the standard HRV metrics [9]. Within this context, the next subsections summarize how nonlinear indices has been applied to HRV analysis in an attempt to understand cardiovascular autonomic regulation before, during and after AF onset and behavior of the AV node during the arrhythmia.

5.1. HRV analysis during SR

The mechanisms leading to the initiation of AF have been under intensive investigation within the last decade. It has been proposed that the autonomic nervous system might have a role in the initiation of this arrhythmia. Precisely, increased vagal tone can predispose to the development of AF [58]. Thereby, several measures of entropy, such as SampEn and ApEn, together with the DFA have been applied to study the HRV complexity evolution in the minutes preceding spontaneous paroxysmal AF onset. To this respect, Vikman et al [59] studied the DFA and ApEn in 20-minutes intervals before 92 episodes of paroxysmal AF in 22 patients without structural heart disease. A progressive decrease in complexity was observed by both indices before the AF episodes. In addition, they also noticed lower complexity values before the onset of AF compared with values obtained from matched healthy control subjects. In a similar way, Tuzcu et al [58] studied via SampEn the HRV complexity of 30 minutes-length segments containing the ECG immediately preceding a paroxysmal AF episode and 30 minutes-length segments of ECG during a period distant, at least 45 minutes, from any episode of AF. Complexity of the HRV was found to be significantly reduced in the segments preceding AF compared with those distant from any AF occurrence. The same study was repeated, but premature atrial complexes were previously removed. In this case, a less pronounced difference was provided. The authors considered that decreased heart rate complexity, for both cases, reflects a change in cardiovascular autonomic regulation that preconditions AF onset. Additionally, the segments preceding AF onset were divided into three successive 10 minutes periods and analyzed with SampEn in order to show the presence of a possible trend. A decreasing complexity trend towards the onset of AF was observed independently on the presence or absence of ectopics, although in the later case the tendency was less pronounced. According to the authors, the decrease in complexity via SampEn before the onset of AF resulted mainly from atrial ectopy. Moreover, the decrease was in consistent agreement with the observed ectopic firing significance, that serves as a trigger of paroxysmal AF, in subjects without evidence of other structural cardiac abnormalities [60].

On the other hand, because of paroxysmal AF has been classified into vagally-mediated and sympathetically-mediated types, based on the autonomic profile and the clinical history, Shin et al [61] analyzed the HRV complexity in these types of AF. In this study, for 44 episodes, divided in three subgroups (vagal, sympathetic and non-related types), the 60 minutes segment of normal sinus rhythm preceding AF onset was divided into 6 periods of 10 minutes. The DFA showed a poor tendency to decrease before the onset of AF and the change of this parameter was divergent according to the AF type. In contrast, ApEn and SampEn revealed a linear decrease of complexity irrespective of AF type. In addition, this result in both ApEn and SampEn before AF onset was not affected whether excluding the ectopic beats or not. In the authors' opinion, the meaning of this progressive entropy reduction before the start of AF was that the heart rate became more orderly before AF; that is, there is a loss of normal "healthy" complexity, thus leading to a cardiac environment vulnerable to the occurrence of AF.

It is interesting note that although nonlinear indices, especially SampEn, have provided to be better predictors than standard HRV measures, their diagnostic ability in paroxysmal AF prediction is far from clinically optimal. Thus, in order to improve their discriminant capability, these nonlinear indices have been combined with other HRV metrics making use of different classification approaches. In this respect, Chesnokov [62] analyzed the combination of spectral features, SampEn and MSE of the HRV by using different artificial intelligent methods. More recently, Mohebbi and Ghassemian have proposed two different combinations of parameters to reach a diagnostic accuracy higher than 95%. Thus, in a first way, they computed a RP of the RR-interval series together with five statistically significant features: recurrence rate, length of longest diagonal segments, average length of the diagonal lines, entropy and trapping time. These parameters were combined making use of a support vector machine (SVM)-based classifier [63]. In the second alternative, a SVM-based classifier was also used to combine spectrum and bispectrum features with SampEn and PP-extracted parameters from the HRV [64].

Finally, several studies have applied nonlinear indices to the HRV after coronary artery bypass graft surgery, i.e. before the onset of AF. Thus, Hogue et al [65] showed that patients who developed AF presented reduced heart rate complexity through ApEn and that standard measures of HRV did not distinguish between these two groups. Logistic regression analysis indicated that only lower complexity via ApEn and higher heart rate were independently associated with AF. In addition, ApEn did not correlate with any other HRV variable, so that the data provide little evidence for a direct relationship between the magnitude of ApEn and the level of autonomic modulation of heart rate. In a similar way, Chamchad et al showed that ApEn provides little complexity in predicting AF after off-pump coronary artery bypass graft surgery [66] and that the CD was independently associated with AF after coronary artery bypass graft surgery, larger values of HRV complexity being associated with the development of post-surgery AF [67].

5.2. HRV analysis during AF

In order to characterize the chaos degree in the ventricular response during AF, Stein et al. [68] implemented an algorithm that uses nonlinear predictive forecasting for the RR-interval series, predicting its future behavior for a few beats by observing other sufficiently similar trajectories in the phase space [69]. Thus, given a RR-interval, the next interval is predicted as the weighed mean of the RR intervals following the three nearest neighbors (found according to Euclidean distance). Results showed that some patients had RR interval series during AF significantly (although weakly) predictable on very short-term scale. This weak predictability, according to the authors, may represent the effect of cyclic oscillations in vagal and/or sympathetic tone at the level of the AV node.

The aforementioned regularity index presented by Mainardi et al [24] has also been applied to the evaluation of exercise effect on ECG recordings from patients with persistent AF [70]. As the autonomic nervous system plays an important role among the factors influencing ventricular response by modulating refractoriness of the AV node, that is mainly dependent on vagal tone, the purpose of the study was to characterize ventricular response during AF to changes of the autonomic balance induced by exercise. The index, reflecting nonlinear series predictability, tended to increase during exercise. It was found that regularity values were very low compared to SR [71], thus the predictability degree of ventricular response is very small during AF. Nevertheless, taking linear and nonlinear dynamics into account, the index succeeded in underlining the increased predictability of ventricular response during exercise. The results highlighted the relevant activity played by the autonomic nervous system in patients with AF, as time domain parameters decreased and predictability indices increased. On the other hand, note that the same regularity index has also been used in order to assess different characteristics in spontaneous paroxysmal AF termination [71]. Thus, the index tried to discriminate between paroxysmal AF episodes that terminate immediately (within 1 second) and others that were not observed to terminate for the duration of the long-term recording, at least for an hour. Results showed higher regularity values for non-terminating than terminating paroxysmal AF episodes, suggesting in agreement with aforementioned works a decrease in the HRV complexity prior to the SR restoration [58, 59, 61].

Sun and Wang have also presented two different alternatives from the HRV analysis to predict spontaneous termination of paroxysmal AF. Thus, in a first way [72], they characterized RR-interval series and its PP extracting eleven features from statistical and geometric viewpoints, respectively. A sequential forward search algorithm was utilized for feature selection and a fuzzy SVM was applied for AF termination prediction. The second alternative [73] was based on the sign sequence of differences of RR intervals. More precisely, this sequence of differences was transformed into the sign sequence based on a threshold. Next, the complexity of the sign sequence and ShEn of probability distribution of substring length were taken as the features of AF signals. Finally, a fuzzy SVM was used to predict AF termination. Although a notably high diagnostic accuracy was reached by both algorithms, the complex combination of multiple parameters in both cases makes difficult the clinical interpretation of the results. In this sense, clinical meaning of each individual parameter is blurred within the classification approach.

On the other hand, Yamada et al [74] analyzed the prognostic significance of ApEn by quantifying intrinsic unpredictability of the RR patterns and found reduced entropy of beat-to-beat fluctuations being predictive of cardiac mortality after adjustment for left ventricular ejection fraction and ischemic etiology of AF. In a similar way, Platonov et al [75] examined the regularity via ApEn of the RR-interval series during AF using short ECG tracings in a subgroup of patients enrolled in the MADIT-II study. However, contrary to the previously mentioned work, ApEn was not predictive of clinical outcome in the MADIT-II subgroup. Nonetheless, there were important differences in the clinical profile of the ischemic patients with congestive heart failure enrolled in the MADIT-II study and the patients with permanent AF with mostly preserved left ventricular ejection fraction studied by Yamada et al [74].

Finally, PPs were used to determine the ventricular response to AF and quinidine-induced changes in its variability in an in vivo study in horses [76]. Results showed a distinct shape in the RR-interval series distribution, suggesting that each RR-interval is determined by the previous one. This, together with the demonstration that there was a negative correlation between consecutive RR intervals and that the standard deviation of the mean of RR intervals was reduced as the AF frequency decreases in the course of quinidine administration, supported the suggestion that, although in the long-term the ventricular response may seem unpredictable, in the short term, the beat-to-beat changes in RR intervals follow deterministic laws established by the frequency-dependent conduction properties of the AV node. On the other hand, by adding the number of occurrences of RR-interval pairs, a 3-D PP can be constructed in which clusters of RR intervals can be identified. Interestingly, in AF patients with clustering of RR intervals, ECV was more effective to restore SR, and, of greater clinical interest, SR persisted for a longer period than in patients without clustering [77].

5.3. HRV analysis to distinguish between AF and SR

Automated detection of AF in heart beat interval time series is useful in patients with cardiac implantable electronic devices that record only from the ventricle. To this respect, PPs have been widely applied to the RR-interval series. Thus, Kikillus et al [78] estimated density of points in each segment of PP and calculated an indicator of AF from standard deviation of temporal differences of the consecutive inter-beat intervals. Thuraisingham [79] used a wavelet method to obtain a filtered time series from the input ECG. He calculated the standard deviation of the time series and the standard deviation of successive differences, and the length of the ellipse that characterized the PP. These indicators were used to discriminate AF from SR. Esperer et al [80] analyzed PP of 2700 patients with atrial and/or ventricular tachyarrhythmias and 200 controls with pure SR. Each plot obtained was categorized according to its shape and basic geometric parameters. Thus, results provided that different shapes were associated with AF and SR, both rhythms being accurately distinguished. Finally, Park et al [81] extracted three measures from PP characterizing AF and SR: the number of clusters, mean stepping increment of inter-beat intervals and dispersion of the points around a diagonal line in the plot. They divided distribution of the number of clusters into two, calculated mean value of the lower part by *k*-means clustering method and classified data whose number of clusters was more than one and less than this mean value as SR data. In the other case, they tried to discriminate AF from SR using SVM with the other feature measures: the mean stepping increment and dispersion of the points in the PP.

Although previous algorithms reached a high classification ability in long heart rate records, their performance was notably reduced for sort data sets. Similar behavior was appreciated for MSE measures [23]. Thus, in long RR time series, when matches abound, entropy metrics can distinguish AF well from SR [23]. However, there is a challenge, though, in assuring a sufficient number of matches when the data sets are short [82]. Thereby, Lake and Moorman [82] optimized the SampEn, developing general methods for the rational selection of the template length m and the tolerance matching r. The major innovation was to allow r to vary so that sufficient matches are found for confident entropy estimation, with conversion of the final probability to a density by dividing by the matching region volume, $2r^m$. The optimized SampEn estimate and the mean heart beat interval each contributed to accurate detection of AF in as few as 12 heartbeats. The final algorithm, called the coefficient of SampEn (COSEn), provided high degrees of accuracy in distinguishing AF from SR in 12-beat calculations performed hourly. The most common errors were atrial or ventricular ectopy, which increased entropy despite SR, and atrial flutter, which can have low or high entropy states depending on dynamics of atrioventricular conduction.

Finally, Segerson et al [83] showed that measures of short-term HRV during SR correlate with measures of cycle length entropy during paroxysms of AF. More precisely, two measures of short-term HRV in SR, such as the root mean square of the differences between consecutive normal intervals (RMSSD) and the inter-beat correlation coefficient (ICC), correlated with well-established measurements of entropy during AF, such as ShEn and ApEn. Recognizing that RMSSD and ICC are known measures of parasympathetic function in SR, authors' claimed that their results suggest a role for vagal regulation of cycle length entropy during AF.

5.4. HRV analysis to characterize the AV node

During AF, the fibrillatory impulses continuously bombard and penetrate the AV node to varying degrees (concealed conduction), creating appreciable variability on the AV nodal refractoriness [84]. Since the AV node is the structure responsible for the conduction of atrial impulses to the ventricles, the strategy of rate control during AF deals with efforts to utilize and adjust the propagation properties of the node [84]. Characteristics of AV conduction have been widely investigated during the last years by using different techniques and, especially, PP analysis. In this graph, it is possible to identify the lower envelope, which have been used to characterize the functional refractory period and the rate dependence of AV node conduction [85, 86]. In addition, the degree of scatter of the PP, calculated as the root mean square difference of each RR-interval and the lower envelope, has been presented as a measure of concealed conduction in the AV node [86].

By applying PP analysis to 24-h Holter recordings of 48 patients with chronic AF, it was suggested that both AV node refractoriness and the degree of concealed AV conduction during AF may show a circadian rhythm, but also that circadian rhythms may be attenuated in patients with heart failure [86]. These findings point to the possibility of obtaining information concerning altered autonomic control of the RR intervals in patients with AF (and heart failure or other disease) with this simple technique.

On the other hand, Oka et al [87] showed that for some PPs computed from 24-h recordings exhibited two separate sectors of RR intervals. When this occurred, the RR-interval histogram disclosed a bimodal distribution in approximately 40% of patients. It should be noted,

http://dx.doi.org/10.5772/53407

however, that these RR-interval histograms were not stratified for different average heart rates. Nonetheless, authors suggest that PPs with two sectors could hold information of the functional refractory periods of each of the two conduction routes that can present the AV node [87]. Interestingly, the circadian variability of the fast pathway functional refractoriness was more pronounced than that of the slow pathway. More recently, Climent et at [88] have presented a method to automatically detect and quantify preferential clusters of RR-intervals. This method, named Poincaré surface profile (PSP), uses the information of histographic PPs to filter part of the AV node memory effects. PSP detected all RR populations present in RR interval histograms in 55 patients with persistent AF and also 67% additional RR populations. In addition, a reduction of beat-to-beat dependencies allowed a more accurate location of RR populations. This novel PP-based analysis also allowed monitoring of short-term variations of preferential conductions, which was illustrated by evaluating the effects of rate control drugs on each preferential conduction.

6. Conclusions

Different pathophysiologic processes control heart's behavior during AF in opposite directions, making difficult the understanding of the mechanisms provoking onset, maintenance and termination of this arrhythmia. Nonetheless, the state of the art summarized in the present work suggests that the use of modern methods of nonlinear analysis can facilitate the understanding of cardiovascular function during AF, in a complementary way to the traditional linear techniques. Thus, nonlinear indices have provided robust estimates of AF organization able to reveal information about several aspects of the arrhythmia. In this respect, clinically relevant information related to the arrhythmia state and its progression after pharmacological and electrical cardioversion has been shown by different researches. In addition, nonlinear analysis has shown to play an important role in the analysis of the ventricular response provoked by the arrhythmia, thus being able to reflect cardiovascular autonomic regulation changes before, during and after AF onset.

7. Acknowledgements

This work was supported by the projects TEC2010–20633 from the Spanish Ministry of Science and Innovation and PPII11–0194–8121 and PII1C09–0036–3237 from Junta de Comunidades de Castilla-La Mancha.

Author details

Raúl Alcaraz[1,*] and José Joaquín Rieta[2]

* Address all correspondence to: raul.alcaraz@uclm.es

[1]Innovation in Bioengineering Research Group, University of Castilla-La Mancha, Cuenca, Spain
[2]Biomedical Synergy, Universidad Politécnica de Valencia, Gandía, Spain

References

[1] Alberto Porta, Marco Di Rienzo, Niels Wessel, and Juergen Kurths. Addressing the complexity of cardiovascular regulation. *Philos Transact A Math Phys Eng Sci*, 367(1892):1215–8, Apr 2009.

[2] Donald M Bers and Eleonora Grandi. Human atrial fibrillation: insights from computational electrophysiological models. *Trends Cardiovasc Med*, 21(5):145–50, Jul 2011.

[3] José Joaquín Rieta, Francisco Castells, César Sánchez, Vicente Zarzoso, and José Millet. Atrial activity extraction for atrial fibrillation analysis using blind source separation. *IEEE Trans Biomed Eng*, 51(7):1176–86, Jul 2004.

[4] Raul Alcaraz and Jose Joaquin Rieta. A review on sample entropy applications for the non-invasive analysis of atrial fibrillation electrocardiograms. *Biomed Signal Process Control*, 5:1–14, 2010.

[5] M A Allessie, W J E P Lammers, F I M Bonke, and J Hollen. *Experimental evaulation of Moe's multiple wavelet hypothesis of atrial fibrillation*. In: EP Zipes and J Jalife (eds.), Cardiac Electrophysiology and Arrhythmias, Grune & Stratton Inc., Orlando, 1985.

[6] K. T. Konings, C. J. Kirchhof, J. R. Smeets, H. J. Wellens, O. C. Penn, and M. A. Allessie. High-density mapping of electrically induced atrial fibrillation in humans. *Circulation*, 89(4):1665–80, Apr 1994.

[7] Luca T Mainardi, Valentina D A Corino, Leonida Lombardi, Claudio Tondo, Massimo Mantica, Federico Lombardi, and Sergio Cerutti. Linear and nonlinear coupling between atrial signals. Three methods for the analysis of the relationships among atrial electrical activities in different sites. *IEEE Eng Med Biol Mag*, 25(6):63–70, 2006.

[8] J L Wells, Jr, R B Karp, N T Kouchoukos, W A MacLean, T N James, and A L Waldo. Characterization of atrial fibrillation in man: studies following open heart surgery. *Pacing Clin Electrophysiol*, 1(4):426–38, Oct 1978.

[9] Buccelletti Francesco, Bocci Maria Grazia, Gilardi Emanuele, Fiore Valentina, Calcinaro Sara, Fragnoli Chiara, Maviglia Riccardo, and Franceschi Francesco. Linear and nonlinear heart rate variability indexes in clinical practice. *Comput Math Methods Med*, 2012:219080, 2012.

[10] Simona Petrutiu, Jason Ng, Grace M Nijm, Haitham Al-Angari, Steven Swiryn, and Alan V Sahakian. Atrial fibrillation and waveform characterization. A time domain perspective in the surface ECG. *IEEE Eng Med Biol Mag*, 25(6):24–30, 2006.

[11] L. Sörnmo and P. Laguna. *Bioelectrical Signal Processing in Cardiac and Neurological Applications*. Elsevier Academic Press, 2005.

[12] Raúl Alcaraz and José Joaquín Rieta. Adaptive singular value cancelation of ventricular activity in single-lead atrial fibrillation electrocardiograms. *Physiol Meas*, 29(12):1351–69, Dec 2008.

[13] M Stridh and L Sörnmo. Spatiotemporal QRST cancellation techniques for analysis of atrial fibrillation. *IEEE Trans Biomed Eng*, 48(1):105–11, Jan 2001.

[14] Mathieu Lemay, Jean-Marc Vesin, Adriaan van Oosterom, Vincent Jacquemet, and Lukas Kappenberger. Cancellation of ventricular activity in the ECG: evaluation of novel and existing methods. *IEEE Trans Biomed Eng*, 54(3):542–6, Mar 2007.

[15] William G Stevenson and Kyoko Soejima. Recording techniques for clinical electrophysiology. *J Cardiovasc Electrophysiol*, 16(9):1017–22, Sep 2005.

[16] S Shkurovich, A V Sahakian, and S Swiryn. Detection of atrial activity from high-voltage leads of implantable ventricular defibrillators using a cancellation technique. *IEEE Trans Biomed Eng*, 45(2):229–34, Feb 1998.

[17] José Joaquín Rieta and Fernando Hornero. Comparative study of methods for ventricular activity cancellation in atrial electrograms of atrial fibrillation. *Physiol Meas*, 28(8):925–36, Aug 2007.

[18] V Barbaro, P Bartolini, G Calcagnini, S Morelli, A Michelucci, and G Gensini. Automated classification of human atrial fibrillation from intraatrial electrograms. *Pacing Clin Electrophysiol*, 23(2):192–202, Feb 2000.

[19] Luca Faes, Giandomenico Nollo, Renzo Antolini, Fiorenzo Gaita, and Flavia Ravelli. A method for quantifying atrial fibrillation organization based on wave-morphology similarity. *IEEE Trans Biomed Eng*, 49(12 Pt 2):1504–13, Dec 2002.

[20] A Paraschiv-Ionescu, E Buchser, B Rutschmann, and K Aminian. Nonlinear analysis of human physical activity patterns in health and disease. *Phys Rev E Stat Nonlin Soft Matter Phys*, 77(2 Pt 1):021913, Feb 2008.

[21] Holger Kantz and Thomas Schreiber. *Nonlinear time series analysis*. Cambrigde University Press, 2003.

[22] J S Richman and J R Moorman. Physiological time-series analysis using approximate entropy and sample entropy. *Am J Physiol Heart Circ Physiol*, 278(6):H2039–49, Jun 2000.

[23] Madalena Costa, Ary L Goldberger, and C-K Peng. Multiscale entropy analysis of biological signals. *Phys Rev E Stat Nonlin Soft Matter Phys*, 71(2 Pt 1):021906, Feb 2005.

[24] L T Mainardi, A Porta, G Calcagnini, P Bartolini, A Michelucci, and S Cerutti. Linear and non-linear analysis of atrial signals and local activation period series during atrial-fibrillation episodes. *Med Biol Eng Comput*, 39(2):249–54, Mar 2001.

[25] Jack Waddell, Rhonda Dzakpasu, Victoria Booth, Brett Riley, Jonathan Reasor, Gina Poe, and Michal Zochowski. Causal entropies–A measure for determining changes in the temporal organization of neural systems. *J Neurosci Methods*, 162(1-2):320–32, May 2007.

[26] K T Konings, J L Smeets, O C Penn, H J Wellens, and M A Allessie. Configuration of unipolar atrial electrograms during electrically induced atrial fibrillation in humans. *Circulation*, 95(5):1231–41, Mar 1997.

[27] Maria S Guillem, Andreu M Climent, Francisco Castells, Daniela Husser, Jose Millet, Arash Arya, Christopher Piorkowski, and Andreas Bollmann. Noninvasive mapping of human atrial fibrillation. *J Cardiovasc Electrophysiol*, 20(5):507–13, May 2009.

[28] Daniela Husser, Martin Stridh, David S Cannom, Anil K Bhandari, Marc J Girsky, Steven Kang, Leif Sörnmo, S Bertil Olsson, and Andreas Bollmann. Validation and clinical application of time-frequency analysis of atrial fibrillation electrocardiograms. *J Cardiovasc Electrophysiol*, 18(1):41–6, Jan 2007.

[29] Raúl Alcaraz, Fernando Hornero, and José J Rieta. Assessment of non-invasive time and frequency atrial fibrillation organization markers with unipolar atrial electrograms. *Physiol Meas*, 32(1):99–114, Jan 2011.

[30] Raúl Alcaraz, Fernando Hornero, Arturo Martínez, and José J Rieta. Short-time regularity assessment of fibrillatory waves from the surface ECG in atrial fibrillation. *Physiol Meas*, 33(6):969–84, Jun 2012.

[31] Raúl Alcaraz and José Joaquín Rieta. The application of nonlinear metrics to assess organization differences in short recordings of paroxysmal and persistent atrial fibrillation. *Physiol Meas*, 31(1):115–30, Jan 2010.

[32] Giovanni Calcagnini, Federica Censi, Antonio Michelucci, and Pietro Bartolini. Descriptors of wavefront propagation. Endocardial mapping of atrial fibrillation with basket catheter. *IEEE Eng Med Biol Mag*, 25(6):71–8, 2006.

[33] Raúl Alcaraz, José Joaquín Rieta, and Fernando Hornero. Non-invasive atrial fibrillation organization follow-up under successive attempts of electrical cardioversion. *Med Biol Eng Comput*, 47(12):1247–55, Dec 2009.

[34] M C Wijffels, C J Kirchhof, R Dorland, and M A Allessie. Atrial fibrillation begets atrial fibrillation. A study in awake chronically instrumented goats. *Circulation*, 92(7):1954–68, Oct 1995.

[35] Raúl Alcaraz, Fernando Hornero, and José Joaquín Rieta. Surface ECG organization time course analysis along onward episodes of paroxysmal atrial fibrillation. *Med Eng Phys*, 33(5):597–603, Jun 2011.

[36] Raul Alcaraz and Jose Joaquin Rieta. Central tendency measure and wavelet transform combined in the non-invasive analysis of atrial fibrillation recordings. *Biomed Eng Online*, 11:46, 2012.

[37] Tsair Kao, Yueh-Yun Su, Chih-Cheng Lu, Ching-Tai Tai, Shih-An Chen, Yi-Chen Lin, and Han-Wen Tso. Differentiation of atrial flutter and atrial fibrillation from surface electrocardiogram using nonlinear analysis. *Journal of Medical and Biological Engineering*, 25(3):117–122, 2005.

[38] Rongrong Sun and Yuanyuan Wang. Predicting termination of atrial fibrillation based on the structure and quantification of the recurrence plot. *Med Eng Phys*, 30(9):1105–11, Nov 2008.

[39] F Gaita, L Calò, R Riccardi, L Garberoglio, M Scaglione, G Licciardello, L Coda, P Di Donna, M Bocchiardo, D Caponi, R Antolini, F Orzan, and G P Trevi. Different

patterns of atrial activation in idiopathic atrial fibrillation: simultaneous multisite atrial mapping in patients with paroxysmal and chronic atrial fibrillation. *J Am Coll Cardiol*, 37(2):534–41, Feb 2001.

[40] B P Hoekstra, C G Diks, M A Allessie, and J DeGoede. Nonlinear analysis of epicardial atrial electrograms of electrically induced atrial fibrillation in man. *J Cardiovasc Electrophysiol*, 6(6):419–40, Jun 1995.

[41] Bart P. T. Hoekstra, Cees G. H. Diks, Maurits A. Allessie, and Jacob DeGoede. Nonlinear analysis of the pharmacological conversion of sustained atrial fibrillation in conscious goats by the class Ic drug cibenzoline. *Chaos*, 7(3):430–446, Sep 1997.

[42] L T Mainardi, A Porta, G Calcagnini, F Censi, P Bartolini, A Michelucci, and S Cerutti. Discrimination of atrial rhythms by linear and non-linear methods. *Ann Ist Super Sanita*, 37(3):335–40, 2001.

[43] Luca T Mainardi, Valentina D A Corino, Leonida Lombardi, Claudio Tondo, Massimo Mantica, Federico Lombardi, and Sergio Cerutti. Assessment of the dynamics of atrial signals and local atrial period series during atrial fibrillation: effects of isoproterenol administration. *Biomed Eng Online*, 3(1):37, Oct 2004.

[44] Jason Ng, Aleksey I Borodyanskiy, Eric T Chang, Roger Villuendas, Samer Dibs, Alan H Kadish, and Jeffrey J Goldberger. Measuring the complexity of atrial fibrillation electrograms. *J Cardiovasc Electrophysiol*, 21(6):649–55, Jun 2010.

[45] Atul Verma, Paul Novak, Laurent Macle, Bonnie Whaley, Marianne Beardsall, Zaev Wulffhart, and Yaariv Khaykin. A prospective, multicenter evaluation of ablating complex fractionated electrograms (CFES) during atrial fibrillation (AF) identified by an automated mapping algorithm: acute effects on AF and efficacy as an adjuvant strategy. *Heart Rhythm*, 5(2):198–205, Feb 2008.

[46] H F Pitschner, A Berkovic, S Grumbrecht, and J Neuzner. Multielectrode basket catheter mapping for human atrial fibrillation. *J Cardiovasc Electrophysiol*, 9(8 Suppl):S48–56, Aug 1998.

[47] A Berkowitsch, J Carlsson, A Erdogan, J Neuzner, and H F Pitschner. Electrophysiological heterogeneity of atrial fibrillation and local effect of propafenone in the human right atrium: analysis based on symbolic dynamics. *J Interv Card Electrophysiol*, 4(2):383–94, Jun 2000.

[48] H F Pitschner and A Berkowitsch. Algorithmic complexity. A new approach of non-linear algorithms for the analysis of atrial signals from multipolar basket catheter. *Ann Ist Super Sanita*, 37(3):409–18, 2001.

[49] Raquel Cervigón, Javier Moreno, César Sánchez, Richard B Reilly, Julián Villacastín, José Millet, and Francisco Castells. Atrial fibrillation organization: quantification of propofol effects. *Med Biol Eng Comput*, 47(3):333–41, Mar 2009.

[50] R Cervigón, J Moreno, R B Reilly, J Millet, J Pérez-Villacastín, and F Castells. Entropy measurements in paroxysmal and persistent atrial fibrillation. *Physiol Meas*, 31(7):1011–20, Jul 2010.

[51] F Censi, V Barbaro, P Bartolini, G Calcagnini, A Michelucci, and S Cerutti. Non-linear coupling of atrial activation processes during atrial fibrillation in humans. *Biol Cybern*, 85(3):195–201, Sep 2001.

[52] Valentina D A Corino, Massimo Mantica, Federico Lombardi, and Luca T Mainardi. Assessment of spatial organization in the atria during paroxysmal atrial fibrillation and adrenergic stimulation. *Biomed Tech (Berl)*, 51(4):260–3, Oct 2006.

[53] F Censi, V Barbaro, P Bartolini, G Calcagnini, A Michelucci, G F Gensini, and S Cerutti. Recurrent patterns of atrial depolarization during atrial fibrillation assessed by recurrence plot quantification. *Ann Biomed Eng*, 28(1):61–70, Jan 2000.

[54] Michela Masè, Luca Faes, Renzo Antolini, Marco Scaglione, and Flavia Ravelli. Quantification of synchronization during atrial fibrillation by shannon entropy: validation in patients and computer model of atrial arrhythmias. *Physiol Meas*, 26(6):911–23, Dec 2005.

[55] Prashanthan Sanders, Omer Berenfeld, Mélèze Hocini, Pierre Jaïs, Ravi Vaidyanathan, Li-Fern Hsu, Stéphane Garrigue, Yoshihide Takahashi, Martin Rotter, Fréderic Sacher, Christophe Scavée, Robert Ploutz-Snyder, José Jalife, and Michel Haïssaguerre. Spectral analysis identifies sites of high-frequency activity maintaining atrial fibrillation in humans. *Circulation*, 112(6):789–97, Aug 2005.

[56] Luca T Mainardi. On the quantification of heart rate variability spectral parameters using time-frequency and time-varying methods. *Philos Transact A Math Phys Eng Sci*, 367(1887):255–75, Jan 2009.

[57] Task Force of the European Society of Cardiology and the North American Society of Pacing and Electrophysiology. Heart rate variability: standards of measurement, physiological interpretation and clinical use. *Circulation*, 93(5):1043–1065, Mar 1996.

[58] Volkan Tuzcu, Selman Nas, Tülay Börklü, and Ahmet Ugur. Decrease in the heart rate complexity prior to the onset of atrial fibrillation. *Europace*, 8(6):398–402, Jun 2006.

[59] S Vikman, T H Mäkikallio, S Yli-Mäyry, S Pikkujämsä, A M Koivisto, P Reinikainen, K E Airaksinen, and H V Huikuri. Altered complexity and correlation properties of R-R interval dynamics before the spontaneous onset of paroxysmal atrial fibrillation. *Circulation*, 100(20):2079–84, Nov 1999.

[60] M. Haïssaguerre, P. Jaïs, D. C. Shah, A. Takahashi, M. Hocini, G. Quiniou, S. Garrigue, A. Le Mouroux, P. Le Métayer, and J. Clémenty. Spontaneous initiation of atrial fibrillation by ectopic beats originating in the pulmonary veins. *N Engl J Med*, 339(10):659–666, Sep 1998.

[61] Dong-Gu Shin, Cheol-Seung Yoo, Sang-Hoon Yi, Jun-Ho Bae, Young-Jo Kim, Jong-Sun Park, and Geu-Ru Hong. Prediction of paroxysmal atrial fibrillation using nonlinear analysis of the R-R interval dynamics before the spontaneous onset of atrial fibrillation. *Circ J*, 70(1):94–99, Jan 2006.

[62] Yuriy V Chesnokov. Complexity and spectral analysis of the heart rate variability dynamics for distant prediction of paroxysmal atrial fibrillation with artificial intelligence methods. *Artif Intell Med*, 43(2):151–165, Jun 2008.

[63] Maryam Mohebbi and Hassan Ghassemian. Prediction of paroxysmal atrial fibrillation using recurrence plot-based features of the RR-interval signal. *Physiol Meas*, 32(8):1147–62, Aug 2011.

[64] Maryam Mohebbi and Hassan Ghassemian. Prediction of paroxysmal atrial fibrillation based on non-linear analysis and spectrum and bispectrum features of the heart rate variability signal. *Comput Methods Programs Biomed*, 105(1):40–9, Jan 2012.

[65] C W Hogue, Jr, P P Domitrovich, P K Stein, G D Despotis, L Re, R B Schuessler, R E Kleiger, and J N Rottman. RR interval dynamics before atrial fibrillation in patients after coronary artery bypass graft surgery. *Circulation*, 98(5):429–34, Aug 1998.

[66] Dmitri Chamchad, Jay C Horrow, Louis E Samuels, and Lev Nakhamchik. Heart rate variability measures poorly predict atrial fibrillation after off-pump coronary artery bypass grafting. *J Clin Anesth*, 23(6):451–5, Sep 2011.

[67] Dmitri Chamchad, George Djaiani, Hyun Ju Jung, Lev Nakhamchik, Jo Carroll, and Jay C Horrow. Nonlinear heart rate variability analysis may predict atrial fibrillation after coronary artery bypass grafting. *Anesth Analg*, 103(5):1109–12, Nov 2006.

[68] K M Stein, J Walden, N Lippman, and B B Lerman. Ventricular response in atrial fibrillation: random or deterministic? *Am J Physiol*, 277(2 Pt 2):H452–8, Aug 1999.

[69] G Sugihara and R M May. Nonlinear forecasting as a way of distinguishing chaos from measurement error in time series. *Nature*, 344(6268):734–41, Apr 1990.

[70] V D A Corino, L T Mainardi, Daniela Husser, Helmut U Klein, and Andreas Bollmann. Ventricular response during atrial fibrillation: Evaluation of exercise and flecainide effects. *Proc. Comput. Cardiol.*, 33:145–148, 2006.

[71] L. T. Mainardi, M. Matteucci, and R. Sassi. On predicting the spontaneous termination of atrial fibrillation episodes using linear and non-linear parameters of ECG signal and RR series. *Proc Comput Cardiol*, 31:665–668, 2004.

[72] R R Sun and Y Y Wang. Predicting spontaneous termination of atrial fibrillation based on the RR interval. *Proc Inst Mech Eng H*, 223(6):713–26, Aug 2009.

[73] Rongrong Sun dan Yuanyuan Wang. Predicting termination of atrial fibrillation based on sign sequence of RR interval differences. *Chinese Journal of Scientific Instrument*, 2009.

[74] A Yamada, J Hayano, S Sakata, A Okada, S Mukai, N Ohte, and G Kimura. Reduced ventricular response irregularity is associated with increased mortality in patients with chronic atrial fibrillation. *Circulation*, 102(3):300–6, Jul 2000.

[75] Pyotr G Platonov and Fredrik Holmqvist. Atrial fibrillatory rate and irregularity of ventricular response as predictors of clinical outcome in patients with atrial fibrillation. *J Electrocardiol*, 44(6):673–7, 2011.

[76] A R Gelzer, N S Moïse, D Vaidya, K A Wagner, and J Jalife. Temporal organization of atrial activity and irregular ventricular rhythm during spontaneous atrial fibrillation: an in vivo study in the horse. *J Cardiovasc Electrophysiol*, 11(7):773–84, Jul 2000.

[77] Maarten P Van Den Berg, Trudeke Van Noord, Jan Brouwer, Jaap Haaksma, Dirk J Van Veldhuisen, Harry J G M Crijns, and Isabelle C Van Gelder. Clustering of RR intervals predicts effective electrical cardioversion for atrial fibrillation. *J Cardiovasc Electrophysiol*, 15(9):1027–33, Sep 2004.

[78] Nicole Kikillus, Gerd Hammer, Steven Wieland, and Armin Bolz. Algorithm for identifying patients with paroxysmal atrial fibrillation without appearance on the ECG. *Conf Proc IEEE Eng Med Biol Soc*, 2007:275–8, 2007.

[79] Ranjit Arulnayagam Thuraisingham. An electrocardiogram marker to detect paroxysmal atrial fibrillation. *J Electrocardiol*, 40(4):344–7, Oct 2007.

[80] Hans D Esperer, Chris Esperer, and Richard J Cohen. Cardiac arrhythmias imprint specific signatures on lorenz plots. *Ann Noninvasive Electrocardiol*, 13(1):44–60, Jan 2008.

[81] Jinho Park, Sangwook Lee, and Moongu Jeon. Atrial fibrillation detection by heart rate variability in poincare plot. *Biomed Eng Online*, 8:38, 2009.

[82] Douglas E Lake and J Randall Moorman. Accurate estimation of entropy in very short physiological time series: the problem of atrial fibrillation detection in implanted ventricular devices. *Am J Physiol Heart Circ Physiol*, 300(1):H319–25, Jan 2011.

[83] Nathan M Segerson, Michael L Smith, Stephen L Wasmund, Robert L Lux, Marcos Daccarett, and Mohamed H Hamdan. Heart rate variability measures during sinus rhythm predict cycle length entropy during atrial fibrillation. *J Cardiovasc Electrophysiol*, 19(10):1031–6, Oct 2008.

[84] Youhua Zhang and Todor N Mazgalev. Ventricular rate control during atrial fibrillation and AV node modifications: past, present, and future. *Pacing Clin Electrophysiol*, 27(3):382–93, Mar 2004.

[85] Junichiro Hayano, Shinji Ishihara, Hidekatsu Fukuta, Seiichiro Sakata, Seiji Mukai, Nobuyuki Ohte, and Genjiro Kimura. Circadian rhythm of atrioventricular conduction predicts long-term survival in patients with chronic atrial fibrillation. *Chronobiol Int*, 19(3):633–48, May 2002.

[86] J Hayano, S Sakata, A Okada, S Mukai, and T Fujinami. Circadian rhythms of atrioventricular conduction properties in chronic atrial fibrillation with and without heart failure. *J Am Coll Cardiol*, 31(1):158–66, Jan 1998.

[87] T Oka, T Nakatsu, S Kusachi, Y Tominaga, S Toyonaga, H Ohnishi, M Nakahama, I Komatsubara, M Murakami, and T Tsuji. Double-sector lorenz plot scattering in an R-R interval analysis of patients with chronic atrial fibrillation: Incidence and characteristics of vertices of the double-sector scattering. *J Electrocardiol*, 31(3):227–35, Jul 1998.

[88] Andreu M Climent, María de la Salud Guillem, Daniela Husser, Francisco Castells, Jose Millet, and Andreas Bollmann. Poincaré surface profiles of RR intervals: A novel noninvasive method for the evaluation of preferential AV nodal conduction during atrial fibrillation. *IEEE Trans Biomed Eng*, 56(2):433–42, Feb 2009.

Section 4

Anticoagulation Therapy

Chapter 9

New Oral Anticoagulants in Atrial Fibrillation

Lucía Cid-Conde and José López-Castro

Additional information is available at the end of the chapter

http://dx.doi.org/10.5772/53614

1. Introduction

Atrial fibrillation (AF) is the most common cardiac arrhythmia in clinical practice with a strong impact on public health. The prevalence in the general population is 0.4% and their incidence increases markedly with age to reach 4-5% in patients over 65 years and 9% in patients older than 80 years [1]. The main complication associated with this disease is the development of an embolic event, peripheral or cerebral, strokes being caused by the AF the most serious and worse prognosis. The risk that a patient suffers a stroke with AF is related to the presence of other cardioembolic risk factors: hypertension, diabetes mellitus, heart failure or left ventricular systolic dysfunction, moderately severe, age over 75 years, female, vascular disease or stroke have shown a previous cerebral (transient or established). These risk factors are reflected in the scales $CHADS_2$ or $CHA_2DS_2\text{-}VAS_C$ used today to evaluate this type of patient.

In the management of patients with AF, the most important to improve prognosis is correct indication of anticoagulant therapy. For over 60 years using vitamin K antagonists (VKAs), especially warfarin and acenocoumarol, have been shown in several studies a reduction of 70% risk of stroke in AF patients correctly anticoagulated compared with only 22% reduction of antiplatelet drugs, or a nonsignificant 19% reduction with acetylsalicylic acid. Thus, oral anticoagulants (OACs) are recommended in AF patients at moderate-high risk for sroke and tromboembolism [2]. The VKAs are drugs with proven efficacy, specific antidote in case of bleeding, possibility of discontinuing medication urgently and low cost. However, VKAs have limitations that affect the quality of life of patients and increase morbidity: narrow therapeutic window (International normalized ratio, INR 2.0-3.0) [3], unpredictable response, systematic control of bleeding, frequent dose adjustments and numerous food and drug interactions. Also, scenarios such as intercurrent infections and other medical conditions can also modify the values of the INR [4]. These results indicate that it is important to stratify each patient, both the risk of stroke such as bleeding, to individually assess what the best therapeutic approach in each case.

Due to the complexity of the use of VKAs in routine clinical practice in the last decade has developed an extensive research activity and has seen the introduction of new oral anticoagulants (NOACs): The direct thrombin inhibitors (dabigatran) and factor Xa (rivaroxaban and apixaban) that do not possess the disadvantages of the VKAs. These drugs are characterized by rapid onset of action, low potential for drug and food interactions and a predictable anticoagulant effect that avoids the need to monitor coagulation (Table 1) [5-7].

Comparative features of VKAs and NOACs	
Advantage	**Clinical implications**
The rapid onset of action	No bridge therapy required
Predictable anticoagulant effect	No routine coagulation monitoring required
Diana enzymatic cascade specific clotting	Low risk of adverse effects related to its mechanism of action
Low potential for interactions with food	No dietary restrictions
Low potential for drug interactions	Few drugs restrictions

Table 1. Comparative features of VKAs and NOACs

2. Evaluation of the risk of tromboembolism and bleeding to recommend anticoagulant therapy in the AF

Currently, there have been scales for assessing the risk of stroke and bleeding in patients with AF. The risk of stroke is classified into low, moderate and high, depending on the factors set out in the $CHADS_2$ scale (Table 2) [8]. A higher score greater risk. Patients at high risk should receive OACs and low risk, acetylsalicylic acid or nothing (prefer no treatment). In intermediate-risk patients should consider any of the two treatments.

$CHADS_2$ acronym	**Score**
Congestive Heart failure (CHF)	1
Hypertension	1
Aged ≥ 75 years	1
Diabetes mellitus	1
Stroke or transient ischemic attack (TIA)	2
Maximum score	**6**

Table 2. Stroke risk stratification with the $CHADS_2$ score

Given the limitations of $CHADS_2$ scale, a large proportion of patients are classified as intermediate risk and to the omission of potential risk factors for thromboembolism, there is the scale CHA_2DS_2-VASc [9,10]. This new scale is more comprehensive as additional risk factors: the presence of vascular disease, a younger age range than the $CHADS_2$ and female category (Table 3). The patients with a grade of 0 are at low risk and should not be treated. The rest should be considered for oral anticoagulation, establishing the risk of bleeding by HAS-BLED scale (Table 4) [11]. In patients with a HAS-BLED score ≥3, caution and regular review are recomended and to correct the potentially reversible risk factors for bleeding. A high HAS-BLED score per se should not be used to exclude patients from OAC therapy.

CHA_2DS_2-VASc acronym	**Score**
CHF or LVEF ≤ 40%	1
Hypertension	1
Aged ≥ 75 years	2
Diabetes mellitus	1
Stroke / TIA / Thromboembolism	2
Vacular disease	1
Aged 65-74 years	1
Sex category (Female)	1
Maximum score	**9**

Table 3. Stroke risk stratification with the CHA_2DS_2-VASc score

HAS-BLED risk criteria	**Score**
Hypertension	1
Abnormal renal or liver function (1 point each)	1 or 2
Stroke	1
Bleeding	1
Labile INRs	1
Elderly (age > 65)	1
Drugs or alcohol (1 point each)	1 or 2

Table 4. HAS-BLED risk criteria

If a patient has a rating of less than 2 on the $CHADS_2$ scale, it also assesses the amendment CHA_2DS_2-VASc, although this could be applied directly: if the score is zero, who are at low risk, with none of the risk factors, no antithrombotic treatment is indicated and if the score is

1, is preferred to administer OACs (VKAs or NOACs) based upon an assessment of the risk of bleeding complications and patient preferences. If CHA_2DS_2-VASc score equal to or greater than 2, the treatment is with OACs (VKAs or NOACs) is recommended, unless contraindicated. When the patients refuse the use of OACs (VKAs or NOACs), antiplatelet therapy should be considered (combination therapy with acetylsalicylic acid plus clopidogrel).

In patients with CHA_2DS_2-VASc score of 1, apixaban and both doses of dabigatran (110 mg twice daily and 150 mg twice daily) had a positive net clinical benefit while, in patients with CHA_2DS_2-VASc score ≥2, all three NOACs were superior to warfarin, with a positive net clinical benefit, irrespective of bleeding risk. The patients with CHA_2DS_2-VASc equal to 0 have a lower risk of stroke and could be left with acetylsalicylic acid or no treatment, preferring the latter option, as it has not shown any benefit in this group without treatment.

When using dabigatran, the dose is 150 mg administered twice daily in patients with low risk of hemorrhage (HAS-BLED scale of 0 to 2) and 110 mg twice daily in patients with increased risk hemorrhage (HAS-BLED ≥ 3), elderly patients, concomitant use of interacting drugs and moderate renal impairment (creatinine clearance (CrCl) 30-49 mL/min) [12].When using rivaroxaban, the dose is 20 mg daily in the most patients and 15 mg daily en high bleeding risk (HAS-BLED ≥ 3) and moderate renal impairment (CrCl 30-49 mL/min) [13].

3. Objectives of anticoagulant therapy

Anticoagulant therapy is recommended in patients with AF with risk factors for systemic embolism. The choice of treatment is based on the absolute risk of stroke, the risk of bleeding and the risk/benefit ratios for each patient [14]. The recent development of NOACs, with innovative mechanisms of action of therapeutic targets in the coagulation could change the current standard anticoagulant drug treatment [15]. The NOACs are orally administered drugs that directly inhibit the coagulation steps defined by decreasing or inhibiting thrombin generation of the final enzyme, thrombin. Thrombin (factor IIa) is the end effector of the coagulation cascade that catalyzes the formation of fibrin from plasma fibrinogen. Is the most potent physiological agonist of platelet activation, so it is considered a key therapeutic target in the development of NOACs. The Factor Xa acts as a point of convergence of the intrinsic and extrinsic pathways of coagulation and catalyzes the conversion of prothrombin to thrombin [16,17]. A single molecule of factor Xa can generate more than 1.000 molecule of thrombin, as a consequence the inhibition of factor Xa can block this process by reducing the activation of coagulation and platelet thrombin mediated. Whether the coagulation cascade is inhibited at the level of thrombin and factor Xa, or even above the sequence, the net result is a decreased activity of thrombin.

The NOACs are characterized by specific inhibition of one of the two key factors in the coagulation system, factor Xa and thrombin. Dabigatran, MCC977 and AZD0837 acts by directly inhibiting thrombin thus interfere with the first phase (initial phase) and late (amplification / propagation phase) the model based on the coagulation system. Rivaroxaban, apixaban, edoxaban, betrixaban, eribaxaban, LY517717, YM150, TAK-442 and bind to either factor Xa or factor Xa without bound in the prothrombinase complex thus blocking the conversion of prothrombin to thrombin in the early stage (stage start) and end (amplification / propagation phase) the model based on the coagulation system.

4. New oral anticoagulants

The search of ideal anticoagulant is one of the most active fields of investigation in lasts years. The ideal anticoagulant would be one that fulfilled the following characteristics: Oral administration, effective in the treatment of AF and low bleeding risk, predictable kinetics, which does not require monitoring of coagulation and platelet count, which is not necessary to adjust the dose, wide therapeutic range, low drug interaction, cost effective and availability of an effective antidote.

With these premises have been developed more specific inhibitors of coagulation factors: factor Xa and factor II (thrombin). In Table 5, inspired by Phillips and Ansell collected some of the most relevant pharmacological characteristics of NOACs (dabigatran, ribaroxaban and apixaban) compared with VKAs (warfarin and acenocoumarol) [18].

	Warfarin	**Acenocoumarol**	**Dabigatran**	**Rivaroxaban**	**Apixaban**
Target	VKOR and factors II,VII,IX, X	VKOR and factors II, VII,IX,X	Factor IIa (Thrombin)	Factor Xa	Factor Xa
Time to peak concentration	72-96 h		1,5-3 h	2-4 h	1-3 h
Vol. of dist.			60-70 l	50 l	Reported as low
Half-life	40 h	8-11 h	12-14 h	9-13 h	9-14 h
Metabolism	Liver-CYP2C9	Liver- CYP2C9	Conjugation	Liver-CYP3A4 and CYP2J2	Partially through CYP3A4
Elimination	Bile and urine	Bile and urine	80% renal, 20% faecal	66% faecal, 33% renal	75% faecal, 25% renal
Administration	Once Daily	Once Daily	Once or Twice daily	Once daily	Twice daily
Monitoring	INR	INR	Not needed	Not needed	Not needed
Antidote or potencial therapy for bleedind	Vitamin K, FFP, PCC or rFVIIa	Vitamin K, FFP, PCC or rFVIIa	FFP, PCC or rFVIIa	FFP, PCC or rFVIIa	FFP, PCC or rFVIIa
Assay	PT/INR	PT/INR	Experimental	Experimental	Experimental
Drug interactions	CYP2C9		PPIs decrease absorption and potent P-gp inhibitors	Potent CYP3A4 inhibitors and P-gp inhibitors	Potent CYP3A4 inhibitors

VKOR: vitamin K oxidase reductase; CYP: cytochrome P450; PCC: prothrombin complex concentrates; PPIs: proton pump inhibitors; P-gp: P-glycoprotein; h: hour.

Table 5. Summary of pharmacokinetics and pharmacodynamics of VKAs and NOACs

The following describes the characteristics of each one of them:

4.1. Dabigatran

It is a potent, selective and reversible thrombin [19]. Has been authorized, among other indications, in preventing stroke and systemic embolism in adult patients with non-valvular AF with one or more risk factors: stroke, transient ischemic attack or previous systemic embolism, left ventricular ejection fraction <40 %, symptomatic heart failure class ≥ 2 scale New Cork Heart Association (NYHA), age ≥ 75 years, age ≥ 65 years associated with diabetes mellitus, coronary artery disease or hypertension.

It is administered orally as a prodrug (dabigatran etexilate), which is rapidly transformed by intestinal bioconversion by esterases to its active form. With a bioavailability of 6.5% for adequate absorption requires an acidic microenvironment, provided by multiple tartaric acid microspheres present in the composition of the capsules. It reaches its peak plasma concentration 2 hours after administration, with slight delays in the presence of food (up to 4 hours) or in the postoperative period (up to 6 hours). Elimination half life is about 12-14 hours. Approximately 20% of the drug is metabolized in the liver and excreted by the biliary system, independent of cytochrome P450. Most of dabigatran (about 80%) is eliminated renally as unchanged, so that his administration is contraindicated in patients with severe renal impairment (CrCl <30 mL/min), requiring administered with caution (setting dose) in patients with CrCl 30-49 mL/min. No other adjustments are required, except in patients over 75 years, which should decrease the dose. Administration is not recommended if liver enzymes are elevated (transaminases 2 times baseline). Are recommended a baseline measurement before starting treatment, in patients with severe renal impairment (CrCl <30 mL/min) or in cases of concomitant quinidine. The main adverse event of dyspepsia is related to the pharmaceutical formulation. Dabigatran need a daily oral dose and fixed (in two doses), independent of age, weight and race, with predictable effects and constant, without significant interactions with food or other drugs without coagulation controls. The absorption of dabigatran administration is reduced by approximately 25% with the co-administration of proton pump inhibitors. Dabigatran is contraindicated if the patient is treated with systemic ketoconazole, cyclosporine, itraconazole and tacrolimus, and should be used with caution if the patient is receiving other potent inhibitors of P-glycoprotein (P-gp): amiodarone, quinidine or verapamil.

4.2. Rivaroxaban

It is a potent and selective inhibitor of factor Xa [20], having peak plasma levels approximately 3 hours after oral ingestion. As dabigatran, is indicated for the prevention of stroke and systemic embolism in adult patients with non-valvular AF, with one or more risk factors: congestive heart failure, hypertension, age ≥75 years, diabetes mellitus, stroke or attack transient ischemic. Bioavailability is 80-100% for the dose of 10 mg. Rapidly absorbed and reaches peak concentrations at 2-4 hours after ingestion. Its plasma half-life is 5 to 9 hours but increases markedly in people over 75 years from 9 to 13 hours. Not recommended for use in patients with CrCl <15 mL/min. The intensity of inhibition and, therefore, the generation of thrombin, is dose dependent, meaning that high doses could compromise coagulation. Has a dual route of elimination: 1/3 of the drug is eliminated via the kidney and 2/3 of the drug has hepatic metabolism. No interaction was observed with drugs such as acetylsalicylic acid, aluminum hydroxide and magnesium, ranitidine or naproxen. Its bioavailability increases with inhibitors of CYP3A4 and P-gp, such as ketoconazole and ritonavir, and diminishes with rifampicin. The bioavailability increases only marginally with food.

4.3. Apixaban

It is an oral potent inhibitor reversible and highly selective direct factor Xa [21]. Has greater affinity for factor Xa attached to clot which is free. Inhibits and delays the generation of thrombin without significantly affecting platelet aggregation. The oral bioavailability is approximately 50%. Rapidly absorbed and reaches peak concentrations at 3-4 hours after ingestion. Food intake does not affect the area under the curve or maximum concentration, and can be taken with or without food. The binding to plasma proteins is 87%. The half-life is 12 hours and is metabolized with CYP3A4/5. It is also a substrate binding proteins, P-gp. Not recommended for use with potent CYP3A4 inhibitors and P-gp and that may increase exposure to apixaban twice. With the administration of inductors opposite happens. Aproximately 25% of the drug is excreted in the urine and more than 50% in the feces. The multiple elimination pathways suggest that even patients with moderate hepatic or renal impairment may be suitable for this anticoagulant. No need to monitor renal function.

4.4. Oral anticoagulants under investigation

Currently, there are other investigational drugs: direct thrombin inhibitor (AZD0837 and MCC977), direct inhibitors of factor Xa (betrixaban, YM150, edoxaban, eribaxaban, LY517717, TAK-442, otamixaban (parenteral) [22].

5. Monitoring of NOACs

The NOACs not require routine monitoring. However, there are situations where it is advisable to monitor selected patients as those with extreme weights, kidney failure or those who suffer thrombotic complications being treated with these drugs.

As a result of the occurrence of serious adverse effects, including severe gastrointestinal bleeding (81 cases) and deaths (260 cases) of bleeding in patients treated with dabigatran were published safety ratings by the rating agencies worldwide drug advising monitoring of renal function in patients with moderate renal impairment (30-50 mL/min) receiving dabigatran and in patients over 75 years. Rivaroxaban is contraindicated if CrCl <15 mL/min, and should be used with caution if is 15-30 mL/min.

Monitoring is also useful to evaluate the adherence to treatment (the omission of one or more doses puts the patient at risk of complications at an early stage) or when the patient needs to undergo an invasive procedure. When subjecting a patient to an invasive procedure, it is important to note that the drug half-life (12-14 hours dabigatran, rivaroxaban 9-13 hours and apixaban 9-14 hours). If the invasive procedure has a low bleeding risk, it is sufficient to suspend the drug 24-36 hours before surgery and if no complications arise, resume anticoagulant treatment at 36-48 hours [23].

The ideal test for monitoring of direct thrombin inhibitors is the coagulation time of ecarin, with a linear relationship, and a good slope and discriminate levels of dabigatran in plasma. The problem is that it is non-standardized and few laboratories possess it.

The studies suggest that dabigatran monitoring will be done with a variant of thrombin time (TT). TT is very sensitive, with a linear relationship, but with a high slope, so that at low concentrations of dabigatran, TT extends above the detection limit of the coagulometer. It is a very good from a qualitative point of view, to assess adherence to treatment, but cannot quantify levels. The thrombin time will be a diluted thrombin time, marketed as Hemoclot®, which manages to improve the linear relationship with respect to TT and discriminate between low, intermediate and high dabigatran in plasma [24].

Monitoring of rivaroxaban will be done by a method chromogenic anti-factor Xa. This test is marketed as anti-Xa assay. Is a sensitive and accurate, useful to measure the maximum and minimum plasma concentrations of rivaroxaban [25,26].

6. Bleeding complications and antidotes

The fear of bleeding complications is one of the most prevalent obstacles in anticoagulant treatment in AF, especially cerebral hemorrhage.

These drugs have no specific antidotes which is a problem in patients who are at high risk of bleeding or hemorrhagic. Dabigatran is a dialyzable drug, which can eliminate up to 60% of the molecule in serum. Other possibilities include the use of activated coal and of neutralizing antibodies but are lacking in vivo experience. With respect to rivaroxaban is working in a variant of factor Xa would compete with the normal to factor Xa when joining rivaroxaban and thus the effect would be reversed.

In order to reverse the effect of NOACs designed a crossover trial, randomized, double-blind, placebo-controlled study included 12 healthy male volunteers. Received rivaroxaban 20 mg/12h or dabigatran 15 mg/12h for 2.5 days followed by a single bolus of 50 IU/kg of prothrombin complex concentrate (PCC) or similar volume of saline. The results concluded that the PCC completely and immediately reversed the anticoagulant effect of ribaroxaban but had no influence on the effect of dabigatran at the doses used in this study. These results should be analyzed with caution due to small sample size (12 patients) and the characteristics of the population that was part of the study (only male patients and healthy). [27]. Another study found the low doses of non-specific reversal agents (anticoagulant anti-inhibitor complex with non-activated factors II, IX and X and activated factor VII) appear to be able to reverse the anticoagulant activity of rivaroxaban or dabigatran. However, clinical evaluation is needed regarding haemorrhagic situations, and a meticulous risk-benefit evaluation [28]. The absence of normalization of coagulation tests not necessarily correlate with the absence of anti-haemorrhagic effect, as demonstrated in animal models [24].

http://dx.doi.org/10.5772/53614

Thus, in a patient treated with dabigatran and rivaroxaban that presents a mild bleeding complication, it is advisable to delay the next drug administration or discontinuation. If bleeding is moderate or severe, symptomatic treatment is indicated as mechanical compression standard, surgical hemostasis bleeding control procedure, blood products and hemodynamic support (packed red cells or fresh frozen plasma). In the case of very severe bleeding will require charcoal filtration or haemodialysis or administration of an agent for reversing the specific procoagulant effect, such as prothrombin complex, the prothrombin complex concentrate or activated recombinant factor VIIa. In this case, experience is limited.

7. Evaluation of scientific evidence, relevance and limitations of the study

It will analyze the scientific evidence, the limitations of design and the clinical relevance of the results of published clinical trials (RE-LY, ROCKET AF, AVERROES and ARISTOTLE). In general, these new drugs are at least equally effective and safer than warfarin, with the advantage of inducing a lesser extent intracerebral hemorrhages (Table 6).

	Dabigatran	Rivaroxaban	Apixaban	
	(RE-LY)	(ROCKET AF)	(AVERROES)	(ARISTOTLE)
Study design	Randomized open label	Multicenter, randomized, double-blind, double-dummy	Multicenter, randomized, double-blind, double-dummy	Multicenter, randomized, double-blind, doble-dummy
Number of patients	18.113	14.264	5.599	18.201
Mean age	71.5 years	73 years	70 years	70 years
Male:female ratio	63.6%: 36.4%	60%:40%	58.5%: 41.5%	64.7%: 35,30%
Follow-up period, years	2 years	1.9 years	1.1 years	1.8 years
Randomized groups	Dose-ajusted WA vs. blinded doses of DA (150 mg BID, 110 mg BID)	Dose-ajusted WA vs. RI 20 mg OD	AAS 81-324 mg OD vs. API 5 mg BID	Dose-ajusted WA vs. API 5 mg BID
Mean $CHADS_2$ score	2.1	3.5	2.1	2.1
Primary endpoint: stroke and systemic embolism (in % per year)	1.71% WA 1.54% DA 110mg 1.11% DA 150mg	2.42% WA 2.12% RI	3.9% AAS 1.7% API	1.60% WA 1.27% API
Major bleeding events	3.57% WA 2.87% DA 110mg 3.32% DA 150mg	3.45% WA 3.6% RI	1.2% AAS 1.4% API	3.09% WA 2.13% API

BID: twice daily; OD: once daily; WA: warfarin; DA: dabigatran; RI: rivaroxaban; API: apixaban; AAS: acetylsalicylic acid

Table 6. Summary of the main clinical trials with NOACs

7.1. Dabigatran

The RE-LY is the largest study of AF (Randomized Evaluation of Long term anticoagulant therapy) [29]. The primary endpoint was to establish non-inferiority of dabigatran etexilate compared with warfarin for a minimum of 1 year follow-up to a maximum 3 years, median follow-up of 2 years in 18.113 patients with nonvalvular AF (mean age 71 years) with at least one of the following risk factors for stroke: previous stroke or transient ischemic attack, left ventricular ejection fraction <40%, symptoms of heart failure class 2 or higher NYHA, age >75 years or 65-74 years associated with diabetes mellitus, hypertension or coronary artery disease. Meanwhile, we excluded patients with: severe valvular disease, recent stroke, (a condition that increases the risk of bleeding), CrCl <30mL/min, active liver disease and pregnancy.

Patients were randomized into three treatment arms: 110 mg dabigatran twice daily, dabigatran 150 mg twice daily and adjusted dose warfarin (INR 2.0-3.0). In patients randomized to receive warfarin, the average percentage of time within therapeutic range (INR = 2.0-3.0) were 64.4%. Dabigatran was administered in a blinded fashion in both treatment arms; the administration of warfarin was opened. In all branches were allowed concomitant use of acetylsalicylic acid or other antiplatelet agent. Also allowed the concomitant use of quinidine with dabigatran during the first two years of the study, when it was prohibited by the possibility of interaction with dabigatran.

The primary endpoint studied was the appearance of stroke or systemic embolic event and the primary safety outcome was the occurrence of serious bleeding. The criterion for non-inferiority was established that the upper limit of confidence interval (CI) 97.5% of the relative risk of occurrence of stroke or systemic embolism with dabigatran compared to warfarin was <1.46. The non-inferiority margin was established from the results of a meta-analysis with VKAs against a control treatment in patients with AF. The value of 1.46 represents half of the 95% CI relative risk estimated effect on warfarin control. All analyzes were by intention to treat (ITT).

The results for the primary endpoint were: onset of stroke or systemic embolism in 182 patients in the group treated with dabigatran 110 mg (1.53% per year), in 134 patients with dabigatran 150 mg (1.11% per year) and 199 patients with warfarin (1.69% per year). The two treatment groups dabigatran meet the criteria for non-inferiority to be the upper limit of 95% relative risk less than 1.46 (1.11 in the first case and 0.82 in the second), but only dabigatran 150 mg was associated with lower rate of stroke and embolic events than warfarin (RR = 0.66, 95% CI 0.53 to 0.82), dabigatran 110 mg was similar to warfarin.

Regarding security, in the RE-LY study, the treatment with dabigatran was associated with an "annual rate" of major bleeding (defined as bleeding associated with a decrease in hemoglobin of at least 2g/dL, transfusion of at least 2 units of whole blood or symptomatic bleeding in a critical organ or area (intraocular, intracranial, intraspinal or intramuscular with compartment syndrome, retroperitoneal bleeding, bleeding or intra-articular pericardial bleeding). Severe bleeding was divided in turn into intracranial hemorrhage (intracerebral or subdural) and extracranial (gastrointestinal or not gastrointestinal). The major bleeds were categorized as critical if they met one or more of the following criteria: fatal bleeding, symptomatic intracranial bleeding, reduced hemoglobin of at least 5g/dL, transfusion of at least 4 units of whole blood or packed red cells, bleeding associated with hypotension requiring the use of intravenous inotropic agents, bleeding required surgery) of 2.71% for dabigatran 110 mg, 3.11% for dabigatran 150 mg and 3.36% for warfarin. No significant difference in major bleeding between dabigatran 150 mg twice daily and warfarin; on the contrary, dabigatran 110 mg twice daily resulted in less major bleeding, RR 0.80 (95% CI: 0.69 to 0.93) p = 0.003. As for minor bleeding (defined as all non-major bleeding definition, previously expressed) annual rates were 13.16%, 14.84% and 16.37% for dabigatran 110 mg, dabigatran 150 mg and warfarin, respectively. In this case, the risk was significantly lower for dabigatran 110 mg [RR = 0.79 (95% CI: 0.74 to 0.84)] and dabigatran 150 mg [RR = 0.91 (95% CI: 0.85 to 0.97)] with respect to warfarin and was higher for dabigatran 150 mg versus dabigatran 110 mg [RR = 1.16 (95% CI: 1.08 to 1.24)]. Similarly, the risk of intracranial hemorrhage was significantly lower for dabigatran 110 mg [RR = 0.31 (95% CI: 0.20 to 0.47)] and for dabigatran 150 mg [RR = 0.40 (95% CI: 0.27 to 0.60)] against warfarin and no significant differences between the two doses of dabigatran. However, the risk of bleeding severe gastrointestinal was significantly higher in the group treated with dabigatran 150 mg versus warfarin [RR = 1.50 (95% CI: 1.19 to 1.89)] and versus dabigatran 110 mg [RR = 1.36 (95% CI: 1.09 to 1.70)]. The overall mortality (4%) showed no significant differences (p=0.051) between dabigatan 150 mg twice daily and warfarin, although the rate of deaths from vascular causes was significantly lower in the group treated with dabigatran 150 mg twice daily (p=0.04).

The results of dabigatran 150 mg dose showed that the benefit is somewhat larger than warfarin in $CHADS_2 \geq 2$ while the hemorrhagic risk is similar in both groups. In $CHADS_2$ = 0-1 the benefit is also somewhat higher than warfarin while the hemorrhagic risk is somewhat lower. A dose of 110 mg the benefit and bleeding risk is similar in every category of $CHADS_2$ except for the category $CHADS_2$ = 0-1 where the risk is somewhat lower.

Dropout rates were higher with dabigatran: 14.5% with dabigatran 110 mg, 15.5% with 150 mg dabigatran and 10.2% with warfarin the first year and 20.7% with dabigatran 110 mg, 21.2% with dabigatran 150 mg and 16.6% with warfarin the second year. There were more withdrawals due to serious adverse events with dabigatran (2.7%) than with warfarin (1.7%).

The incidence of myocardial infarction was higher with dabigatran 110 mg twice daily (0.72%, p = 0.07) and dabigatran 150 mg twice daily (0.74%, p = 0.048) than warfarin (0.53%), having calculated that myocardial infarction could occur for every 500 patients treated with dabigatran. With the correction of the results of RE-LY study the differentiation in the apparition of the myocardial infarction no longer statistically significant. However, a meta-analysis of 7 trials published recently concluded that the use of dabigatran is associated with an increased risk of myocardial infarction or acute coronary syndrome in a broad spectrum of patients compared with VKAs, antiplatelet or placebo [30]. Although the absolute risk may be low, it is necessary to closely monitor patients and the importance of improving pharmacovigilance systems [31].

7.2. Rivaroxaban

The ROCKET AF study (Rivaroxaban Once daily, oral, direct factor Xa inhibition Compared with vitamin K for prevention of stroke Antagonism and Embolism Trial in Atrial fibrillation) compared the clinical outcomes of rivaroxaban at doses of 20 mg/day (15 mg/day for those with estimated CrCl 30-49 mL/min) with warfarin dose-adjusted INR in patients with AF. It is a prospective, randomized, double-blind, parallel group, multicenter, event-based and non-inferiority which involved 14.264 patients. The patients had high risgo of stroke ($CHADS_2$ score >2 in 90%) [32, 33]. It was shown that the new anticoagulant was non-inferior to warfarin in the combined primary endpoint, which included stroke and systemic embolism. Embolic events were presented to the central nervous system or systemic 1.7% per year in the rivaroxaban group compared with 2.2% in the warfarin group, which has met the criterion for non-inferiority. However, ITT analysis showed that superiority failed. The incidence rates of primary safety outcome (major bleeding episodes and no clinically relevant non-major bleeding) were similar in both treatment groups but, with rivaroxaban, there was a significant reduction in fatal bleeding, as well as an increase in gastrointestinal bleeds and bleeds requiring transfusion. Premature discontinuation of treatment was more common with rivaroxaban (23.9%) than with warfarin (22.4%). The duration of follow-up was 12-32 months.

7.3. Apixaban

The AVERROES study is a multicenter, randomized, double-blind and double-dummy (Apixaban Versus Stroke Acetylsalicylic Acid to Prevent Stroke in Atrial Fibrillation Patients Who Have Failed or Are Unsuitable for Vitamin K Antagonist Treatment) comparing apixaban 5 mg twice daily (2.5 mg twice daily in patients ≥80 years, weight ≤60 kg or with a serum creatinine ≥1.5 mg/dL) versus acetylsalicylic acid 81-324 mg daily in 5.599 patients with AF at high risk of stroke and without indication for treatment with VKAs or by difficulties in anticoagulation or because the patient refused anticoagulation therapy.

The trial was stopped early, after about a year after intermediate analysis showed a significant reduction of 50% in the risk of stroke. There were 1.6% of cerebral and systemic embolic events in the apixaban group compared to 3.5% in the acetylsalicylic acid group. The frequency of bleeding was similar (1.4 versus 1.2% per year); there was no difference between patients treated with apixaban and acetylsalicylic acid on the incidence of major bleeding, intracranial hemorrhage, or gastrointestinal bleeding even if appreciate a significant increase of the total number of bleeding (major and minor). Mortality was lower in the apixaban group (3.5% per year) than acetylsalicylic acid (4.4% per year), results that corroborate the greatest benefit of anticoagulant therapy in AF. In patients with AF for whom therapy is inadequate VKAs, apixaban reduces the risk of stroke or systemic embolism without increasing the risk of major bleeding or intracranial hemorrhage [34].

The ARISTOTLE study is a multicenter, randomized, double-blind and double-dummy (Apixaban for Reduction in Stroke and Other Events in Atrial Fibrillation thromboembolic) comparing apixaban 5 mg orally twice daily (2.5 mg twice daily in patients ≥80 years, weight ≤60 kg or with a serum creatinine ≥1.5 mg/dL) versus adjusted-dose warfarin (INR

2.0-3.0). The study was designed to demonstrate non-inferiority of apixaban compared to warfarin. Analysis is performed of non-inferiority trial and after an analysis of superiority. The primary efficacy endpoint was the composite of stroke and systemic embolism. The primary safety outcome was major bleeding. The mean duration of follow-up was 1.8 years. The study included 18.201 patients with AF at high risk of systemic and cerebral embolism. Cerebrovascular events were 1.27% per year in the apixaban group versus 1.60% in the warfarin group ($p < 0.001$ for non-inferiority and $p = 0.01$ for superiority), bleeding of 2.13% versus 3.09% for year ($p < 0.001$), respectively. Significantly decreased the incidence of any type of bleeding, major bleeding and intracranial bleeding and not change the frequency of appearance of gastrointestinal bleeding. Mortality from all causes was 3.52% versus 3.94%, demonstrating the superiority of apixaban compared to warfarin in preventing stroke or central nervous system systemic fewer bleeding complications and lower mortality. Cerebrovascular events in patients with $CHADS_2 \geq 3$ were 1.9% per year in patients treated with apixaban compared to 2.8% per year in patients treated with warfarin; $CHADS_2$ = 0-1, 0.7% per year versus 0.9% per year and $CHADS_2$ = 2, 1.2% per year versus 1.4% per year. In patients under 65 years no difference in efficacy between both groups, but in patients over 65 years the difference is 0.9%.

In conclusion, treatment with apixaban compared to warfarin in AF patients with more than one risk factor reduces the incidence of stroke and systemic embolism by 21% ($p = 0.01$), reduced major bleeding by 31% ($p < 0.001$) and reduces mortality by 11% ($p = 0.047$) [35].

7.4. Methodological limitations of studies

Taking into account the results of the studies so far mentioned, there are some differences in patients enrolled in the RE-LY, the ROCKET AF, the AVERROES and the ARISTOTLE. The study population ARISTOTLE included subjects both with a $CHADS_2$ score of 1 point and those of scores. In the RE-LY incorporated population according to the $CHADS_2$ score was mild-moderate risk (32% of patients with a $CHADS_2$ of 3 to 6 points) and the ROCKET-AF population included was moderate to severe (87% patients had a $CHADS_2$ risk score (of 3 to 6 points) which makes comparisons difficult between these studies. RE-LY and ARISTOTLE have similar characteristics on patient demographics (age, gender...) and in the risk of stroke (average $CHADS_2$ score of 2.1). However, ROCKET AF patients were slightly older (median age 73 years), were at high risk of stroke (mean $CHADS_2$ score of 3.5), and 55% were a secondary prevention population [36]. Exclusion criteria of patients pose leave out AF patients eligible for treatment with VKAs, as those who have suffered a recent stroke or those with liver enzyme elevations 2 times the upper limit of normal.

They are non-inferiority studies. The European Medicines Agency (EMEA) recommended in these studies an ITT and per protocol analysis (PP). In the RE-LY is not a PP (which could favor dabigatran) and also the non-inferiority margin has questionable clinical relevance. The superiority analysis showed more effectively to the highest dose of dabigatran. The ROCKET AF results PP were slightly significant in favor of rivaroxaban while ITT results demonstrate the non-inferiority of rivaroxaban with warfarin. ARISTOTLE and AVERROES studies also reflect the non-inferiority of apixaban versus warfarin however, the results were better in the Asian population and whether they may be due to different effectiveness of the drug in this population or whether there was any element related to the study design to justify these differences. In addition 35% of patients with warfarin were outside the therapeutic range, implying poor control within the clinical trial.

In the RE-LY treated with warfarin branch has an open design which favors the appearance of bias. It would be necessary to make a double-blind design with warfarin (this limits the internal validity of the test. Both the ROCKET AF as ARISTOTLE was double blind). Dabigatran is necessary to take it twice a day. This helps to foster low compliance. Only in the RE-LY study, where patients are monitored closely, the dropout rate was 20.7% with dabigatran 110 mg and 21.2% with dabigatran 150 mg at two years. The same can happen with rivaroxaban and apixaban, the absence of regular checks can relax patients. Poor adherence to treatment would leave the patient exposed because the anticoagulant effect almost completely disappear (are drugs with short half-life). Unlike NOACs, with VKAs is necessary to periodically checks to confirm that are within the therapeutic range, a fact that is achieved in 58-65% of cases. The compliance rate is not always the desired (30% dropout) [37]. A subgroup analysis and an FDA report further notes that the benefit of dabigatran is significant only in those centers where patients have poorer control with warfarin. The results of the centers with better INR control with warfarin did not show superiority of dabigaran 150 mg versus warfarin. Improving the monitoring of the INR, the benefits seen for dabigatran compared to warfarin decreased. The ARISTOTLE study showed no superiority of apixaban in terms of INR control. The ROCKET AF study the level of INR of warfarin group was very low which has reduced the conviction to conclusions (55% versus 64.4% of RE-LY and 62% of ARISTOTLE).

Regarding the dose to be administered there are disputes between the position of the FDA (Food and Drug Administration) and EMEA. FDA has approved only high doses of dabigatran (150 mg/12h). Argued that low doses of dabigatran (110 mg/12h), the demonstration of non-inferior to warfarin, is not as conclusive as with higher doses. In addition to high doses reduces episodes of stroke but increase bleeding. The lower dose may be indicated in patients with increased risk of bleeding. The RE-LY study could not identify a subgroup of patients who would benefit from low dose.

Recently has been published a study that try to perform an indirect comparison analysis of NOACs regarding its efficacy and safety [36]. Despite the limitations of indirect comparison study (differences in patient population, differences in definition of major bleeding and unblended versus nonblinded/double-blinded comparisons), no profound significant differences were found in efficacy between apixaban and dabigatran (both doses) or rivaroxaban. Dabigatran 150 mg twice daily was superior to rivaroxaban for efficacy (with less stroke and systemic embolism (by 26%), as well as less hemorrhagic stroke (by 56%, p=0.039 and non-disabling stroke (by 40%, p=0.038). There were no significant differences in preventing stroke and systemic embolism for apixaban versus dabigatran (both doses) or rivaroxaban, or rivaroxaban versus dabigatran 110 mg twice daily. For the ischemic stroke, there were no significant differences between the NOACs. Major bleeding was significantly lower with apixaban versus dabigatran 150 mg twice daily (by 26%) and rivaroxaban (by 34%), but was not significantly different from dabigatran 110 mg twice daily. There were no significant differences between apixaban and dabigatran 110 mg twice daily. Apixaban had lower major or clinically relevant bleeding (by 34%) versus ribaroxaban. When compared with rivaroxaban, dabigatran 110 mg twice daily was associated with less mayor bleeding (by 23%) and intracranial bleeding (by 54%). No significant differences myocardial infarction events between dabigatan (both doses) and apixaban. However, only a head-to-head direct comparison of the different NOACs would be able to answer the question of efficacy/safety differences between them in the prevention of stroke in AF.

An advantage of the NACOs proposes absence monitoring. Instead, experts recommend that in chronic treatment with narrow therapeutic window and potentially serious complications (stroke/hemorrhage), lack of control is much more harmful than adequate control. The regular monitoring to adjust and correct the treatment regimen and distinguish, if complications, treatment failure or lack of adherence.

Are emerging post-marketing data on major bleeding and death with dabigatran: Japan (5 deaths and 81 cases of severe reactions), Australia (7 deaths and 24 serious reactions) and Europe (21 deaths). In the subsequent reanalysis of data from the RE-LY was a higher incidence of stroke, myocardial infarction and major bleeding compared to those initially reported, in those over 75 years more extracranial bleeding [38].

No specific antidote proved effective, which hinder the resolution of bleeding emergencies. In addition, the high cost compared to VKAs is a major limitation. Have been published some cost-effectiveness data for dabigatran, and dabigatran appears to be cost-effective for most patients, except in those with very well-controlled INRs [39,40].

8. Current recommendations - Caution

With the entry into force of the NOACs is emerging a new era in anticoagulant therapy. These drugs are proving to be at least as effective as VKAs without coagulation monitoring, with a reduction of more serious bleeding (intracranial) and with far fewer potential drug interactions and food.

But not all advantages. These drugs also have drawbacks and uncertainties about their safety, and to their clinical evaluation is needed before definitive recommendations on its use. Lack of specific antidotes which is a problem in patients who are at high risk of bleeding or hemorrhage (to negate the effect is included prothrombin complex or factor specifying of hospitalization and increasing costs associated with treatment), contraindicated in patients with renal impairment, short half-life (limits its use in patients with poor adherence), with higher incidence of gastrointestinal bleeding and high cost. In addition, there are no safecy data long-term selected populations and are generating security alerts.

In the initial euphoria, with the placing on the market NOACs, it is necessary to proceed with caution. A few years ago, another promising thrombin inhibitor, ximelagatran, which showed that it was at least as effective and safe as warfarin for stroke prevention in AF patients, had to be withdrawn by its liver toxicity after creating many expectations [41].

All this raises questions: Is it appropriate to change oral anticoagulation with warfarin or acenocoumarol to a patient controlled? Can these NOACs impact in preventing thromboembolism, especially stroke, in patients with AF? Will we monitor patients? Is it acceptable despite the cost of not requiring monitoring? How do we assess adherence?

The Canadian Cardiovascular Society (CCS) [41], the European Society of Cardiology (ESC) [13,42,43], the American College of Cardiology Foundation (ACCF), the American Heart Association (AHA) and the Heart Rhythm Society (HRS) recently updated their guidelines for the treatment of patients with AF. The guidelines report that when OAC is recommended, one of NOACs should be considered rather than adjusted-dose VKAs (INR 2.0-3.0) for most patients with AF, when studied in clinical trials to date. The NOACs provide better efficacy, safety and comfort compared to the OAC with VKAs. There is insufficient evidence to recommend one over another NOACs, although some patient characteristics, drug tolerability and compliance and the cost may be important factors in the choice of agent. As experience with NOACs is still limited, strict adherence to the recommended indications approved and aftercare marketing.

The short half-lives of NOACs compared with that do not require routine monitoring of coagulation, causes adherence is very relevant. Poor adherence increase morbidity, mortality, and in turn, overall health costs. Poor compliance can be a particular problem in patients with AF who often has no symptoms. Warfarin has a half life of 40 hours, so that a slight failure of the patient will have a negligible effect on clotting compared to a drug with short half life.

In this context it is useful to provide a meta-analysis of clinical trials in patients treated with VKAs. The results showed that patients who achieved a treatment well stabilized, the determination home ("self") for the same patient resulted in a significant reduction in mortality and morbidity from thromboembolism without increasing the risk of serious bleeding in a selected group of motivated adults [44]. The results of a subsequent meta-analysis showed a reduced risk of thromboembolic disease, but no major bleeding or mortality [45].

The NOACs will not replace the classical therapy of oral anticoagulant therapy automatically. As a general rule, you should not change the anti-clotting drug to patients who are currently well controlled with acenocoumarol or warfarin and have an INR within the therapeutic range. The NOACs be reserved for those who have not attained regular values (between 2.0 and 3.0) the INR by more than 60% of the determinations despite good adherence to the prescription by the patient (for drug interactions that hinder the anticoagulation control, special dietary or digestive disorders that affect the pharmacokinetics of VKAs. Should not switch to dabigatran in patients with inadequate control of INR and nonadherence) [46], for those with mobility problems or difficulties traveling to determine the INR and for which have allergies or intolerance to the adverse effects of OACs. An anticoagulant is, by definition, a drug of high risk. And a patient with AF generally well. The fact that new drugs is involved uncertainty about their safety in the short and long term. You have to define more precisely the role of new drugs, considered as therapeutic innovations, and they are accompanied by a careful evaluation of their efficacy and toxicity in actual practice.

http://dx.doi.org/10.5772/53614

The experience of use and new studies will determine the profile of patient who may benefit most from these new therapies. Be taken into account: stage of disease, the left atrial size, presence and severity of underlying disease, therapeutic approaches and patient preferences. It also assessed the patients' age, presence of comorbidities and polypharmacy. Advanced age increases the impact of AF on the embolic risk. The elderly population is particularly vulnerable to stroke in AF. In addition, stroke patients with AF have increased mortality and the consequences are devastating.

9. Conclusions

Clinical trials available to date show that NOACs are at least as effective and safe as VKAs. However, although the evidence is a useful tool, it should await the development of major clinical studies in different populations to see the real benefit of these drugs. The main problems are lacking proven methods of monitoring, so that in certain patients (elderly, low weight, renal or liver impairment...) fixed dose may not be therapeutic. There are no conclusive data on its long-term safety and are already generating security alerts in different countries. No studies support the use of an antidote in case of overdose with bleeding. There is no justification to replace the current oral anticoagulant treatment by the NACOs in patients that conventional treatment is well tolerated and its controls are stable. Its high cost limits the use of these drugs. Independent trials are needed to precisely define the role of new drugs in patients with non-valvular AF.

Author details

Lucía Cid-Conde[1] and José López-Castro[2]

1 Department of Pharmacy, Hospital Comarcal Valdeorras, Sergas, Spain

2 Department of Internal Medicine, Hospital Comarcal Valdeorras, Sergas, Spain

Not have any conflict of interest relating to the information in this article.

References

[1] Fuster V, Rydén LE, Cannom DS, Crijns HJ, Curtis AB, Ellenbogen KA, et al. ACC/AHA/ESC 2006 Guidelines for the Management of Patients with Atrial Fibrillation: A report of the American College of Cardiology/American Heart Association Task Force on Practice Guidelines and the European Society of Cardiology Committee for Practice Guidelines (Writing Committee to Revise the 2001 Guidelines for the Management of Patients With Atrial Fibrillation): Developed in collaboration with

the European Heart Rhythm Association and the Heart Rhythm Society. Circulation. 2006; 114(7):e257–e354.

[2] Hart RG, Pearce LA, Aguilar MI. Meta-anaysis: anti-thrombotic therapy to prevent stroke in patients who have nonvalvular atrial fibrillation. Ann Intern Med. 2007: 146(12):857-67.

[3] Hylek EM, Go AS, Chang Y, Jensvold NG, Henault LE, Selby JV et al. Effect of intensity of oral anticoagulation on stroke severity and mortality in atrial fibrillation. N Engl J Med. 2003; 349:1019-26.

[4] Ansell J, Hirsh J, Hylek E, Jacobson A, Crowther M, Palareti G; American College of Chest Physicians. Pharmacology and management of the vitamin K antagonists: American College of Chest Physicians Evidence-Based Clinical Practice Guidelines (8th Edition). Chest. 2008; 133(6):160S-198S.

[5] Eriksson BI, Quinlan DJ, Eikelboom JW. Novel oral factor Xa and thrombin inhibitors in the management of thromboembolism. Annu Rev Med. 2011; 62:41–5.

[6] Ordovás Baines JP, Climent Grana E, Jover Botella A, Valero García I. Pharmacokinetics and pharmacodynamics of the new oral anticoagulants. Farm Hosp. 2009; 33:125:33.

[7] Escobar C, Barrios V, Jiménez D. Atrial fibrillation and dabigatran: has the time come to use new anticoagulants? Cardiovasc Ther. 2010; 28(5): 295-301.

[8] Hughes M, Lip GY. Stroke and thromboembolism in atrial fibrillation: a Systematic Review of Stroke Risk Factors, risk stratification data schema and Cost Effectiveness. Thromb Haemost. 2008; 99:295-304.

[9] Lip GY, Nieuwlaat R, Pisters R, Lane DA, Crijns. Refining clinical risk stratification for predicting stroke and thromboembolism in atrial fibrillation using a novel risk factor-based approach: the Euro Heart Survey on atrial fibrillation. Chest. 2010; 137: 263-272.

[10] Olesen JB, Lip GY, Hansen PR, Tolstrup JS, Lindhardsen J, Selmer C, et al. Validation of risk stratification schemes for predicting stroke and thromboembolism in patients with atrial fibrillation: nationwide cohort study. BMJ. 2011; 342: d124.

[11] Pisters R, Lane DA, Nieuwlaat R, De Vos CB, Crijns HP, Lip GY. A novel user-friendly score (HAS-BLED) to assess 1-year risk of major bleeding in patients with atrial fibrillation: the Euro Heart Survey. Chest. 2010; 138 (5): 1093-1100.

[12] Wann L, Curtis AB, Ellenbogen KA, et al. 2011 ACCF/AHA/HRS Focused Update on the Management of Patients With Atrial Fibrillation (Update on Dabigatran): A Report of the American College of Cardiology Foundation. JACC. 2011; 57 (11):1330-7.

[13] Camm AJ, Lip GY, De Caterina R, Savelieva I, Atar D, Honloser SH et al. 2012 focused update of the ESC Guidelines for the manegement of atrial fibrillation. An update of the 2010 ESC Guidelines for the management of atrial fibrillation * Developed

with the special contribution of the European Heart Rhythm Association. Eur Heart J. 2012. Avaliable http://www.ncbi.nlm.nih.gov/pubmed/22922413.

[14] Fuster V, Rydén LE, Cannom DS, Crijns HJ, Curtis AB, Ellenbogen KA et al. American College of Cardiology Foundation / American Heart Association Task Force. 2011 ACCF/AHA/HRS focused updates incorporated into the ACC/AHA/ESC 2006 guidelines for the management of patients with atrial fibrillation: a report of the American College of Cardiology Foundation/American Heart Association Task Force on practice guidelines. Circulation. 2011;15:123(10): e269-36.

[15] Desai SS, Massad MG, DiDomenico RJ, Abdelhady K, Hanhan Z, Lele H, et al. Recent developments in antithrombotic therapy: will sodium warfarin be a drug of the past? Recent Pat Cardiovasc Drug Discov. 2006;1:307-16.

[16] Mann KG, Brummel K, Butenas S. What is all that thrombin for? J Thromb Haemost. 2003; 1:1504-14.

[17] Mann KG, Butenas S, Brummel K. The dynamics of thrombin formation. Arterioscler Thromb Vasc Biol. 2003; 23:17-25.

[18] Phillips KW, Ansell J. The Clinical Implications of new oral anticoagulants: the potential Advantages Hill be Achieved? Thromb Haemost. 2010; 103:34-3.

[19] Pradaxa ®, SPC. Available http://www.emea.europa.eu

[20] Xarelto ®, SPC. Available http://www.emea.europa.eu

[21] Eliquis ®, SPC. Available http://www.emea.europa.eu

[22] Garcia D, Libby E, Crowther MA . The new oral anticoagulants. Blood. 2010; 115:15-20.

[23] Lecumberri R. Practical Management of the new oral anticoagulants. Haematological. 2012, 97(2): 14-17.

[24] Van Ryn J, Stangier J, Haertter S, Liesenfeld KH, Wienen W, Feuring M, Clemens A. Dabigatran etexilate—a novel, reversible, oral direct thrombin inhibitor: interpretation of coagulation assays and reversal of anticoagulant activity. Thromb Haemost. 2010; 103:1116–27.

[25] Tripodi A. Measuring the anticoagulant effect of direct factor Xa inhibitors. Is the anti-Xa assay preferable to the prothrombin time test? Thromb Haemost. 2011; 105:735–6.

[26] Barrett YC, Wang Z, Frost C, Shenker A. Clinical laboratory measurement of direct factor Xa inhibitors: anti-Xa assay is preferable to prothrombin time assay. Thromb Haemost. 2010; 104:1263-71.

[27] Eerenberg ES, Kamphuisen PW, Sijpkens MK,Meijers JC, Buller HR, Levi M. Reversal of rivaroxaban and dabigatran by prothrombin complex concentrate: a randomized,

placebo-controlled, crossover study in healthy subjects. Circulation. 2011; 124(14): 1573-9.

[28] Marlu R, Hodaj E, Paris A, Albaladejo P, Crackowski JL, Pernod G. Effect of nonspecific reversal agents on anticoagulant activity of dabigatran, rivaroxaban. A randomised crossover ex vivo study in healthy volunteers. Thromb Haemost. 2012;108:217–24.

[29] Ezekowitz MD, Connolly S, Parekh A, Reilly PA, Varrone J, Wang S, et al. Rationale and design of RE-LY: Randomized evaluation of long-term anticoagulant therapy, warfarin, compared with dabigatran. Am Heart J. 2009; 157(5):805-10.

[30] Uchino K, AV Hernandez. Dabigatran Association with Higher Risk of acute coronary events. Meta-analysis of randomized controlled noninferiority trials. Arch Intern Med. 2012; 172:1-6.

[31] Jacobs JN, Stessman J. Dabigatran: do we Have Sufficient data? Arch Intern Med. 2012; 172:2-3.

[32] ROCKET AF Study Investigators. Rivaroxaban – once daily, oral, direct factor Xa inhibition compared with vitamin K antagonism for prevention of stroke and Embolism Trial in Atrial Firbrillation: rationale and design of the ROCKET AF study. Am Heart J. 2010; 159(3): 340.e1-347.e1.

[33] Patel MR, Mahaffey KW, Garg J, Pan G, Singer DE, Hacke W, Breithard G, Halperin JL, Hankey GJ, Piccini JP, Becker RC, Nessel CC, Paolini JP, Berkowitz SD, Fox KAA, Califa RM, for the ROCKET AF investigators. Rivaroxaban versus warfarin in nonvalvular atrial fibrillation. N Engl J Med. 2011; 365: 883-91.

[34] Connolly SJ, Eikelboom J, Joyner C, Diener H-C, Hart R, Golitsyn S, Flaker G, Avezum A, Hohnloser SH, Parkhomenko R, Jansky P, Commerford P, Tan RS, Sim K-H, Lewis BS, Van Mieghem W, Lip GYH, Kim JH, Lanas Zanetti F, González-Hermosillo A, Dans AL, Munawar M, for the AVERROES Steering Committee and Investigators. Apixaban in patients with atrial fibrillation. N Engl J Med. 2011; 364:806-17.

[35] Granger CB, Alexander JH, McMurray JJ, Lopes RD, Hyek EM, Hanna M, et al. ARISTOTLE Committees and Investigators. Apixaban versus warfarin in patients with atrial fibrillation. N Engl J Med. 2011; 365:981-92.

[36] Lip GY, Larsen TB, Skjøth F, Rasmussen LH. Indirect Comparisons of New Oral Anticoagulants Drugs for Efficacy and Safety When Used for Stroke Prevention in Atrial Fibrillation. J Am Coll Cardiol. 2012; 60(8): 738-46.

[37] Connolly SJ; Pogue J, Eikelboom J, et al. Benefit of oral anticoagulant over antiplatelet therapy in atrial fibrillation depends on the quality of international normalized ratio control achieved by centers and countries as measured by time in therapeutic range. Circulation. 2008; 118(20): 2029-37.

[38] Connoy S, Ezekowitz MD, Yusuf S, et a. Newy identified events in the RE-LY trial. N Engl J Med. 2011; 365: 2039-40.

[39] Sorensen SV, Kansal AR, Connolly S, Peng S, Linnehan J, Bradley-Kennedy C, Plumb JM. Cost-effectiveness of dabigatran etexilate for the prevention of stroke and systemic embolism in atrial fibrillation: a Canadian payer perspective. Thromb Haemost. 2011;105:908–19.

[40] Shah SV, Gage BF. Cost-effectiveness of dabigatran for stroke prophylaxis in atrial fibrillation. Circulation. 2011;123:2562–70.

[41] SPORTIF Executive Steering Committee for the SPORTIF V Investigators. Ximelagatran vs warfarin for stroke prevention in nonvalvular atrial fibrillation Patients with: a randomized trial. J Am Med Assoc. 2005, 293:690-8.

[42] Skanes AC, Healey JS, Cairns JA, Dorian P, Gillis AM, McMurtry MS, Mitchell LB, Verma A, Nattel S; Canadian Cardiovascular Society Atrial Fibrillation Guidelines Committee. Focused 2012 Update of the Canadian Cardiovascular Society Atrial fibrillation Guidelines: recommendations for stroke prevention and rate/rhythm control. Can J Cardiol. 2012; 28:125–36.

[43] Wann LS, Curtis AB, Ellenbogen KA, et al. 2011 ACCF/AHA/HRS focused update on the management of patients with atrial fibrillation (update on dabigatran): a report of the American College of Cardiology Foundation/American Heart Association Task Force on Practice Guidelines. Heart Rhythm. 2011; 8:e1-e8.

[44] Camm AJ, Kirchhof P, Lip GY, et al. Guidelines for the management of atrial fibrillation: the Task Force for the Management of Atrial Fibrillation of the European Society of Cardiology (ESC). Eur Heart J. 2010; 31: 2369–429.

[45] Bloomfield HE, Krause A, Greer N, Taylor BC, MacDonald R, Rutks I, Reddy P, Wilt TJ. Meta-analysis: effect of patient self-testing and self-management of long-term anticoagulation on major clinical outcomes. Ann Intern Med. 2011; 154:472-8.

[46] Heneghan C, Ward A, Perera R, and the Self-Monitoring Trialists Collaboration. Self-monitoring of oral anticoagulation: Systematic review and meta-analysis of an individual patient data. Lancet. 2012, 379:322-34.

[47] Amouyel P, P Mismetti, LK Langkilde, Jasso-Mosqueda G, K Nelander, Lmarque H. INR variability in atrial fibrillation: a Risk Model for cerebrovascular events. Eur J Intern Med. 2009; 20(1):63-9.

Chapter 10

Anticoagulant Therapy in Patients with Atrial Fibrillation and Coronary Artery Disease

Atila Bitigen and Vecih Oduncu

Additional information is available at the end of the chapter

http://dx.doi.org/10.5772/54147

1. Introduction

Atherosclerotic cardiovascular disease and atrial fibrillation (AF) are causes of increased mortality and morbidity all over the world. Coexistence of both leads to even higher rates of mortality and morbidity. In AF, the main reason responsible for increased mortality and morbidity is thromboembolisation and consequently the development of a stroke [1]. Among patients with atrial fibrillation, the incidence of atherosclerotic cardiovascular disease has been reported to be 20-30% [2]. Thus, development of an acute coronary syndrome (ACS) requiring percutaneous coronary intervention is very probable in patients with atrial fibrillation. Despite a 17% reduction in the incidence of stroke with aspirin compared to placebo, vitamin K antagonist (VKA) warfarin is superior to both aspirin and aspirin plus clopidogrel combinations due to its preventing AF patients from thromboemboli [3]. While triple antithrombotic therapy (VKA+aspirin+clopidogrel) lowers the risk of stroke in stent implanted patients with AF, it increases the risk of bleeding at long- term. Thus careful judgement of the risk of emboli and bleeding, the stent type (drug eluted or bare metal) to be implanted and the duration of appropriate treatment regimen is important.

2. The evaluation of embolic risk

In patients with atrial fibrillation the main goal of antithrombotic therapy is to prevent stroke. In patients with non-valvular AF, the atherosclerotic cardiovascular disease (especially a history of myocardial infarction) has been found to be associated with an increased incidence of stroke. Other important risks factors are diabetes, hypertension, previous stroke/ transient ischemic attack and age. In patients with non valvular AF $CHADS_2DS_2$-

Vasc-Score [6] derived from a European Heart Survey were found to be beneficial for estimation of the risk of stroke. This scoring system is suggested for risk stratification in both the European Society of Cardiology (ESC) [7] and the American College of Cardiology/ American Heart Association (ACC/AHA) [8] guidelines. (Table1). According to this scoring system, the patients are stratified into three risk groups as low (0), medium (1 – 2) and high (>2). While the risk of emboli is 1.3 % at score 1, the risk increases to 15.2 % at score 9. While previous embolism/TIA/stroke and age ≥75 are the major risk factors, the other clinical situations are classified as the non-major risk factors. Not only previous myocardial infarction but also complex atheroma plaques and peripheral vascular disease have also been included in the definition of vascular disease.

Letter	Clinical Condition and age	Points
C	Congestive heart failure†	1
H	Hypertension	1
A	Age≥75 years	2
D	Diabetes mellitus	1
S	Stroke/TIA/Thromboembolism	2
V	Vascular disease*	1
A	Age 65 – 74	1
S	Female sex	1
		max. 9 points

†Heart failure or moderate to severe left ventricular systolic dysfunction (e.g. LV EF < 40%)

*Prior myocardial infarction, peripheral artery disease, aortic plaque. TIA =transient ischaemic attack.

Table 1. CHA_2DS_2-Vasc-Score for determining embolic risk

3. Bleeding risk evaluation

In choosing the antithrombotic therapy regime, both the risk of bleeding and the evaluation of thromboembolic risk are important. The use of VKA causes a more meaningful decrease in embolic risk compared to aspirin alone or DAPT (dual antiplatelet therapy) in patients with a medium and high risk. However the use of VKA increases the risk of major bleeding especially when used with DAPT. Therefore, determining the risk of bleeding is important before starting the therapy. Although various risk scores evaluating the risk of bleeding have been obtained, they were all developed to estimate the risk of major bleeding and they can be classified into three groups as low, medium and advanced. ESC guidelines recommend using HAS-BLED scoring [Table 2] (hypertension, abnormal renal/liver function, stroke, bleeding history or predisposition, labile INR, elderly (>65), drugs/alcohol concomitantly) in the estimation of bleeding risk [9]. HAS-BLED≥3 was found to be related to high risk of bleeding. However, parameters such as a history of stroke, old age, and hypertension also affect the risk of emboli estimated by using the CHA2DS2-Vasc-Score,. Thus, patients with a high bleeding risk must be carefully managed.

Letter	Clinical characteristic*	Point
H	Hypertension	1
A	Abnormal renal or liver function (1 point each)	1 or 2
S	Stroke	1
B	Bleeding history	1
L	Labile INR	1
E	Elderly ("/>65 years)	1
D	Drugs or alcohol comsumption (1 point each)	1 or 2
		Max 9 poits

*Hypertension' is defined as systolic blood pressure >160 mmHg. 'Abnormal kidney function' is defined as the presence of chronic dialysis or renal transplantation or serum creatinine ≥200 mmol/L. 'Abnormal liver function' is defined as chronic hepatic disease (e.g. cirrhosis) or biochemical evidence of significant hepatic derangement (e.g. bilirubin >2 x upper limit of normal, in association with aspartate aminotransferase/alanine aminotransferase/alkaline phosphatase >3 x upper limit normal, etc.). 'Bleeding' refers to previous bleeding history and/or predisposition to bleeding, e.g. bleeding diathesis, anaemia, etc. 'Labile INRs' refers to unstable/high INRs or poor time in therapeutic range (e.g., 60%). Drugs/alcohol use refers to concomitant use of drugs, such as antiplatelet agents, non-steroidal anti-inflammatory drugs, or alcohol abuse, etc. INR = international normalized ratio. Adapted from Pisters et al (9).

Table 2. HAS-BLED bleeding score

4. Choosing antithrombotic therapy

In coronary artery disease, DAPT has been found superior to aspirin plus oral anticoagulant (OAC) therapy in preventing recurrent ischemic events [10]. Although, in a long term period, OAC therapy has been found superior to DAPT in AF patients, this therapy, especially in situations when it must be combined with DAPT, has a major bleeding incidence of up to 4.7 %. This bleeding usually happens within the first month and has been fatal in almost half of the patients [11]. Therefore, the management of patients with nonvalvular AF who require PCI (percutaneous coronary intervention) is very important for many clinicians.

Nowadays, therapy guidelines include a therapy of low aspirin dose or no therapy for low risk patients, OAC or aspirin for medium risk patients, and a therapy of OAC in patients with a high risk. In medium risk patients, DAPT has been found inequivalent to VKA in studies conducted on DAPT therapy (aspirin+ clopidogrel). VKA is related to lower bleeding and stroke. Therefore, in medium and high thromboli risk patients, if the risk of hemorrhage is high, because of the high incidence of intracranial and extra cranial bleeding incidence, the option of DAPT should not be preferred.

In the abovementioned patients the low dose dabigatran option must be considered and if they are treated with VKA, a lower INR (1.8-2.5) target should be chosen. However according to the studies made, patients with an INR <2 have double the risk of stroke compared to patients whose INR is > 2.

5. Choosing therapy following elective percutaneous coronary intervention

In elective percutaneous coronary interventions (PCI), if there is no obligatory indication (long lesion, small vessel, diabetes, etc.) the intervention must be limited to a bare metal stent (BMS). Because after the implantation of a drug eluting stent (DES), there is a requirement for a triple antiplatelet for a longer time (3 months for sirolimus, 6 months for paclitaxel) and this may lead to a higher mortality rate associated with increased bleeding risk. While the post BMS triple anti platelet therapy is limited to a 4 week period, it has to be used longer following DES. In patients with low-medium bleeding risk but low embolic risk, during the first four weeks after BMS, triple anti platelet therapy is suggested. After 4 weeks, lifelong OAC (INR=2-3) should be preferred. As an approach, there is a difference between ESC guidelines and USA clinical practice [12]. In patients with low-medium hemorrhagic risk both the ESC and the USA approaches suggest triple anti platelet therapy for BMS and DES, but in the USA approach, only DAPT is suggested in patients with a high bleeding risk. However, in ESC guidelines, despite the high bleeding risk, during the 2-4 week interval after BMS elective implantation, triple anti platelet therapy is advised.

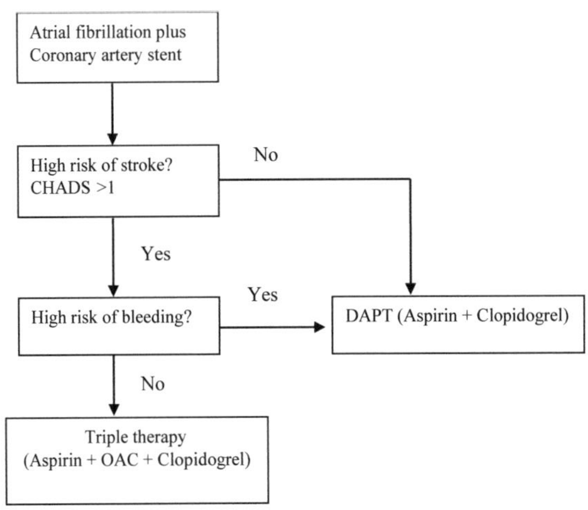

Figure 1. US Approach-Adapted from Paikin et al [12}

http://dx.doi.org/10.5772/54147

As a therapy regime, OAC (INR=2 – 2.5), aspirin daily ≤100 mg and clopidogrel 75 mg daily is included. In patients with a high risk of bleeding, it has been stressed in both guidelines that DES should be avoided and if possible BMS should be implanted. Among patients having a low and medium bleeding risk, for those who have been implanted BMS, 1 month of triple anti platelet therapy is advised. Among those patients who are DES implanted, for the limus group, 3 months of triple antiplatelet therapy is advised while for the paclitaxel group, 6 months of DAPT is advised. Furthermore, in DES implanted patients, a dual therapy of OAC plus aspirin up to 1 year or OAC plus clopidogrel is advised and after 1 year only OAC mono therapy is advised. Therefore, DES implantation should be avoided because it requires long term dual and triple therapy (Table3).

Hemorrhagic risk	Clinic	Stent type	Anticoagulation regime
Low-Medium HAS-BLED (0 – 2)	Elective	BMS	1 month: triple therapy of warfarin (INR 2.0–2.5) + aspirin ≤ 100 mg/day + clopidogrel 75 mg/day Lifelong: warfarin (INR 2.0–3.0) alone
	Elective	DES	3 (-olimus group) to 6 (paclitaxel) months: triple therapy of warfarin (INR 2.0–2.5) + aspirin ≤ 100 mg/day + clopidogrel 75 mg/day Up to 12 months: combination of warfarin (INR 2.0–2.5) + clopidogrel 75 mg/day (or aspirin 100 mg/day)* Lifelong: warfarin (INR 2.0–3.0) alone
	ACS	DES/BMS	6 months: triple therapy of warfarin (INR 2.0–2.5) + aspirin ≤ 100 mg/day + clopidogrel 75 mg/day Up to 12 months: combination of warfarin (INR 2.0–2.5) + clopidogrel 75 mg/day (or aspirin 100 mg/day)* Lifelong: warfarin (INR 2.0–3.0) alone
High HAS-BLED (≥3)	Elective	BMS	2–4 weeks: triple therapy of warfarin (INR 2.0–2.5) + aspirin ≤ 100 mg/day + clopidogrel 75 mg/day Lifelong: warfarin (INR 2.0–3.0) alone
	ACS	BMS	4 weeks: triple therapy of warfarin (INR 2.0–2.5) + aspirin ≤ 100 mg/day + clopidogrel 75 mg/day Up to 12 months: combination of warfarin (INR 2.0–2.5) + clopidogrel 75 mg/day (or aspirin 100 mg/day); mg/day)* Lifelong: warfarin (INR 2.0–3.0) alone

ACS=Acute coronary syndrome, BMS=Bare metal stent, DES=Drug eluted stent, INR=International normalized ratio

*Combination of warfarin (INR 2.0–2.5) + aspirin ≤ 100 mg/day may be considered as an alternative.

Drug-eluting stents should be avoided.Adapted from Lip et al

Table 3. ESC suggestions for anticoagulation in patients with coronary stent who have medium and high emboli risk

6. Acute coronary syndrome

In patients with non-valvular AF who have acute coronary syndrome (ACS), the puncture site for PCI is important. In anti- coagulated patients, how the therapy will be conducted in the hospital and choosing the right type of stent bears an importance. As for those patients who are not anti coagulated, the antithrombotic therapy during discharge is important. In anticoagulated patients, femoral intervention is an independent predictor for major hemorrhage and other vascular complications and therefore in those patients radial intervention is preferred because it causes less bleeding and better results [13,14].

In patients with ACS, especially those in whom primary PCI have been applied, BMS should be preferred because it requires a shorter duration triple antithrombotic therapy. OAC should be given to non-STEMI patients when they are hospitalized and DAPT and heparin should be given to those patients who have no therapy. If the thromboembolic risk is too high, OAC therapy might as well be started in those patients during in-hospital period. There are two approaches for patients who receive OAC during hospitalization. The first and mostly used approach in clinical practice is the bridge therapy which involves stopping OAC therapy and starting heparin. The second approach is to continue OAC therapy so that INR will be in the 2-2.5 interval. The main drawback of the bridge therapy is when the therapy is stopped and then restarted, Protein –C and –S are not suppressed, and they increase embolic complications paradoxically in patients with a very high emboli risk [15]. Therefore, in patients with ACS having a very high embolic risk, it is advised that DAPT should be added to the therapy without stopping OAC and without adding heparin (if the INR <2, then heparin may be added) [16,17]. In STEMI patients for whom P-PCI is applied, if the INR is within the interval of 2 – 3, then a similar approach is applicable. However, glycoprotein (GP) IIb/IIIa inhibitors may have to be used due to the high thrombus burden. In those patients with a high thrombus burden, if the INR>2, then GP IIb/IIIa inhibitor must not be started, and, if possible thrombectomy should be considered instead. Alternatively, in patients with INR<2, bivaluridin might be considered for use instead of GP IIb/IIIa inhibitor + heparin. Due to high hemorrhagic risks, in patients using OAC and having optimal INR, additional heparin should not be used. In patients whose bleeding risk is high, triple therapy should not be used for more than 1 month. Due to the need for short triple therapy, BMS should always be preferred. Following ACS, triple therapy should be given for 1 month, dual therapy including OAC should be given up to 12 months, and after 12 months only OAC should be given lifelong. The short and long term antithrombotic therapy regimen of the ACS patients is summarized in table 3.

Advice On Decreasing Hemorrhagic Risk:

1. The balance between hemorrhagic risk and embolic risk should be maintained very well.

2. No therapy may be given to patients who are under 65 years of age having a low embolic risk.

3. In combined therapies, the dose of aspirin should be kept low (75 – 100 mg).

4. In patients having a high bleeding risk hypertension should be treated aggressively.
5. Hepatic and renal functions should be followed closely in patients who take OAC.
6. In case of stent requirement, BMS should be preferred as much as possible.
7. During ACS, additional heparin, GP IIb/IIIa inhibitor or bivaluridin should not be given to those patients who have an effective INR and who take OAC.
8. Radial intervention should be applied to patients who take OAC and who are intervened with STEMI.
9. Triple antiplatelet therapy should not be used for more than 1 month in patients whose bleeding risk is high.
10. DAPT should not be given for a long time, instead only OAC should be given in long term therapy.
11. Proton pump inhibitors may be added to the therapy.
12. In long term therapy, dabigatran 110 mg twice a day or rivaroxaban once a day should be considered for use (compared to VKA lower bleeding incidence, equal stroke rates) in patients whose bleeding risk is high (especially in the presence of INR labile).

7. New anticoagulant drugs

In AF patients, oral anticoagulation is traditionally done with VKA. However, due to personal differences in responses, the need for a balance in dose, labile INR and bleeding risk; studies have been made on new drugs which do not require follow-up. With these new drugs such as direct thrombin inhibitor dabigatran, factor Xa inhibitors apixaban and rivaroxaban, the incidence of major bleeding is significantly lower compared to VKA. When Dabigatran 110 mg twice a day is compared with VKA, nonvalvular AF stroke prevention in the RELY study (Randomized Evaluation of Long-term Anticoagulant Therapy) there is no difference between stroke and systemic embolism, but the rate of major hemorrhage is meaningfully less in 110 mg Dabigatran than it is in VKA [18]. In the dose of 150 mg, the rates of major bleeding and stroke were determined to be similar. In patients with non valvular AF whose INR values were labile, if they cannot be followed closely and if they do not have an advanced hepatic and renal problem, dabigatran is an alternative to warfarin. In non- valvular AF patients, in the ARISTOTLE study done with Apixaban, apixaban is related to lower hemorrhage complication and lower mortality compared to warfarin [19]. In the ROCKET-AF [20] study, while there was no difference between the major hemorrhage rates of patients using rivaroxaban and warfarin, the fatal and intracranial hemorrhage rates were lower in patients using rivaroxaban than in those patients using warfarin. The systemic emboli and stroke prevention rates between the two were equal.

The results of this study are hopeful for long term anticoagulation regimes. There is no sufficient clinical evidence regarding the fact that these drugs are appropriate for a combination therapy (DAPT plus OAC). However, regarding these three studies (RELY, ROCKET-AF, and ARISTOTLE), when the dual therapy using VKA is compared with dual therapy using new anticoagulant drugs (apixaban, rivaroxaban, dabigatran), there is no additional difference in terms of hemorrhage rate. Thus, when the combination of DAPT with new drugs is compared to the combination of VKA and DAPT, there is no additional increase in hemorrhage. Nevertheless, in the monotherapy with OAC, the risk of hemorrhage is at its lowest. However, regarding the safety of the combined use of the new anticoagulant drugs with dual antiplatelet therapy, there is no sufficient evidence regarding long-term use and there is a need for further studies.

Author details

Atila Bitigen and Vecih Oduncu

Medikalpark Hospital – Fatih, Istanbul, Turkey

References

[1] Stewart S, Hart CL, Hole DJ, McMurray JJ. A population-based study of the longterm risks associated with atrial fibrillation: 20-year follow-up of the Renfrew/Paisley study. Am J Med 2002;113:359–364.

[2] Nieuwlaat R, Capucci A, Camm AJ, et al. Atrial fibrillation management:a prospective survey in ESC member countries: the Euro Heart Survey on Atrial Fibrillation. Eur Heart J. 2005; 26: 2422-2434.

[3] Heart RG, Pearce LA, Aguilar MI.Meta-analysis:antithrombotic therapy to prevent stroke in patients who have nonvalvular atrial fibrillation. Ann Intern Med 2007;146:857-867.

[4] Connolly S, Pogue J, Hart R, Pfeffer M, Hohnloser S, Chrolavicius S, Yusuf S. Clopidogrel plus aspirin versus oral anticoagulation for atrial fibrillation in the Atrial fibrillation Clopidogrel Trial with Irbesartan for prevention of Vascular Events (ACTIVE W): a randomised controlled trial. Lancet 2006;367:1903–1912.

[5] Gage BF, Waterman AD, Shannon W, Boechler M, Rich MW, Radford MJ. Validation of clinical classification schemes for predicting stroke: results from the National Registry of Atrial Fibrillation. JAMA 2001;285:2864–2870.

[6] Lip GY, Nieuwlaat R, Pisters R, Lane DA, Crijns HJ. Refining clinical risk stratification for predicting stroke and thromboembolism in atrial fibrillation using a novel risk factor-based approach: the Euro Heart Survey on atrial fibrillation. Chest 2010;137:263–272.

[7] Camm AJ, Kirchhof P, Lip GY et al. Guidelines for the management of atrial fibrillation: The Task Force for the Management of Atrial Fibrillation of the European Society of Cardiology (ESC). European Heart Journal. 2010; 31: 2369–2429.

[8] Wann LS, Curtis AB, January CT et al. 2011 ACCF/AHA/HRS focused update on the management of patients with atrial fibrillation (Updating the 2006 Guideline): a report of the American college of cardiology foundation/American heart association task force on practice guidelines. Circulation. 2011; 123: 104–123.

[9] Pisters R, Lane DA, Nieuwlaat R, de Vos CB, Crijns HJ, Lip GY. A novel userfriendly score (HAS-BLED) to assess one-year risk of major bleeding in atrial fibrillation patients: The Euro Heart Survey. Chest. 2010;138:1093-100.

[10] Rogacka R, Chieffo A, Michev I, et al. Dual antiplatelet therapy after percutaneous coronary intervention with stent implantation in patients taking chronic oral anticoagulation. JACC Cardiovasc Interv. 2008; 1: 56-61.

[11] Rubboli A, Milandri M, Castelvetri C, Cosmi B. Meta-analysis of trials comparing oral anticoagulation and aspirin versus dual antiplatelet therapy after coronary stenting. Clues for the management of patients with an indication for long-term anticoagulation undergoing coronary stenting. Cardiology 2005;104:101–106.

[12] Paikin JS, Wright DS, Crowther MA, Mehta SR, Eikelboom JW. Triple antithrombotic therapy in patients with atrial fibrillation and coronary artery stents. Circulation. 2010;121:2067-2070.

[13] Lip GY, Huber K, Andreotti F, Arnesen H, Airaksinen KJ, Cuisset T, Kirchhof P, Marin F. Management of antithrombotic therapy in atrial fibrillation patients presenting with acute coronary syndrome and/or undergoing percutaneous coronary intervention/stenting. Thromb Haemost 2010;103:13–28.

[14] Jolly SS, Amlani S, Hamon M, Yusuf S, Mehta SR. Radial versus femoral access for coronary angiography or intervention and the impact on major bleeding and ischemic events: a systematic review and meta-analysis of randomized trials. Am Heart J 2009;157:132–140.

[15] Palareti G, Legnani C. Warfarin withdrawal. Pharmacokinetic pharmacodynamic considerations. Clin Pharmacokinet. 1996; 30: 300-313.

[16] Karjalainen PP, Vikman S, Niemela M, et al. Safety of percutaneous coronary intervention during uninterrupted oral anticoagulant treatment. Eur Heart J. 2008; 29: 1001-1010.

[17] Lip GY, Huber K, Andreotti Fet al., Antithrombotic management of atrial fibrillation patients presenting with acute coronary syndrome and/or undergoing coronary stenting: executive summary. A Consensus Document of the European Society of Cardiology Working Group on Thrombosis, endorsed by the European Heart Rhythm Association (EHRA) and the European Association of Percutaneous Cardiovascular Interventions (EAPCI). European Heart Journal, 2010;31:1311–1318.

[18] Connolly SJ, Ezekowitz MD, Yusuf S, Eikelboom J, Oldgren J, Parekh A, et al. RE-LY Steering Committee and Investigators. Dabigatran versus warfarin in patients with atrial fibrillation. N Engl J Med. 2009;361:1139-1151.

[19] Connolly SJ, Eikelboom J, Joyner C, Diener HC, Hart R, Golitsyn S, et al. Apixaban in patients with atrial fibrillation. N Engl J Med. 2011;364:806-817.

[20] Patel MR, Mahaffey KW, Garg J, Pan G, Singer DE, Hacke W , et al. ROCKET AF Investigators.Rivaroxaban versus warfarin in nonvalvular atrial fibrillation, New England Journal of Medicine. 2011; 365: 883–891.